Neurology of the Arts

Painting • Music • Literature

Neurology of the Arts

Painting • Music • Literature

Editor

F Clifford Rose

Consulting Neurologist, Regional Neurosciences Centre,
Charing Cross Hospital, London

Founding Director, Academic Unit of Neuroscience,
Charing Cross and Westminster (now Imperial College)
Medical School, University of London

Director, London Neurological Centre

ICP

Imperial College Press

Published by

Imperial College Press
57 Shelton Street
Covent Garden
London WC2H 9HE

Distributed by

World Scientific Publishing Co. Pte. Ltd.
5 Toh Tuck Link, Singapore 596224
USA office: Suite 202, 1060 Main Street, River Edge, NJ 07661
UK office: 57 Shelton Street, Covent Garden, London WC2H 9HE

British Library Cataloguing-in-Publication Data
A catalogue record for this book is available from the British Library.

Cover illustration: *Transfiguration*, by Raphael; from the Vatican Museum.

NEUROLOGY OF THE ARTS: PAINTING, MUSIC, LITERATURE

ISBN 1-86094-368-3

Printed in Singapore by World Scientific Printers (S) Pte Ltd

Preface

The Medical Society of London — the oldest medical society in the world, being founded in 1773 — was left a bequest in the early 1970s by Mrs Florence Alice Mansell. Her husband had been a Fellow of the Society and died in his fifth decade of motor neurone disease. The bequest specifically stated that it should be used to further neurological studies, and the Council of the Society agreed to invest the capital and use the accrued interest to fund symposia related to neurological topics. These meetings were to be restricted to the participants and Fellows of the Society, but the proceedings were to be published.

The first symposium, held in 1976, understandably on motor neurone disease, lasted only one day. Since then, the meetings have been held every two to three years, lasting two days, with 12 speakers each day. On average, 6 speakers would come from North America, 6 from the Continent and elsewhere, and the rest from the UK. The subjects chosen were those not readily accepted by commercial publishers; for example, the proceedings of the motor neurone disease symposium contituted the first book on the subject for 25 years. Other topics have been the first of their kind, such as clinical neuroimmunology and clinical neuroepidemiology (see following table). The present volume, the proceedings of "Neurology of the Arts", is again the first in this field.

The medicine of art has been a hobby of mine since I became a medical student. My preclinical-education school (King's College, London) and medical school (Westminster Hospital) were both a few minutes' walk from several of Britain's most famous art galleries, so these were easy to visit. Looking at pictures has never been a hardship with me, and it is difficult to understand why there are some who do not find it pleasurable. From walking the wards to walking the galleries, it was not unnatural to take note of those paintings which carried some significance for medical studies, possibly because of guilt feelings over the latter being neglected. During the ensuing decades, on frequent lecture tours abroad, I followed this bent whilst visiting art galleries in foreign cities.[1] That this is not an original idea has been pointed out by a famous medical historian: "Whenever a doctor goes on a vacation trip to Europe, accompanied by his wife, who insists on seeing the galleries, he

1. F.C. Rose, The medicine of art: presidential address, *Trans. Med. Soc. London* (1985).

spends his time hunting for pathological subjects, sure to make a 'discovery' and to write a paper about it."[2]

It seemed appropriate to add music and literature (in their broadest sense) in equal measures to painting so as to provide an overview of an area which is extremely large, as indicated by the table of contents, and of wide interest.

2. H.E. Sigerist, The historical aspects of art and medicine, *Bull. Inst. Hist. Med.* **II**, 271–97 (1936).

THE MANSELL BEQUEST SYMPOSIA
OF THE MEDICAL SOCIETY OF LONDON
(Editor: F. Clifford Rose)

Year	Title	Publisher
1977	Motor Neurone Disease	Pitman Medical
1979	Clinical Neuro-immunology	Blackwell Science
1980	Clinical Neuro-epidemiology	Pitman Medical
1981	Metabolic Disorders of the Nervous System	Pitman Medical
1982	Advances in Stroke Therapy	Raven Press
1984	Advances in Aphasiology	Raven Press
1985	Advances in Neuro-oncology (*with W.S. Fields*)	Karger, Basle
1988	Physiological Aspects of Clinical Neuro-ophthalmology (*with C. Kennard*)	Chapman & Hall Medical
1989	The Control of the Hypothalamo-pituitary-adrenocortical Axis	International Universities Press, Chicago
1993	Advances in Neuropharmacology	Smith Gordon
1995	Recent Advances in Tropical Neurology	Elsevier Science
1997	Towards Migraine 2000	Elsevier Science
1999	A Short History of Neurology: The British Contribution 1660–1910	Butterworth-Heinemann
2001	Twentieth Century Neurology: The British Contribution	Imperial College Press

List of Contributors

Geneviève Aubert	Université Catholique de Louvain, Department of Neurology and Service d'EEG, Cliniques Universitaires Saint-Luc, Avenue Hippocrate, 10 (1932) B-1200, Bruxelles, Belgium
Jean-Claude Baron	Department of Neurology, University of Cambridge, UK
Michael E. Charness	Associate Professor of Neurology, Harvard Medical School; Associate Chief, Department of Neurology; Director, Performing Arts Clinic, Brigham and Women's Hospital; Chief, Neurology Service, Boston Healthcare System, MA 02132, USA
Bernt A. Engelsen	Institute of Neurology, University of Bergen, Haukeland Hospital, Sykehus Neurologisk, AVD Poliklinik, N-5021, Bergen, Norway
F. Eustache	Inserm E0218, University of Caen, France
Stanley Finger	Department of Psychology, Washington University Campus, Box 1125, One Brooking's Drive, St Louis, Missouri, 63130-4899, USA
John J. Fino	University of Illinois Medical Center, Chicago, Illinois 60612, USA; Senior Research Specialist, Department of Neurology, Chicago, Illinois 60612, USA
David A. Gallo	Department of Psychology, Washington University, St Louis, Missouri, 63130-4899, USA

Christopher Gardner-Thorpe	Consultant Neurologist, Exeter Neurosciences and Peninsula Medical School, Royal Devon and Exeter Hospital, Barrack Road, Exeter, EX2 5DW, UK
Christopher G. Goetz	Professor of Neurological Sciences and Pharmacology, Rush University, Rush-Presbyterian, St Luke's Medical Center, 1725 West Harrison St, Suite 1106, Chicago, Illinois 60612, USA
John R. Hughes	Professor of Neurology, Director of Clinical Neurophysiology & Epilepsy, University of Illinois Medical Center, M/C T96 912 South Wood Street, Chicago, Illinois 60612, USA
Milo Keynes	Honorary Consultant Surgeon, Radcliffe Infirmary, Oxford, UK and 3 Brunswick Walk, Cambridge, CB5 8DH, UK
Halfdan Kierulf	Consultant Neurologist, Ullevalsveien, 52 N – 0454 Oslo, Norway
John B. Lyons	Professor of the History of Medicine, Royal College of Surgeons in Ireland; formerly Consultant Physician to St Michael's and Mercer's Hospitals, Ireland
E. Wayne Massey	Duke University Medical Center, Durham, North Carolina, 27710, USA
H. Platel	Inserm E0218, University of Caen, France
Paul Robertson	Visiting Professor, University of Kingston and Bournemouth and The Old Farm House, Hermongers Rudgewick, West Sussex, RH12 3AL, UK
Julius Rocca	Honorary Research Fellow, Faculty of Medicine, University of Birmingham, UK; formerly Wellcome Trust Research Fellow in the History of Medicine, University of Cambridge, UK

Frank Clifford Rose	London Neurological Centre, 110 Harley Street, London, W1G 7JG, UK
Gottfried Schlaug	Assistant Professor of Neurology, Harvard Medical School; Director of Neuroimaging, Beth Israel Deaconess Medical Center, Boston MA, USA
C.U.M. Smith	Vision Sciences, Aston University, Birmingham, B4 7ET, UK
David Steinberg	Såa Institute, 15111 Tyler Road, Fiddletown, CA 95629, USA
Ragnar Stien	Department of Neurology, Ulleval Hospital, Oslo, N-0407, Norway
Jason Warren	Senior Research Fellow, Wellcome Unit, National Hospital, Queen Square, London, WC1N 3BG, UK
Peter Wolf	Institute for Interdisciplinary Epilepsy Research, Epilepsy Centre Bethel, Maraweg 21, D-33617 Bielefeld, Germany
George K. York	Department of Neurology, Såa Institute, 21201 Ostrom Road, Fiddletown, CA 95629 and Kaiser Permanente Medical Center, Stockton, CA, USA
Semir Zeki	Wellcome Department of Cognitive Neurology, Institute of Neurology, Queen Square, London, WC1, UK (University College, London)

Contents

Chapter 1

The Cerebral Localization of Creativity

George K. York

This chapter examines the cerebral localization of creative processes from the point of view of the practical neurologist. The appreciation of visual, musical or verbal artistry leads the clinical neurophysiologist to ask whether creativity arises in a discrete part of the nervous system. Modern clinical neurophysiology localizes sensorimotor functions, not mental ones. For a creative induction to be localized, it must be exclusively sensorimotor, yet the artistic process is intrinsically mental. For neurologists, mental processes occur concomitant to physical events leading to doubt that artistry emerges from one or another part of the nervous system. Aesthetic assessment of the creative output of a patient does not help in localizing a lesion—a distressing conclusion for the sensitive neurologist. He or she may take comfort, though, in the realization that neurological diagnosis tests the creative mind of the examiner, if not the patient.

Introduction

Works of art fill the viewer or listener with many feelings, not least of which is a sense of wonder at the source of the artist's achievement. Neurologists compound this amazement by asking the classic neurological question: Where in the brain does the picture, or the symphony, or the poem come from? Most people accept that the creative process arises in the brain, and scientific neurology is based on the premise that different parts of the nervous system have different functions. Thus the neurologist in the art gallery might consider the question where in the brain creative ideas arise. Science has produced conflicting observations on the cerebral localization of artistic processes, and this chapter aims to examine some of these observations from the point of view of a practical clinical neurologist.

In considering this topic, the words and works of John Hughlings Jackson articulate the point of view of a practicing neurologist, which can be summarized as the conviction that it is possible to test the function of the nervous system by bedside examination. Stimulation or destruction of different parts of the nervous system leads to different signs and symptoms. Clinical neurophysiology, the conceptual framework of diagnostic neurology, rests on the principle that stimulating or ablating a part of the brain illuminates that area's function.

The Jacksonian neurologist's point of view is little known in wider circles because scientific medicine strives to be rational and skeptical—characteristics that do not necessarily promote the sensitive appraisal of artistry. However, physicians are privileged to examine people in whom nature has contrived to damage or destroy a part of the nervous system and who are willing to undergo a full range of diagnostic maneuvers in the hope of better health. Therefore, the neurologist is put in the unique position of being able to study neurobiology and human nature simultaneously. In this way the inquiring neurologist may offer a different and enlightening way to look at painting, music, literature and science.

Scientific Cerebral Localization

Clinical neurophysiology begins with the following question: What, precisely, do neurologists localize when they examine a patient? Hughlings Jackson, as a practicing neurologist, declared that neurologists localize symptoms rather than elemental neurological functions.[1] More importantly, he asserted that symptoms are exclusively sensory and motor.[2] At the bedside, to say nothing of the gallery or the symphony hall, the Jacksonian neurologist regards the nervous system as an exclusively sensory–motor machine that works by integrating afferent and efferent electrochemical impulses. Scientific neurology demands rigorous adherence to such matters as thermodynamics and the laws of conservation of energy and mass. As a result, a bedside test may be critically important to the patient even when the sign itself is of dubious scientific significance. It would be disingenuous to say that these signs and symptoms have nothing whatever to do with the presence or absence of elemental neurological functions. For example, hemiparesis seems strongly related to voluntary movement, which is an arguably circumscribed neurological function. Even so, focal signs do not necessarily define a basic neurophysiological function.

Practical clinical neurology relies on the principles of evolutionary neurophysiology, a discipline that has been called the most successful application of evolutionary theory to medicine.[3] Evolutionary neurophysiology considers the nervous system an aggregate of discrete organs, each with a single physiological function.[4] This fundamental neurophysiological idea can be traced to the phrenological movement.[5,6] In developing this phrenological assumption, Hughlings Jackson thought that each neurological organ is organized as a hierarchy of three evolutionary levels. The lowest of these levels comprises a number of nodes or centers, each representing a small part of the body, such as the face, the arm or the leg. At the middle and highest evolutionary levels, each center contains a complete representation of the next lower level, but each is also weighted for a different body part. This weighting is dynamic, so that reweighting after focal brain necrosis results in recovery of function. Superior levels suppress or inhibit the function of subordinate levels. This hierarchical organization means that symptoms of neurological disease are dual in nature, negative symptoms resulting from the loss of higher level function and positive ones from the appearance of function of previously inhibited lower levels. Neurological disease may be focal or diffuse, meaning that it may affect one, many or all centers at one, two or all three levels.[7]

In everyday practice, the principle of weighted ordinal representation allows neurologists to predict the presence and location of pathology with tolerable accuracy.[8–10] Physicians use this diagnostic process to distinguish between focal and diffuse disease of the nervous system, an endeavor which would be absurd if there were no localization of function. They examine patients for negative symptoms due to the loss of higher levels, such as hemiplegia. They also look for the emergence of positive signs due to disinhibition of lower levels, for example pathological hyperreflexia or Babinski's sign. The diagnostic system inherent in Jacksonian neurophysiology becomes second nature to experienced neurologists, who regard it as "thinking neurologically".

Of course, all work and no play makes for a dull neurologist. A visit to the Tate Modern or St. Martin's-in-the-Fields, not to mention a midnight walk in the West End, makes thoughtful neurologists vividly aware of the reality of the mind in health and disease. As medical men and women, they know well the importance of the mind in everyday life, and as cultivated citizens of the world they realize that painting, music, literature and drama emerge from creative minds rather than sensorimotor machines. But there's the rub, because long years of practicing neurology also tell them that mental functions, however precisely defined, do not arise in one lobe or hemisphere. The mind, if it has any physical existence at all, must obey the conservation laws that say that an immaterial agent cannot energize a material system. In the strict medical sense, mental processes can be said to arise anywhere, or everywhere, in the cortex. Mental processes, including creativity, are sensorimotor processes, or they are nothing at all.[11]

It follows that bedside mental tests do not lead to localization of a pathological lesion in the same way that sensorimotor tests do. How, then, are the brain and the creative mind related? A Jacksonian solution to this problem, though perhaps philosophically uninformed, remains a useful clinical approach. In Hughlings Jackson's doctrine of concomitance, there is no causal connection between the brain and the mind at all, that they exist concomitantly.[7] This parallelism has two practical effects. First, it allows neurologists to practice a diagnostically useful form of medicine based on sensorimotor physiology without having to consider the localization of mental symptoms. Second, it suggests an evolutionary structure for the mind analogous to that of the nervous system. Given the undeniable success of evolutionary neurophysiology as a bedside tool, neurologists have regarded the mind as a three-level hierarchy governed by a process of weighted ordinality. Such a structure allows neurologists to characterize mental states and processes, and imposes certain constraints on the products of the mind.[7,11–13]

In hierarchical terms, the mental aspect of art making can be regarded as an inductive process that elevates concepts to conscious awareness. This inductive process appears when a superior and controlling mental state, namely consciousness, stops working temporarily. Paul Klee, an inspired commentator as well as a one-man art movement, wrote that art does not reproduce the visible; rather, it makes the invisible visible.[14] This stands as one of the most profound statements of where art comes from, but a discerning neurologist would hesitate to say where in Klee's nervous system his words, much less his paintings or drawings, arose. Visual artists or musicians may not have the verbal skills to describe precisely what they do, and we ought to be skeptical of reports by artists about the process of their own creativity. Nevertheless, first-person reports provide a primary source, a direct insight into the mind of the artist. Creative people often observe that their own art making requires a certain alteration of consciousness, an exalted state of mind conducive to the creative process. Those with particular insight tell us of a type of hallucination that envelops them when they are doing something artistic. The use of alcohol or other mind-altering substances to artificially produce or prolong this state has been common since the very beginning of art—an experience also well known to many neurologists.

The idea that the creative process brings some ill-defined visual, auditory or verbal image from a subconscious level to conscious awareness implies that the creative state is lower, in evolutionary terms, than a state of conscious awareness. The products of creativity, the paintings and novels and songs, have their origin at a lower evolutionary level, which suggests that everyone possesses this creative ability, and has interesting consequences in regard to the artistic output of other animals. Alternatively, the altered awareness that enhances creative induction might involve a reweighting of conscious elements analogous to the reweighting of sensorimotor elements that occurs in recovery from stroke. This implies that creative states and processes arise at the highest evolutionary levels rather than at a lower, or subconscious, level. However, it might be difficult in practice to distinguish these possibilities.

The Localization of Creativity

The view that art emerges when the mind is in a disinhibited state has been examined scientifically. In a number of well-studied cases, patients show the preservation, or even the appearance, of artistic output in the face of neurological disease. For example, artists with widespread cortical disease may retain their artistic drive. Some continue to paint, draw, or play the trombone despite severe and progressive Alzheimer's disease.[15,16] The abstract painter Willem de Kooning developed Alzheimer's disease, yet he dramatically increased his productivity after being treated for alcoholism, malnutrition and depression. Art critics say that his paintings improved artistically as well.[17]

Patients with frontotemporal dementia were able to continue to paint, draw, or make photographs, which has been interpreted as the emergence of creativity or talent despite frontal and temporal lobe atrophy and substantial cognitive impairment. Investigators characterized their demented patients' artistry as improved or enhanced after the onset of their illnesses, possibly due to a more intense appreciation of visual images. The authors further observed that preservation of the frontal and parietal lobes allowed planning and execution of the work. They concluded that the patients' art arises from the undamaged parietal and occipital lobes when freed from the inhibition of the anterior temporal lobes.[18,19]

Studies of patients with incomplete surgical division of the corpus callosum suggest that the two hemispheres have different cognitive or perceptual experiences, leading to the assertion that the two hemispheres have different experiences in unoperated subjects. This phenomenon has been described as the existence of "divided selves" either in split-brain subjects or, more controversially, in normal individuals.[20,21] Moreover, the right hemisphere is said to be responsible for creativity, that people paint, act or draw with the right side of the brain. Two investigators describe these so-called split-brain subjects as lacking creativity because they cannot transmit nonverbal or emotive signals from one hemisphere to the other.[22] Another investigator calls the signals that must be sent from the right to the left hemisphere "symbols", and says that split-brain subjects lack creativity because they cannot send nonverbal symbols to the left side of the brain.[23]

These studies suggest that uncreative people have marked hemispheric dominance, with the left hemisphere suppressing creative states and processes. By contrast, creative people are said to have less hemispheric dominance. To examine this contention, a group of scientists measured regional cerebral blood flow in groups of normal subjects who were preselected by neuropsychological tests to be either highly creative or poorly creative. When given a verbal task requiring divergent thinking, the creative people showed bilateral activation of the frontal lobes while the uncreative ones activated only the dominant frontal lobe. The authors interpreted this to mean that creativity requires suppression of convergent thinking in the left hemisphere so that the divergent thinking in the right hemisphere might emerge.[24]

The neurologist at the art gallery has an opportunity to test these claims for lateralization of creative effort. The illness of the painter Katherine Sherwood gives a nice illustration. Professor Sherwood was an accomplished artist when, at age 44, she suffered a severe dominant hemisphere stroke. Since then she has painted with her left hand, and has achieved rather more acclaim and financial success after her stroke than she had before it. Neurologists are therefore invited to compare her painting before and after her stroke, looking for diagnostic information. Interviewed today, Sherwood believes that she is a better painter now than she was before her stroke. She describes her early work as constricted, tripped up by conscious intent, and her recent work as unburdened. She also implies that her current work flows freely from her subconscious, uninhibited by consciousness.[25,26]

In commenting on Sherwood's case, neuroscientists have written that the dominant hemisphere contains an interpreter, a mental function that explains to the rest of the brain why things happen.[20] They say that ablating the dominant hemisphere disables this controlling, bullying, overbearing interpreter, allowing the previously submissive nondominant hemisphere to paint, act or make music better than it did before. The neuroscientist Michael Gazzaniga is quoted as saying that the right hemisphere "does not try to interpret its experience and find deeper meaning", but rather "continues to live in the thin moment of the present".[25]

The drawing teacher Betty Edwards supports the claims that art requires a slightly altered state of consciousness and that suppressing the dominant hemisphere in favor of the nondominant one improves drawing skill. She also says that the exercises in her drawing lessons are designed to be impossible for the dominant left hemisphere to perform. What emerges is, therefore, the product of the nondominant right hemisphere. She characterizes the function of the nondominant hemisphere as nonverbal, synthetic, concrete, analogic, nontemporal, irrational, spatial, intuitive and holistic.[27] Edwards' drawing course is a remarkably successful teaching tool, with those who use it reporting a very high rate of learning to draw.

Neurologists do not try to assess the aesthetic merits of a bedside drawing, only its similarity to the model. The parlous nature of modern drawing makes analysis of its artistic content unsuitable as a bedside technique. Neurologists can demonstrate that patients with constructional apraxia are reasonably likely to have nondominant parietal lobe pathology, predicting the results of pathological examination or imaging. It is well to remember, though, that people who are blind cannot accurately reproduce a simple drawing despite a completely normal nondominant parietal lobe, and patients with advanced forms of dementia cannot draw despite diffuse rather than focal pathology. The astute examiner knows well that testing for constructional apraxia may have no meaning in the context of some illnesses, which is why we spend so much time in eliciting the patient's history.

Skeptical neurologists might find it hard to see the clinical value of these kinds of analyses. They take it as self-evident that there is no physical center of the nervous system, no anatomic point at which an afferent impulse necessarily becomes an efferent impulse. Once an impulse disappears into a cortical network, there is no point in space or in time when the impulse becomes motor. Since these networks may reside in one hemisphere or even in one lobe, it is tempting to ascribe certain mental characteristics to them. Giving a name, a gender or a political persuasion to the integration of sensorimotor impulses that occur in the left frontal lobe may appeal to our sense of shared humanity, but these subjective features make reliable diagnosis difficult unless they are reduced to their sensory and motor constituents. The result may be less attractive, but it is at least arguably useful medicine.

Commentary: The Neurologist in the Gallery

Neurologists assume that interpreting the information elicited by bedside testing is medically useful. A wealth of scientific information and the attitudes of most patients support this belief. The practical neurologist's skeptical point of view about the fruitlessness of localizing mental processes may seem psychologically or philosophically impoverished, but it is both scientifically valid and culturally informed. In addition, taking the skeptical neurologist's point of view is to take sides in an ideological conflict with political and economic overtones, a conflict in which cerebral localization is directly opposed to artistic motivation. Indeed, cerebral dominance for language has been used as a metaphor for undesirable political and social trends. Aggrieved people characterize dominant cultural practices as left-brain influences, with the dominant hemisphere a symbol of oppression. Artists are taken to be unconventional, right-brain types, doomed to the underclass, whereas physicians are identified with dominant political elements. A medicalized, dominant, left-brained modern culture is seen as being doomed to inevitable decay in favor of artistic, right-brained or even holistic tendencies. The alliance of radical rhetoric, artistic expression and cerebral localization may attract those with heterodox or even transgressive artistic and political beliefs. However, the avant-garde must be wary of giving a mantle of scientific respectability to undesirable sociopolitical ideologies—a mistake that once led both scientists and artists to embrace National Socialism.[28]

Neurologists are at least as capable of art criticism as anybody else, yet as a practical matter they find it difficult to apply consistent aesthetic judgments to the artistic output produced in the course of bedside diagnosis. This is particularly true if criteria of logic, power, gender or political persuasion are involved. Furthermore, no reliable bedside technique identifies the putative interpreter that is said to reside in the dominant hemisphere. In sensorimotor terms, the interpreter may be redefined as language comprehension, in which case the practical neurologist can localize Wernicke's aphasia with tolerable accuracy. However, this diagnosis seems far removed from assessing the quality of a patient's artistic output, which highly conditioned by social and cultural experiences. Neurologists routinely diagnose patients with language disorders whose first language they do not speak, but they would find it difficult to assess the artistry of a Zambian or a Timorese.

In more general terms, neurologists are reluctant to ascribe artistic, social, political or philosophical qualities to sensorimotor functions because of the practical difficulties in applying them clinically. Most neurologists would find it difficult to assess the artistic, or divergent or intuitive or nonlinear, thinking in a native of Fiji or the Punjab, but they successfully examine patients from these and many other cultures, not to mention those who reside in some of the more out-of-the-way corners of their own culture. This is not to deny that bedside neurology can be illuminating or even beautiful, or that there is artistry involved in spending one's life examining the anatomy and physiology of the nervous system of human beings. However, using artistic criteria diagnostically in an attempt to localize creativity is inherently impossible.

Put another way, it is easier to be a neurologist in the gallery than an artist at the bedside—a distressing state of affairs for the sensitive neurologist. He or she may take comfort, though, in the realization that neurological diagnosis puts their creative minds to the test. Thinking neurologically is a creative act in the same way that thinking artistically, musically or scientifically is creative. The profession of clinical neurology is an intrinsically artistic endeavor. Neurology and art are not only closely linked—they are in a way identical, at least if done properly. Neurologists may not be able to say where the artistic process is located in the brain, but they can at least have the pleasure of knowing what it is to be creative.

References

1. J. Hughlings Jackson, Notes on the physiology and pathology of the nervous system, *Medical Times and Gazette* **2**, 177–9 (1868).
2. J. Hughlings Jackson, On some implications of dissolution of the nervous system, *Medical Press and Circular* **2**, 411–3 (1882).
3. E.H. Ackernecht, *A Short History of Psychiatry*, 2nd edition (Hafner, New York, 1968).
4. G.K. York, Hughlings Jackson's evolutionary neurophysiology. In: F. Clifford Rose, ed., *A Short History of Neurology: The British Contribution 1660–1910* (Butterworth Heinemann, London, 1999), pp. 151–64.
5. R.M. Young, *Mind, Brain and Adaptation in the Nineteenth Century* (Clarendon, Oxford, 1970), reprinted 1990 (Oxford University Press, Oxford).
6. O. Temkin, Gall and the phrenological movement, *Bull. Hist. Med.* **21**, 275–321 (1947).

7. J. Hughlings Jackson, Evolution and dissolution of the nervous system; Croonian Lectures delivered at the Royal College of Physicians, Mar. 1884, *Lancet* **1**, 555–8, 649–52, 739–44 (1884).
8. O. Temkin, *The Falling Sickness: A History of Epilepsy from the Greeks to the Beginning of Modern Neurology*, 2nd edition (Johns Hopkins University Press, Baltimore, 1971).
9. S.H. Greenblatt, The major influences on the early life and work of John Hughlings Jackson, *Bull. Hist. Med.* **39**, 346–76 (1965).
10. G.K. York and D.A. Steinberg, Hughlings Jackson's theory of cerebral localization, *J. Hist. Neurosci.* **3**, 153–68 (1994).
11. G.K. York and D.A. Steinberg, Hughlings Jackson's rejection of the unconscious, *J. Hist. Neurosci.* **2**, 65–78 (1993).
12. C.U.M. Smith, Evolution and the problem of mind: Part II. John Hughlings Jackson, *J. Hist. Biol.* **15**, 241–62 (1982).
13. H.T. Englehardt, John Hughlings Jackson and the mind–body relation, *Bull. Hist. Med.* **49**, 137–51 (1975).
14. P. Klee, *Schöpferische konfession* (Erich Reiss, Berlin, 1920). Translated as: Creative credo. In: N. Guterman, trans., *The Inward Vision: Watercolors, Drawings and Writings of Paul Klee* (Abrams, New York, 1959).
15. J.L. Cummings and J.M. Zarit, Probable Alzheimer's disease in an artist, *JAMA* **258**, 2731–4 (1987).
16. W.W. Beatty, P. Winn, R.L. Adams *et al.*, Preserved cognitive skill in dementia of the Alzheimer's type, *Arch. Neurol.* **51**, 14–1046, 194.
17. C.H. Espinel, de Kooning's late colours and forms: dementia, creativity, and the healing power of art, *Lancet* **347**, 196–1098 (1996).
18. B.L. Miller, J. Cummings, F. Mishkin *et al.*, Emergence of artistic talent in frontotemporal dementia, *Neurology* **51**, 978–82 (1998).
19. B.L. Miller, M. Ponton, D.F. Benson *et al.*, Enhanced artistic creativity with temporal lobe deterioration, *Lancet* **348**, 1744–5 (1996).
20. M.S. Gazzaniga, Consciousness and the cerebral hemispheres. In: M.S. Gazzaniga, ed., *The Cognitive Neurosciences* (MIT Press, Cambridge, Massachusetts, 1995), pp. 1391–404.
21. A. Harrington, *Medicine, Mind and the Double Brain* (Princeton University Press, Princeton, 1987).
22. J.E. Bogen and G.M. Bogen, Creativity and the corpus callosum, *Psychiatric Clin. N. Amer.* **11**, 293–301 (1988).
23. K.D. Hoppe, Hemispheric specialization and creativity, *Psychiatric Clin. N. Amer.* **11**, 303–15 (1988).
24. I. Carlsson, P.E. Wendt and J. Risberg, On the neurobiology of creativity: differences in frontal activity between high and low creative subjects, *Neuropsychologia* **38**, 873–85 (2000).

25. P. Waldman, Tragedy turns a right-handed artist into a lefty—and a star in the art world, *The Wall Street Journal*, May 12, 2000, p. 1.
26. K. Maclay, A painter reinvents herself, *Berkeleyan* **28**, 1–2 (1999).
27. B. Edwards, *Drawing on the Right Side of the Brain: A Course on Enhancing Creativity and Artistic Confidence*, revised edition (Jeremy B. Tarcher, Los Angeles, 1989).
28. A. Harrington and G. Oepen, "Whole brain" politics and brain laterality research, *Eur. Arch. Psychiatry Neurol. Sci.* **239**, 141–3 (1989).

Chapter 2

Neural Concept Formation and Art: Dante, Michelangelo, Wagner

Semir Zeki

Introduction

> "Something, and indeed the ultimate thing, must be left over for the mind to do."
>
> —Arthur Schopenhauer[1]

What is art? What constitutes great art? Why do we value art so much and why has it been such a conspicuous feature of all human societies? These questions have been discussed at length, though without satisfactory resolution. This is not surprising. Such discussions are usually held without reference to the brain, through which all art is conceived, executed and appreciated. Art has a biological basis. It is a human activity and, like all human activities (including morality, law and religion), depends upon, and obeys, the laws of the brain. To understand the biological foundations of art, we must enquire into the biological foundations of knowledge, for art constitutes a form of knowledge—indeed, is knowledge. We are still far from knowing the neural basis of the laws that dictate artistic creativity, achievement and appreciation, but spectacular advances in our knowledge of the visual brain allow us to make a beginning in trying to formulate neural laws of art and aesthetics—in short, to study *neuroaesthetics.* In this essay, I try to discuss the art of three titanic figures in Western culture—Dante, Michelangelo and Wagner—in neurological terms. I try to show that we can trace the origins of their art to a fundamental characteristic of the brain, namely its capacity to form concepts. This capacity is itself the by-product of an essential characteristic of the brain. That characteristic is abstraction, and is imposed upon the brain by one of its chief functions, namely the acquisition of knowledge.

In all three examples that I use, the passion that governed the artists' work is romantic love, one of the most complex and overwhelming of all sentiments. It is in fact not so much love, but the ideal of love that each had created in his brain. None of the three found that ideal in real life, and each was impelled in a different way to create works of art in response to that gap. The ideal of love is of course not the only one that artists have tried to translate into their works. An artist may want to re-create simpler ideals, for example of natural scenery or even a straight line. But in every case, the motive force comes from the creation of ideals and concepts by the brain. I therefore begin by enquiring neurologically into the concept of ideals and their formation by the brain. That there are ideals, and that we have them, is a subject that has been discussed and debated by philosophers for over two millennia. They spoke in terms of the mind, not the brain.[a] I will speak exclusively in terms of the brain, and begin by arguing that the formation of ideals is the necessary and unavoidable by-product of an efficient knowledge-acquiring system, which is what the brain is. But the imperative in terms of efficiency in acquiring knowledge also exacts a high toll, which can be alleviated through art. My approach is dictated by a truth that I believe to be axiomatic—that all human activity is dictated by the organization and laws of the brain; that, therefore, there can be no real theory of art and aesthetics unless it is neurobiologically based, a belief I have developed at greater length elsewhere.[2] This speculative essay is a contribution, however small, towards the neurobiology of aesthetics. Its main thrust is that a basically similar neural process governs the generation of all concepts, be they simple or lofty, and that art is a manifestation of that neural capacity, and reveals to us both the strengths and the weaknesses of the concept-forming systems of the brain.

Abstraction as a Repetitively Applied Innate Cerebral "Concept"

One of the primordial functions of the brain, then, is to obtain knowledge about the world. How it does that is a problem that, today, belongs firmly in the field of neuroscience in its broadest sense. But long before neuroscience

---

a. This is a correct general statement, but it is interesting to draw attention here to a remarkable passage from Plato's *Phaedo* (p. 96, b, c), in which Socrates asks: "Is it with blood that we think, or with the air and fire that is in us? Or is it none of these, but the brain that supplies our sense of hearing, and sight and smell, and from these that memory and opinion arise, and from memory and opinion, when established, that knowledge comes?"

existed as a discipline, the same problem exercised philosophers. Indeed, the problem of knowledge, of how we acquire it and how certain we can be of what we know, has been a cornerstone of philosophical debate ever since the time of Plato. For Plato and his successors in the Western philosophic tradition, the problem revolved critically around the doctrine that Plato ascribed to Heraclitus, which has therefore become known as the Heraclitan doctrine of flux. In general terms, this reflects the reality that things are never the same from moment to moment. The task for the brain thus becomes one of acquiring knowledge about the essential, permanent and constant properties of objects and situations, when the information reaching the brain is never the same from moment to moment and everything is in a continual state of flux. Nor is the importance of mutability restricted to Western culture. A cornerstone of Eastern cultures, for example, is the belief that nothing is permanent except change.

Plato himself believed in a world of Ideas that have an existence independent of man. He supposed that true knowledge can only be knowledge of those Ideas and that the only way of obtaining that knowledge is through a thought process, since Ideas are supra-sensible. There is little doubt that his Ideal Theory went through several stages.[3] These can be traced through the early Socratic discourses and especially *Theaetetus* to the later Platonic dialogues, but this is not the place to trace that development. Suffice it to say that it is arguable whether Plato was ever convinced that he should make Ideas of objects and things such as houses, horses or instruments. In Book X of *The Republic* (p. 598, b, c) he used the example of a couch to question whether art could really give true knowledge, and to therefore express his contempt for it. Art, he thought, could only represent one particular facet of a particular object, not the universal, Ideal, object, which alone could give knowledge about all objects of that category. Even in spite of this, he nevertheless acknowledged his own uncertainty about whether to make Ideas of things (as at p. 130, b, c in *Parmenides*). What is certain is that his main preoccupation was with the idealization of abstract notions such as justice, goodness and, above all, beauty and love (as at the close of *Cratylus* and especially in *Phaedo* and *The Symposium*). The thesis he entertained is that general notions such as beauty, love and goodness exist permanently and are not subject to the changes to which the sensible world is hostage. The neurobiologist would not share Plato's hesitation and would not wish to thus restrict himself. He would want to consider, instead, how the brain constructs abstract representations of particular things, as well as of more general notions such as the ones that preoccupied Plato. Plato believed that there must be some kind of power in the mind which can compare the information provided by the different senses, and that notions such as "smaller" and "larger", or "more beautiful" that enable comparisons must be innate, in order to supply the power for reasoning. Much later, Immanuel Kant[4] proposed that we can never obtain knowledge about the "thing-in-itself" ("*das Ding an sich*"), independently of our experience of it, which includes a thought process. But he supposed that the ingredients of knowledge are provided by the sensory input, read into thought processes of the brain that are governed by the two innate intuitions of time and space. In seeking to understand our knowledge, it is therefore important to understand not only the formal contribution made by the mind (for us, the brain) but also the limitations imposed by it. I have argued that although time and space are critical "intuitions" for obtaining knowledge, they cannot be applied in a uniform way in the acquisition of all knowledge, since the temporal and spatial requirements for constructing even two sub-modalities of vision, for example colour and motion, are significantly different.[5,6] But I believe that there is a formal contribution that is made repetitively by the brain, in every area of the cerebral cortex, and that contribution—abstraction—is not acquired through experience but is innate.[5,6] Thus, contrary to the supposition of Plato, who believed that things are derived from abstractions, most today would probably say that it is the other way round, and that sensory data are submitted to the innately acquired abstractive processes of the brain. By "abstraction" I mean the process by which the particular is subordinated to the general, so that what is represented is applicable to many particulars. I would like to propose not only that all brain systems, however they differ in their functions, are engaged in abstraction and concept formation, because they are all somehow involved in the acquisition of knowledge, but also that a basically similar neural process governs the generation of different ideals by the brain. Art is basically a by-product of this abstracting, concept-forming, knowledge-acquiring system of the brain and can only be understood biologically in that context.

Functional Specialization in the Visual Brain

That different areas of the brain undertake different tasks has been known for a long time, and it is common to speak of a functional localization in the cerebral cortex. More recently, it has been found that even the part of the brain devoted to a single modality consists of many different areas. This has been most extensively studied in the visual brain, and the general picture of the organization of the visual brain that has emerged is worth alluding to briefly, because it gives us insights into the following question: Is there an operation that is performed in each one of the many cortical areas, regardless of what its specialization may be, and what can that operation be?

The most striking picture of the visual brain is one of functional specialization, in that different areas constituting it undertake different tasks.[7–9] There are separate colour and visual motion centres (V4 complex and V5 complex, respectively). In addition, there are areas that are specialized for object recognition, face recognition, and the recognition of position in space. Of these, the most intensively studied are the V4 and V5 complexes, and I will therefore make larger use of them in illustrating the general point, that each one of these areas is capable of abstracting to a certain level of sophistication, in addition to the other functions in which it is specialized. The neurological processes underlying these abstractions are ones that occur automatically; we are not conscious of the processes but are only conscious of their results. If we say that each of the cortical areas is capable of abstractions in the domain in which it is specialized, we are naturally led to asking another question: Do the processes of abstraction that are integral to the physiology of an area result in a conscious correlate, a percept? Or is the processing spatially separate from the perception?

Processing Sites in the Visual Brain Are Also Perceptual Sites

We have recently shown, using a visual stimulation paradigm, that the processing sites in the visual brain are also perceptual sites.[10] The use of dichoptic visual stimulation allows us to arrange the sensory input into the visual brain in such a way that it is sometimes-seen and sometimes not seen, even though the stimulus is identical in the two situations. Thus, when an identical stimulus, such as a house or a face, is presented monocularly to each eye in turn, the presentation to one eye alternating with that to the other eye every 100 ms, the two images are fused into a single image and the subject can report consciously and correctly what the stimulus was. But if the same stimulus is presented to each eye in the same way but with opposite colour contrasts, the two colours cancel each other out in the fusion and the stimulus is no longer perceived and cannot be recognized by the subject, even though the visual input to the brain through the eyes is the same as in the condition where the stimulus was correctly perceived. Brain imaging experiments show that the same stimulus-specific areas are activated regardless of whether the stimulus is perceived or not. Thus when the stimulus is that of a face, the area in the brain specifically implicated in the perception of faces is specifically activated, regardless of whether the stimulus is perceived or not. A similar result obtains with stimuli depicting houses, which activate a different, specialized, part of the visual brain (see also Ref. 11). This is not to deny that other cortical areas may also be involved in the abstractive process, especially where other, more abstract, notions such as beauty and justice are involved. But the above demonstration, which I consider to be of some importance, shows that the cortical perceptual sites are not separate from the cortical processing sites. This, in turn, makes it credible to suppose that each cortical area has an abstractive machinery, a supposition that is much reinforced by the physiological examples given below. We are, in short, not aware of the abstractive process or of the processing in general, though we are aware of its results. There is, therefore, an unconscious "mind" and a conscious "mind". This is of course not a novel idea. It can be traced back at least to Leibniz, who believed that we cannot be conscious of all the process of mind required to acquire knowledge about the world, and that we must therefore suppose that there is an unconscious mind. He wrote in *La Monadologie* (14): "The passing condition, which involves and represents a multiplicity in the unit [*unité*] or in the simple substance, is nothing but what is called *Perception*, which is to be distinguished from Apperception or Consciousness.... In this matter the Cartesian view is extremely defective, for it treats as non-existent those perceptions of which we are not aware".[12] Here, I am equating the unconscious "mind" with the processing that occurs in an area, the processing that leads to a conscious awareness of the results of the operations that the unconscious "mind" performs. Given the specializations in the visual brain and elsewhere, it is plausible that there are many unconscious "minds" (neural processes) that process signals related to the attribute that they are specialized in, each one being centred on a different cortical area. The results of anatomical, physiological and clinical studies seem to point in this direction.[13] Important in this regard is the result of recent psychophysical experiments which show that we do not become conscious of different visual attributes at the same time.[14,15] Instead, we perceive colour, for example, some 80 ms before we perceive motion, an enormously long time in neural terms. Since perceiving something means being conscious of it, it follows that we become conscious of different attributes at different times. Consciousness is therefore distributed in time. Since it is activity in geographically distinct locations that leads to the perception of different attributes, it follows that consciousness is also distributed in space.

Thus each of the parallel, specialized systems of the brain undertakes its own processing. But to what end? The acquisition of knowledge. And since abstraction is the prerequisite of any efficient knowledge-acquiring system, it follows that there are many abstractive systems, each one tied to activity in a particular cortical area. In a system such as the cerebral cortex, where there are multiple specializations, one can conjecture that each one of the specialized systems or sub-systems is capable of constructing, or at least contributing substantially to, the construction of concepts and ideals, the final step in the acquisition of knowledge. Abstraction, in addition to being a mandatory step in the efficient acquisition of knowledge, also frees the brain from enslavement to the particular, for example a particular point of view or a particular occasion or a particular object. Paradoxically this independence from particulars depends upon experience of many particulars. Through it the brain is no longer enslaved to the particular. Abstraction also frees the brain from total dependence upon the memory system, which can fail. If, for example, recognition of a car as a car depended upon a particular car, then the brain would need a fail-safe memory system, which it obviously does not possess. But abstraction and generalization, as a means of acquiring knowledge, are also testaments to the limitations of the brain. As Frazer (1930) has emphasized, "... generalization, while the highest power of the human intellect and a mark of its strength, is no less a mark of its weakness. Generalization is but the compendious and imperfect way in which a finite mind grasps the infinity of particulars. A mind that could grasp at once all the particulars would not generalize... if there is a mind which grasps the totality of things, it... can have no need to have recourse to the summary which the limitation of our minds compels us to make use of."[3] There is also a price to be paid for this. Abstraction leads to an Idea or concept, but our experience remains that of the particular, and the particular that we experience may not always satisfy the Idea formed in and by our brains. One way of obtaining that satisfaction is to "download" the Idea formed in the brain, into a work of art. This is a theme I will return to later in discussing the three artists I have selected for this essay.

In thus endowing individual cortical areas with the power of abstraction, I do not mean to imply that the individual areas do not interact with one another. As Plato saw (*Theaetatus*, pp. 185–6B), each sense (or each submodality of a sense, such as colour or visual motion) gives only the results of its own processings regarding the attribute it is specialized in. It does not process other senses, or other sub-modalities. It cannot therefore view what other senses have processed in connection with what it has processed. There must therefore be some other power that unifies and binds what these different areas have processed, a problem that is currently under study. The point that I emphasize here is that the unification and the binding come after the abstractive processes, which constitute the first step in the knowledge-acquiring system.

Abstraction in the Visual Brain

How the brain abstracts is only partially known, for simpler constructs only. What is clear is that the neurological processes underlying these abstractions are ones that occur automatically; we are not usually conscious of the processes themselves but only of their results. What is also clear is that the capacity to abstract is not a characteristic of higher areas of the brain, or limited to them. It is characteristic even of early visual areas, as becomes evident when one considers the physiological properties of cells in the visual brain which are specialized for lines of specific orientation, or to detect motion in specific directions, or specific colours.

A cell in the primary visual cortex, area V1, that responds to a straight line of specific orientation is in fact abstracting, since it responds to a line of that orientation no matter what its contrast or colour may be.[16,17] These cells are very interesting to study in the laboratory. Once a cell that is responsive to the vertical orientation is isolated, one can establish quickly that it is responsive not only to a vertical line generated from luminance differences (for example, a white bar against a black background) but almost to any straight vertically orientated line or edge. If it is presented in the appropriate part of the field of view, one could elicit a vigorous response from such a cell by presenting a pencil or a ruler held vertically. The cell, in brief, abstracts for verticality, without being concerned about what is vertical. That the properties of such cells are largely innately determined implies that the abstractive process is also innate, even if the selective responses of such cells require visual nourishment during critical periods to maintain their selectivity and hence their abstractive powers as well.[18] Equally, a cell in V5 concerned with the direction of motion is abstracting the motion and its direction since it is indifferent to the colour of the stimulus and usually to its form as well.[19–21] The V4 complex constructs colours in the abstract, in that it is not concerned with the objects that the colours vest. The latter seems to engage other cortical areas.[22,23] Another kind of abstraction is implicit in the behaviour of cells that are capable of responding in a view-invariant manner to visual stimuli.[24] These cells are located in the parietal cortex of the brain, and more specifically in area V6. Their properties are such that they are capable of signalling the position of an object with respect to egocentric space, regardless of where we are looking.

It is worth emphasizing yet again that the neurological processes underlying these abstractions occur automatically; we are not conscious of them but only of their results. As an example, the construction of colour is a complicated process which must involve a comparison of the wavelength composition of the light reflected from the surface that we are looking at with the wavelength composition of the surrounds.[25,26] We know little about the detailed neural implementation that leads to the construction of colours, but we do know that it involves specialized pathways and areas and that, moreover, we are not conscious of these processes but of their end results—colour—only. We know more about the wiring mechanisms that lead to the emergence of cells in the brain that signal lines of specific orientation.[16] But, once again, we are not aware of the processes themselves but only of their end results.

Perhaps even more interesting in this regard are recent experiments on object recognition. When monkeys are trained to look at particular views of "nonsense" objects, which they have never seen before, most cells in the inferior temporal cortex (a visual centre in the brain) respond to only one of the views that the monkey has seen. But there is a minority of cells that respond in a view-invariant way.[27] By some neural mechanism about which we know little, a sort of idea of the object is built into the responses of single cells, such that their responses are no longer determined by a single view. The neural processes involved are almost certainly highly complex,[28] but we are not aware of them.

It is plausible to suppose that the result of this abstractive process is the creation of an "ideal", in which all the sensory experiences have been combined synthetically to generate a construct which, though dependent upon many particulars in its construction, is also independent of a given particular. For Plato, the Ideal meant the universal as opposed to the particular. The sense in which I use the term here is not vastly different, since the ideal does not represent a particular object, but is a construct of all objects of that category that the brain has experienced. From this, it follows that the ideal formed by a brain is dependent upon its neurological machinery (an innate mechanism) as well as the experience acquired by the individual. That neurological machinery, as well as the experience, varies between individuals. Hence the ideals formulated by one brain are not necessarily identical to those formulated by another, even if there is a common element underlying the formulation of ideals. Yet all brains have the common capacity of abstracting and forming ideals.

Can one generalize from these types of abstraction to love, a subject hardly touched upon in neurological studies. The answer must be speculative at present. Yet it is hard to believe that there isn't an abstractive process involved in love too. We do, after all, have special preferences in love, no doubt dictated by a variety of factors, and artists have tried to express their concepts of love in works of art. Moreover, recent imaging studies have shown that the sentiment of love associated with a face correlates with activity in restricted loci of the brain.[29] Above all, artists have formed concepts and ideals of love, which they have translated into their art.

All Ideals Are Brain Constructs

I shall take what some may consider an extreme position, by supposing that the only "ideals" that we have are those constructed by the brain. This is extreme because there are no doubt those who would disagree with the notion that, for example, natural numbers exist only by virtue of the organization of our brains. Roger Penrose is among them. For him, the mathematical world is not a product of our thinking, and hence its laws do not depend upon the structure and functioning of the brain. The existence of that world "rests on the profound, timeless, and universal nature of these concepts, and on the fact that their laws are independent of those who discover them. . . . The natural numbers were there before there were human beings, or indeed any other creatures here on earth, and they will remain after all life has perished."[30] I have no way of refuting Penrose's claim. Yet I wonder what the reaction would be to another, seemingly powerful, advance in mathematics, namely string theory, which, put simply, is an attempt to quantize gravity. To do so, one needs to construct an abstract space with 26 dimensions, which can then be collapsed into 10, and subsequently into 4, giving the conventional space–time dimensions. As I understand it, there is no current scientific evidence for string theory, or at any rate there was none when the theory was first developed. It is therefore a product of the human imagination, dependent upon brain organization. I wonder whether it would have been at all possible to develop string theory without the kind of brain organization that we have. Yet again, I am not in a position to provide a compelling justification for my view that even the mathematical straight line is a product of the human brain. Even allowing for this lapse, there nevertheless remains an important area—for example, of object and shape recognition, of colour perception, of narrative recognition and much else besides—which most would today acknowledge as being a property of the brain and dependent upon the laws of the brain.

Abstraction and its end process, the formation of ideals, are the necessary ingredients of an efficient knowledge-acquiring system, but there is a heavy price that is exacted in return. The experience that we have depends, by necessity, upon the experience of particulars. But the particular may not always satisfy the "ideal" synthesized by the brain from many particulars. A refuge lies in recreating the brain's ideal in art and through art. I repeat again that abstraction and the construction of ideals is a process that is repetitively applied in the brain. This leads not only to the construction of the ideal straight line, but also the ideal house, the ideal representation of a scenery, and the ideal—of love. Let us acknowledge that there are other dimensions to art. Dance and music are commonly collective artistic experiences that depend upon the interaction of many brains. That interaction can also be seen in the strong cultural influences in the creation and appreciation of works of art. The artist's concepts will also change as his work develops and as he *learns* more while creating. But the primordial source of art is the knowledge-acquiring system of the brain, with all its splendours and shortcomings.

Brain Concepts That Are Only Realised in Art

The three artists whom I use to illustrate my general point, in the chronological order of their lives, have much in common. All were men and each occupies a high position in Western civilization. The culture of all three was deeply rooted in the Western, Christian tradition and each one had been deeply influenced by ancient Greek civilization. The ideals formed by all three were therefore dictated by sensory input and inclination, but also by the culture that they had imbibed. And all three had formed an ideal of love in their brains that they never seemed to have attained in life. All three temporarily saw death as a possible relief from the struggle for attaining it. Art was the refuge for all three. Let me emphasize that, in choosing romantic love, I am focusing on an overwhelmingly powerful passion in the service of which man has achieved a great deal but also destroyed much. I do not mean to imply that people have not found the perfect happiness in love. Many have and yet many have not. My purpose in concentrating on love is to show that concept formation by the brain is important even in so complex a sentiment.

Dante and Beatrice

My concern here is with Dante's relationship to Beatrice, the "lady" who inspired all his work. He met her when both were nine, and he was infatuated with her for the rest of his life. She married a banker and died young. His love and desire for her was thus forever to be frustrated, leading him into deep depression but at the same time unlocking his creative genius.

Dante was to marry later and raise a family. But his wife does not figure in any of his writings, and we can only presume that this was a marriage of convenience and convention, not of passion. In fact, there is only one other female figure that takes a prominent place in Dante's work—Donna Gentile. She appears in the second half of the *Vita Nuova* as a real person, creating a tension in him between his love of Beatrice and her. But she remains an ambiguous figure. In the *Convivio*, written some ten years after the *Vita Nuova*, Dante equates her with Lady Philosophy, who instils in him the philosophical virtues of Wisdom, and consoles him for Beatrice's death. Her existence as a real person has been doubted.[31]

Dante's work is written in the vernacular Italian. It displays deep knowledge of theology, astronomy and philosophy as known at the time. In steps through the *Vita Nuova*, the *Convivio* and the *Paradiso*, his unsatisfied and unfulfilled love for Beatrice is sublimated into love of philosophy and wisdom, which leads into Heaven. Beatrice herself is metamorphosed in the work, from a beautiful woman into Wisdom itself, and thus becomes the most precious of all beauties for Dante. It is she who leads him in steps to the highest reaches of Paradise, the Empyrean. In a sense, therefore, his concept of love itself changes as we follow his writings through the three works, as indeed concepts generally do through the accretion of experience. There is a distinctly Platonic flavour to this metamorphosis. In both *Phaedo* and *The Symposium*, arguments are made in favour of love beginning as attraction and desire and metamorphosing gradually into the philosophical virtues of Wisdom, Truth and Universal Beauty. For Dante, this metamorphosis was probably much aided when the vernaculars, starting with Provençal, came to use the word "*amor*" or "*amore*" in both sexual and sacred senses, its previous use in the sacred sense having been frowned upon as being compromised by its use in the other sense. This dual use of the word "can be said to have facilitated Dante's extraordinary enhancement of his angel-like lady, Beatrice, and his exaltation of her and his love for her".[32] Furthermore, however individual Dante's work is, it is nevertheless worth recalling that idealization of a woman, usually someone other than a wife, was common in the culture to which Dante belonged.[33] This emphasises the importance not only of the cultural context within which Dante worked, but of cultural contexts in general in the formulation of concepts. It also raises the question of why this kind of idealization should have occurred so commonly in literature.

The metamorphosis starts in the *Vita Nuova*, where, interestingly from a neuroaesthetic point of view, Dante begins by writing of the "glorious lady of my mind" ("*la gloriosa donna de la mia mente*"), thus acknowledging that even though his love of her had been triggered by an encounter with a real person, she was very much a construction of his mind, someone whom he loved from a distance. Dante was acquainted with the ingenious view of Greek philosophers that objects take their form by virtue of what the observer vests in them. In the *Convivio* (Tractate III, ix), he writes: "In truth, Plato and other philosophers affirmed that our vision was brought about, not because the object of sight came to the eye, but because the visual power went out to the object," though he adds that "this opinion is censured as false by the Philosopher [Aristotle] in his book *On Sense and the Object of Sense* (Dante, 1304? See Ref. 34). Evidently, however, the Aristotelian view prevailed because when he first sees Beatrice, "the animal spirit, the one abiding in the high chamber [*la secretissima camera*] to which all the senses bring their perceptions, was stricken with amazement, and speaking directly to the spirits of sight said these words, 'Now your bliss has appeared.' " But though metamorphosed in *The Divine Comedy*, and especially in the *Paradiso*, into an object of Wisdom and Truth, the relationship has an early erotic component, acknowledged through its denial. In his commentary to Canzone XVIII of the *Vita Nuova* he writes: "I speak of certain beauties pertaining to her whole body [and then] I speak of certain beauties pertaining to particular parts of her body." But "so that here and now every perverse thought may be extinguished, let him who reads this remember what has been mentioned previously concerning this lady's greeting, which is an act performed by her mouth; namely that it was the goal of all my desire so long as I was able to receive it", from which one may conclude that the thought of kissing her never crossed his mind!

There are erotic allusions in the *Convivio* too. There he says: "The sight of this lady was so generously ordained for us—not just to see her face, which she shows us, but to long to win what she keeps hidden" (Tractate xiv, 13). Writing long before Freud had started to profane the secrets of fantasy, he was able to convey unashamedly the idea of Beatrice as the "mother" and himself as a "child" who falls asleep "like a little boy crying from a spanking", since he was protected from having to acknowledge the source of his phantasms.

Dante's writing thus leaves little doubt that, though she was to be metamorphosed into Truth and Wisdom by him in his work, culminating in the Paradiso, his love of her was the love of a woman. There is acknowledgement, too, that the complete joy one desires in a relationship with a woman may never happen. In the *Convivio*, (Tractate III, xii) he writes: "In other intelligences she exists in a lesser fashion, as it were *like a mistress in whom no lover can take complete joy*, but contents his longing by looking at her" (my emphasis). Death was a solution to this predicament earlier in his life. In Canzone XXIII of *Vita Nuova* comes the surprising dream, possibly even the wish, of her death, which in fact anticipates her real death. In the introduction to his translation of the work, Musa[34] has emphasized that this Canzone occupies the important, central, part of the *Vita Nuova*, whereas her actual death is mentioned in passing later, without comment, as if the death in the mind were the more important event. Realizing that such a heavenly love, much of it created by the mind and of the mind, is not in reality possible, he writes: "And so it seemed to me that when I went to see the body in which that most worthy and blessed soul had dwelt... so strong was the hallucination that it actually showed me this lady dead." Perhaps also anticipating the death wish of Tristan and Isolde, to whom romantic love was also an illusion, he wishes his own death (before her real death), writing:

ch'io dicea: "Morte, assai dolce ti tegno;	I said, "Death, I hold you very dear;
tu dei omar esser cosa gentile,	by now you ought to be a gracious thing
poi ché tu se' ne la mia donna stata	and changed your scorn for sympathy
e dei aver pietate e non disdegno	since in my lady you have been at home
Vedi che si desideroso vegno	I yearn so to become one of your own
d'esser de' toi, ch'io ti simiglio in fede	that I resemble you in every way
Vieni, ché 'l cor te chiede."	My heart begs you to come."

His realization in the *Vita Nuova* that his desire can never be fulfilled leads him in a different direction. Since true happiness cannot come from something as changeable as the lady to whom he is devoted, he looks for something less mutable, more certain—of dedicating himself to her praises and of saying of her what has not been said of any woman ("*io spero di dicer di lei quello che mai no fue detto d'alcuna*"). And thus through his unfulfilled desire he creates a great work of art. Into that art he disgorges the ideals in his brain, as they are metamorphosed through his life. In the end, Beatrice, the earthly woman whom he could never love as a woman, herself changes from being an earthly and desirable, but unattainable, woman to the embodiment of beauty, wisdom and virtue. Thus transformed, she leads him in successive stages through Hell, Purgatory and Paradise to the Empyrean.

The *Non-finito* of Michelangelo

If Dante's work was inspired by a brain concept that could, he knew, never be realized in life (which is presumably why he killed Beatrice off in the *Vita Nuova* before she actually died), and could therefore only be lived in a great work of art, it is not at all obvious that the same is true of the mighty Michelangelo. Yet it is plausible to argue that what made Michelangelo leave so much of his work unfinished can be traced to the same source as that which made Dante create his art—the impossibility of realizing the ideals formed by the brain in the experience of particulars in real life.

All his life, Michelangelo had been dominated by the overwhelming desire to represent not only physical but also spiritual beauty and divine love. There is little doubt that in his Platonic culture, physical and spiritual beauty were entwined and not easily separable, that he formed amorous relations with men, that he yearned for a physical and spiritual dimension to these relationships and that what he experienced had left him largely unsatisfied. The most enduring of these relationships was with Tommaso de' Cavalieri, the young Roman nobleman who had overwhelmed him with his physical and intellectual beauty and who had come to dominate his emotional life in his later years. Yet for all the brilliant work that the relationship unleashed, he felt a prisoner—"*resto prigion d'un Cavalier armato*" ("I remain the prisoner of an armed Knight"). The conflict within him is expressed in one of his *Rime*:

S'un ardente desir mortal bellezza	If mortal beauty be the food of love,
ferma del tutto, non discese insieme	it came not with soul from heaven, and thus
dal ciel con l'alma, e dunque umana voglia:	that love itself must be a mortal fire:
ma se pass' oltre, amor tuo non me sprezza	but if love reaches to nobler hopes above,
ch'altro Dio cerca; e di quell più non teme	thy love shall scorn me not nor dread desire
ch' a lato vien contro a sì bassa spoglia.	That seeks a carnal prey assailing us.

It is against this background of Michelangelo's ideal of love that I want to approach his unfinished work. These constitute three fifths of his sculptures and thus are not a negligible part of his work. This may seem surprising in a man who despised unfinished works in others, and the reason for it has been debated. There may have been technical reasons for this. A correspondent, Anna Winestein, has pointed out to me the difficulties of working with marble, especially of restituting what has been chipped away, thus making it difficult to have many tries. While acknowledging these difficulties, I find it hard to believe that they alone can account for the unfinished status of so many of his works. Like Michelangelo's disciple, Condivi, Giorgio Vasari believed that "Michelangelo's *non-finito* reflects the sublimity of his ideas, which again and again lay beyond the reach of his hands".[36] I would modify that statement somewhat and say that time and again he felt that he could not represent in a single work the inseparable concept of love and beauty that had formed in his brain. His solution was to leave the work unfinished. For Michelangelo, leaving a work unfinished was perhaps an improvement on another characteristic—not undertaking a work at all for fear that he would be incapable of representing on canvas or in sculpture the same ideal that had formed in his brain. We know that this was the reason for his general refusal to execute portraits, two exceptions being those of Andrea Quaratesi and Tomasso de' Cavalieri. In another one of his *Rime*, he wrote:

Se ben concetto ha la divina parte	When that which is divine in us does try
il volto e gli atti d'alcun, po' di quello	to shape a face, both brain and hand unite
doppio valor con breve e vil modello,	to give, from a mere model frail and slight,
dà vita a'sassi, e non è forza d'arte.	life to the stone by Art's free energy.

I interpret "*forza d'arte*" to mean the unhindered concept formed in the artist's brain. But the difficulty of translating all the concepts of love and beauty formed by his brain makes Michelangelo yearn for death, just as Dante saw death as a solution in *Vita Nuova* and Wagner's Tristan and Isolde see death as the salvation for the unrealizable state of the perfect union in love that they yearn for (see below). In one of his *Rime*, Michelangelo wrote:

Deh quando fia, Signor, quell che s'aspetta	When will that day dawn, Lord, for which he waits
per chi ti crede? Ch'ogni troppo indugio	who trusts in Thee? Lo, this prolonged delay
tronca la speme, e l'alma fa mortale	destroys all hope and robs the soul of life
Che val che tanto lume altrui prometta,	Why streams the light from these celestial gates,
s'anzi vien morte, e senz' alcun' rifugio	if death prevent the day of grace, and stay
ferma per sempre in che stato altri assale?	our souls forever in the toils of strife?

There is little doubt that many of his unfinished sculptures were not left unfinished through haste. They were instead brought to a certain state of completion and not continued beyond, even though Michelangelo sometimes kept working on them. A notable example is the Rondanini *Pietà*

(Palazzo Sforzesca, Milan), which Michelangelo was still working on when he died. Charles De Tolnay wrote that, in the Rondanini *Pietà*, "Michelangelo subordinates the representation of physical beauty to the feeling of emotional life [through the use of] flat surfaces, straight lines and the inertia of an amorphous mass lacking contrasts of light and shade". The work, he believed, "comes to represent in the personal life of the artist the fulfilment of his longings, that state of beatitude toward which his unsatisfied soul aspired".[37] Though the work is unfinished, its evocative power is such that, read without reference to its subject, this is really a description of a finished work. What Michelangelo has done, without acknowledging it, is to leave it to the brain of the spectator to complete it. And De Tolnay has done so in his fashion while others may complete the work in a different way, by seeing in it other qualities and evocative powers.

In fact, Michelangelo himself alluded in one of his last sonnets to his belief that the concepts of beauty translated into works of art may pale into insignificance when compared to concepts of beauty formed in the brain. This, among other reasons, led one of the greatest artists the world has produced to turn against art:

Onde l'affettuosa fantasia,	Now I know how fraught with error was that fantasy
Che l'arte mi fece idol' e monarca	That made art my idol and my king
Né pinger né scolpir fia più che quieti	No brush, no chisel can quieten the soul
l'anima volta a quell'Amor divino	Once it turns to the Divine love of Him who from the Cross,
ch'aperse, a prender noi, in croce le braccia.	Outstretched his arms to take us unto Himself.

Ambiguity

It is interesting to introduce here ambiguity, which constitutes another way of leaving a work unfinished. I use the term "ambiguity"—a characteristic of all great art—in a neurological sense, not in the dictionary sense of vagueness and uncertainty. By it I mean that a work of art is "unfinished" enough to offer several solutions, all of equal validity, so that there is no right answer to the puzzle offered by the work of art. It may fit any of the concepts in the viewer's brain. Indeed, the more of the concepts it approximates, the greater the work of art. "Something," Schopenhauer wrote, "and indeed the ultimate thing must be left over for the mind to do." Leaving a work unfinished or making it ambiguous engages the brain more intensly. That is precisely what Michelangelo's unfinished Rondanini *Pieta* and Vermeer's ambiguous *Girl with a Pearl Earring*, among his other works, do. Marcel Proust's just description of Vermeer as "*un artiste à jamais inconnu*"("an artist who is forever unknown") applies to more than just the scanty details of his life. It applies with even greater force to his great paintings, in which the spectator can find many solutions, but none which is dominant or more valid than the others.

Here we can come to a definition of art, and to speculating about what, in neurobiological terms, constitutes great art. The translation of concepts in the artist's mind onto canvas, or into music or literature, constitutes art. Great art is that which corresponds to as many different concepts in as many different brains over as long a period of time as possible. Ambiguity is such a prized characteristic of all great art because it can correspond to many different concepts. Its close affinity with the unfinished is easy to understand, for they both offer the spectator the luxury of choosing from many alternatives, and even picking the alternative that best fits brain concepts at any given time. It was Wagner who combined both ambiguity and the unfinished, or unresolved, as never before. Through the use of this dual but linked device (linked in terms of brain mechanisms), he produced one of the supreme artistic achievements of our culture—his romantic opera *Tristan und Isolde*. A highlight of the opera is the use of what has been called "premeditated irresolvability".[38]

The Unrealizable in Wagner's Art

Dante's solution to his unfulfilled desires and his unfinished earthly love was to metamorphose that love into spiritual and philosophic dimensions in a work of literature. Michelangelo, deprived of the ability to experience that combination of spiritual and physical beauty that he yearned for, and finding it difficult to combine and portray the concepts of love, and of spiritual and divine beauty formed in his brain in a single work of art, found a solution in leaving many of his sculptures unfinished. Wagner, the great womanizer, understood that the concepts of romantic love formed in his brain were not even realizable in life, and this led him to convey the message in a work of art. But that work of art was achieved because of the realization that an unrealizable concept had formed in his brain, though of course Wagner did not think or write about the brain.

Wagner wrote *Tristan und Isolde* relatively late in life. The opera has unmistakable roots in an earlier work, *Wesendonk Lieder*. The latter had been composed when Wagner was staying in Zurich to work in the home of a banker,

Otto von Wesendonk. There he developed a passion for Wesendonk's wife, Mathilde. The relationship had marked Wagner deeply, even though, or perhaps because, it was probably never consummated. But whether it was or not is immaterial to the argument. It is quite evident that the ideal of romantic love as it had developed in his brain is not one that he had actually encountered. Why else would he describe *Tristan und Isolde* as the greatest of all monuments to the greatest of all illusions, romantic love? An illusion is, after all, a creation of the brain.

This may seem surprising. By external appearance at any rate, Wagner did have passionate attachments and, for a time at least, a more or less happy domestic life. Unlike the total silence of Dante on his wife, Wagner seems to have delighted in his second wife, Cosima, and composed music for her. But if his statement above and the message of his opera are to be believed, he craved for something that he was unable to attain and decided in the end that it was unattainable in life. In fact, in a letter to Liszt, he wrote: "Since never in my whole life have I tasted the real happiness of love, I mean to raise a monument to that most beautiful of dreams".[39] In his work, he conveyed the idea that the brain concept—at least as it relates to romantic love—has no counterpart in the experience of particulars.

The legend of Tristan and Isolde, probably born in Wales or Cornwall, had had much currency throughout Europe. Virgil, Dante's guide in the *Inferno*, points Tristan out to him:

Vedi Paris, Tristano: e più di mille	See Paris, Tristan: and more than a thousand
ombre mostrommi e nominommi a dito	shades he pointed out to me and named
ch'amor di nostra vita dipartille	who were parted from our life by love

his presence in hell being presumably the consequence of his amorous escapades.

Wagner dispenses with many of the legend's details in his opera. In his hand, the relationship of Tristan and Isolde becomes entirely ascetic, possibly the most ascetic love relationship ever described. Right from the start, in the *Prelude*, the impossibility of the "dream" of love finds musical expression. Wagner stated in his own programme notes that "it expresses the incessant projection and recoil upon itself of a single emotion—that of longing without satisfaction and without end".[39] The *Prelude* was in fact originally referred to as the *Liebestod* ("love death") by Wagner, who described it as a progression from "the first timidest lament of unappeasable longing, the tenderest shudder, to the most terrible outpouring of an avowal of hopeless love", the music

The Tristan Chord

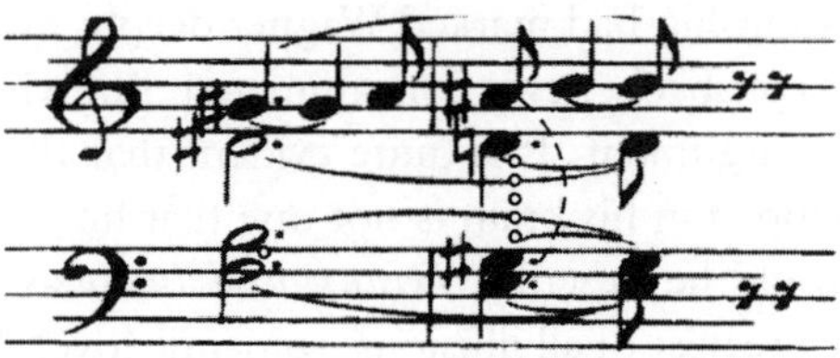

Fig. 1. Diabolic intervals are shown with circles; *appogiatura* to the diabolic interval is shown with dashes.

"traversing all phases of the vain struggle against the inner ardour, until this, sinking back powerless upon itself, seems to be extinguished in death".[39]

Musically, the *Prelude* and especially the dissonant Tristan chord (see Figure 1), which is left unresolved, introduces a much-commented-on ambiguity.[b] When musicians and musical theoreticians speak of dissonance and irresolvability in the music, they imply that there is something dissonant and irresolvable in the music. Even those sympathetic to the importance of incorporating brain studies in theorizing about music follow this trend. Benzon[40] writes: "I believe memes—such as music— reside in the external world", memes being a term introduced by Richard Dawkins to signify the cultural counterpart of the biological gene. My view is that the music, the dissonance, the consonance, the tonality, and the ambiguity all reside in the brain, and are indeed a manifestation of brain activity. It is the brain that is incapable of resolving the chords, or of determining them as irresolvable or, better still, resolving them in a number of different ways. The situation is not vastly dissimilar to that obtaining in colour vision. Colour is a property of the brain, not of the world outside, though of course the brain makes use of different wavelengths of light to construct colour. This was recognized by Newton,[41] who wrote: "For the Rays, to speak properly, have no Colour. In them there is nothing else than a power and disposition to stir up a sensation of this Colour or that."

It is sometimes claimed that in the *Prelude* Wagner destroyed tonality, even against the protestations of musicians like Wilhelm Furtwängler that in *Tristan*

b. John Langerholc has pointed out to me that the ambiguity of the Tristan harmony resides in the progression of the four four-note chords. However, the first chord in itself, generally referred to as *the* Tristan chord, is one of the least ambiguous in all tonal music, being diatonic (i.e. without chromatic alteration) in only one minor key, the "hidden" key of D#/E*b*-minor, and in its parallel F#-major, after enharmonic respelling. This respelling is necessary as the chord is nowhere endemic. On its entrance, this chord abruptly contradicts the seeming A-minor of the beginning, which makes the expectation and curiosity of the listener all the greater.

und Isolde, "so often cited as a crown witness for musical progress, there is not one note which is not to be understood tonally".[42] Langerholc[38,43] is right to draw attention to the similarity, in terms of brain organization, of the effects produced by the "dissonant" and "unresolved" chords of *Tristan*, the impossible figures of Escher and ambiguous bi-stable images such as the Necker cube or the Rubin vase, that grace every textbook of vision. The latter have two equally compelling perceptual interpretations[44] and are therefore being increasingly used to study the neural basis of perception. The question asked in the physiological experiments is simple: To what extent do the cells' responses follow the perceived interpretation? The answer to date has been that there are cells in all visual areas whose responses correlate with the perceived figure, the largest number being observed in the temporal lobe. Equally striking is the number of cells in early visual areas that remain active when the stimulus is "suppressed".[45] Taken together, these results suggest that the conscious perception of a stimulus may be mediated by only a subset of cells in any given area, which is not to say that the others do not contribute to the responses of what we may loosely call the "perceptual cells". Human brain imaging experiments suggest that the perceptual dominance of one image over another in bi-stable images is controlled by a network of cortical areas, which includes the frontal and parietal cortex.[46,47] What this really means is that the brain has a perceptual machinery which is labile enough to allow it to interpret an image in more than one way, and that there is an additional neural machinery that dictates, supervises, or governs which of the two images holds sway. It needs to be emphasized yet again that we are not at all aware of the processes in the brain that result in the perception of one of the two images at any one time, but only conscious of the image that we perceive at a given time. In general, however, one of the two images is not given absolute dominance, and hence the bi-stability and hence, too, the ambiguity.

It must be a neural process of a similar kind that allows for the ambiguity in the music of Wagner. That musical theoreticians should not have been able to agree even on which key or how many are used in the Tristan chord merely serves to emphasize that Wagner, knowledgeable about the operations of the brain without knowing anything about the brain, was able to construct the chord so ambiguously that different musicians found different keys in it. Wagner in fact combined the ambiguous with the unfinished by tapping this brain organization which, though studied best in the visual brain, is not unique to it. He introduced the *appogiatura* into the chord and the diabolic interval into both the harmony and the chord, thus achieving ambiguity, and fortified the effect by leaving it unresolved until the last Act. He thus left it initially to the listener to complete the chord, and it is significant that the chords are followed by long silences which in fact engage the listener's brain, leading one musical expert to write that no one "has ever composed silence as eloquently as Wagner".[48] Nor is this ambiguity and irresolvability limited to the progression of the Tristan chord; the irresolution continues right to the end and is finally resolved in the coda of the last Act, in the *Liebestod*. In creating this remarkable work, Wagner was thus really following the potentialities of the brain, except that in this case he left it to the brain of the listener to complete the chord progression, while he himself only completed it at the very end of the last Act. And, in that sense, Wagner too was a neurobiologist, who had a profound understanding of the workings of the musical brain, without knowing anything about the brain. It is for this reason that I have argued elsewhere that artists are also neurobiologists who study the brain with techniques that are unique to them.[2,5] Langerholc[38] is right when he says: "Escher and Wagner both relied on ancient laws of perspective and tonality *deriving from the nature of our perceptive mechanisms* [our brains] to draft their illusions. Otherwise they would not have worked" (my emphasis). Probably the only way to understand the mysteries of the Tristan chord progression, about which so much has been written, is to understand the neural mechanisms underlying musical perception. And since Wagner was able to instil the "unfinished" quality into the progression of the chord, this in itself becomes the musical metaphor for something that can only be finished in annihilation, when final salvation and the dream of romantic love are achieved in death.

While Wagner furnished his music with qualities that fully engage the listener, his libretto is no less compelling in conveying the idea of a frustrated brain concept, one that has no hope of being satisfied in reality. For our purposes here, it is sufficient to look at Act 2 and the coda of the work. It is here that Wagner relays his message in music and in language that only in death and annihilation can the ideal of romantic love be found. In other words, the ideal constructed by the brain is remote from reality. The music of Act 2 is orchestrally humid and fervid, but throughout the libretto Tristan and Isolde remain indifferent to a physical consummation or a happy outcome on earth, which they indeed consider to be unattainable. The Act begins with an exaltation of the night, where the imagination reigns supreme, and fear of the day, where the reality intrudes:

dem tückischen Tage	for spiteful day
dem härtesten Feinde	the most bitter foe,
Hass und Klage!	hatred and grievance!

Wie du das Licht	Just as you extinguished the light
o könnt' ich die Leuchte	would that I could
der Liebe Leiden zu rächen	extinguish the light of insolent Day
dem frechen Tage verlöschen!	to avenge the pangs of love!
Gibt's eine Not	Is there any distress,
Gibt's eine Pein	is there any anguish
die er nicht weckt	which it does not revive
mit seinem Schein	with its beams
in lichten Tages Schein	in the bright light of Day
wie war Isolde mein?	how could Isolde be mine?

Together they sing, each wishing for the "Night of love to descend and grant oblivion, that I may live" ("*O sink hernieder/Nacht der Liebe/gib Vergessen/dass ich lebe*"). When Tristan longs for death, Isolde asks. "Must Day then waken Tristan?"—as if the reality would shatter the hoped-for perfect bliss. The preoccupation with night and death echoes similar sentiments expressed earlier by Michelangelo in one of his *Rime*:

O nott', o dolce tempo benchè nero	O night, a sweet though sombre span of time
e dall'infima parte all più alta	often by thee in dreams upborne, I wend
in sogno spesso porti ov'ire spero.	from earth to heaven, where yet I hope to climb.
O ombra del morir, per cui sì ferma	O shade of death, through whom the soul at length
ogni miseria l'alma al cor nemica,	shuns pain and sadness hostile to the heart,
ultimo degli afflitti e buon rimedio;	whom mourners find their last and sure relief;
tu rendi sana nostra carn'inferma	You restore our suffering flesh to strength,
rasciug'i pianti, e posi ogni fatica,	driest our tears, assuagest every smart,
e furi a chi ben vive ogni'ir' e tedio.	Purging the spirits of the pure from grief.

And, Isolde goes on, if Tristan were to die, what would become of her and *their* love?

Doch unsre Liebe,	But our love,
Heißt sie nicht Tristan	is it not Tristan
<u>Und</u> – Isolde?	*and* Isolde?

But it is precisely because the ideal of love cannot be attained even with Tristan *and* Isolde that Tristan yearns for her death as well, for only in that way can the illusion be annihilated:

So starben wir	Thus might we die,
um ungetrennt,	that together,
ewig einig	ever one,

ohne End'	without end,
ohn' Erwachen,	never waking,
ohn' Erbangen,	never fearing,
namenlos	namelessly
in Lieb' umfangen	enveloped in love
ganz uns selbst gegeben,	given up to each other,
der Liebe nur zu leben	to live only for love

There is, in Act 3, a brief moment of doubt, for both Tristan and Isolde. He longs to see her. But that joyful anticipation is tempered by the realization of the fearful consequences that the love draught that he was given to drink in Act 1 have had:

da ward der zehrendste	then was the most searing
Zauber erlesen:	magic unleashed:
daß nie ich solte sterben,	that I might never die
mich ew'ger Qual vererben!	But inherit eternal torment!

For Isolde too, the longing for life and the disorienting delights of love are still there:

Nur eine Stunde	Just for one hour
bleibe mir wach!	Stay awake for me!
betrügt Isolden	Will Tristan
betrügt sie Tristan	deny Isolde
um dieses einzige	this single
ewig kurze	eternally brief
letzte Weltenglück?	Final worldly joy?

And if Tristan must die, it must be for love, not from the physical wounds inflicted on him:

an der Wunde stirb mir nicht:	do not die from the wound.
uns beiden vereint	Unite us both,
erlösche das Lebenslicht!	Extinguish the light of life!

At the end of the opera, in the famous *Liebestod*, Isolde ends by singing:

in des Weltatems	in the universal stream
wehendem All—	of the world-breath—
ertrinken,	to drown,
versinken—	to founder—
unbewusst—	unconscious—
höchste Lust!	utmost rapture!

The opera conveys clearly the notion that the ideal of love can never be lived in this life, and that the only hope left is in its annihilation through death. Some producers have tried to resurrect Tristan and Isolde at the end of a performance. Peter Konwitschny did this in his Munich production. In his Covent Garden production of the opera in the 1970s, Peter Hall had Tristan and Isolde rise at the end of the opera and leave the stage holding hands. A Wagner purist in the audience shouted: "Disgusting!", presumably believing that it was a negation of what Wagner had intended. In fact, Wagner had originally referred to the present *Liebestod* as the "*Verklärung*" ("Transfiguration"), and the Tristan legends speak of Tristan and Isolde being buried side by side, with a vine growing from one grave and an ivy from the other, the branches of the two intertwining.

It is of course well known that Wagner had been deeply influenced by his reading of Schopenhauer, the great successor to Kant. Schopenhauer had been led to his highly pessimistic view of life through his philosophical studies, and above all through considering the foundations of knowledge. Through these studies, he had come to the conclusion that much was unattainable, to which one needs to add that much is unattainable because of the constant clash between concepts formed by the brain from the experience of many particulars and the continual experience of particulars. This of course is not the only source of his pessimism, but it is an important one. It was left to Wagner to translate that pessimism into a work of art, using his own experience of the unattainable and his profound knowledge of the mechanisms of the brain and its potentials.

Conclusion

In the past, I have tried to account for the characteristics of some works of art, for example kinetic art,[39] in relatively simple neurobiological terms, basing my analysis on the physiology of visual areas in the cerebral cortex. The account I give here goes beyond and tries to explore the relationship between artistic creativity and appreciation on the one hand, and what I believe to be a ubiquitous operation performed throughout the cerebral cortex on the other. Here, I have approached one of the most complex sentiments that we are capable of, that of romantic love, and tried to show that, exalted though it is, there is a sense in which it, too, obeys a universal rule of brain activity, namely the formation of ideals, a product of the abstractive powers of the brain. Taken together with my exploration of the neurological basis of simpler works of art, we can perhaps see that the neurological motive force for the two is the same and can be traced to a necessary stage in the brain's quest for knowledge. That operation is abstraction and its consequence is the formulation of ideals. In trying to understand the biological foundations of art we have, I think, to first try to understand the biological foundations of knowledge, since art is one means of acquiring that knowledge. I have thus based my analysis of art not on psychology but on the organizing principles that dictate the functioning of the brain. I have tried to show that we can, even today, and even in our imperfect state of knowledge about the brain, try to comprehend even the most exalted works of art by reference to the functions and functioning of the brain. I have of course been vague about the precise neurological way through which ideals are constructed by the brain. But this represents only a beginning in an enquiry which I hope will grow in scope and stature as we learn more about the brain and as we begin to accept that there is merit and intellectual profit in considering art as a product of the brain, determined by it and obeying its rules.

Acknowledgements

The work of this laboratory is supported by The Wellcome Trust, London.

I would like to record my gratitude to colleagues who have read the manuscript and commented on it. I owe special thanks to Anna Winestein, who corresponded with me about several aspects of the manuscript; John Langerholc, who illuminated me about the Tristan chord; and Per Aage Brandt, who discussed it with me extensively. It is hardly worth mentioning that what errors and weaknesses remain are entirely mine.

For my discussion of Plato, I have used *The Collected Dialogues of Plato*, edited by E. Hamilton and H. Cairns (Princeton University Press, 1961) for the Bollingen Foundation. I have used W.W. Jackson's translation of Dante's *Convivio* (The Clarendon Press, Oxford, 1909) and for the *Vita Nuova* I have used M. Musa's translation (Oxford University Press, Oxford, 1992) and the original Italian edition, edited by J. Petrie and J. Salmons (Belefield Italian Library, 1994). I have used J.A. Symonds's translation of Michelangelo's *Sonnets*, but changed them here and there to modernize the translations (*The Sonnets of Michelangelo*, translated by J.A. Symonds, Vision Press, London, 1950). Finally, for the English version of the *Tristan und Isolde* libretto, I have used that accompanying the 1972 recording by the Berliner Philharmoniker, conducted by Herbert von Karajan.

This article was first published in the *Journal of Consciousness Studies* in 2003 and is reprinted here with minor corrections.

References

1. A. Schopenhauer, *Die Welt als Wille und Vorstellung* (1859), Vol. 1, 3rd edn. Translated by E.F.J. Payne as *The World as Will and Representation* (Dover, New York, 1969).
2. S. Zeki, *Inner Vision: An Exploration of Art and the Brain* (Oxford University Press, Oxford, 1999).
3. J.G. Frazer, *The Growth of Plato's Ideal Theory* (Macmillan & Co., London, 1930).
4. I. Kant, *Kritik der reinen Vernunft* (1781), translated by W.S. Pluhar as *Critique of Pure Reason* (Hackett, Indianapolis, 1996).
5. S. Zeki, Splendours and miseries of the brain, *Philosophical Transactions of the Royal Society of London B* **354**, 2053–65 (1999).
6. S. Zeki, Localization and globalization in conscious vision, *Annual Review of Neuroscience* **24**, 57–86 (2001).
7. S. Zeki, Functional specialization in the visual cortex of the monkey, *Nature* **274**, 423–8 (1978).
8. M.S. Livingstone and D.H. Hubel, Segregation of form, color, movement, and depth—anatomy, physiology, and perception, *Science* **240**, 740–9 (1988).
9. S. Zeki, J.D.G. Watson, C.J. Lueck, K.J. Friston, C. Kennard and R.S.J. Frackowiak, A direct demonstration of functional specialization in human visual cortex, *Journal of Neuroscience* **11**, 641–9 (1991).
10. K. Moutoussis and S. Zeki, The relationship between cortical activation and perception investigated with invisible stimuli, *Proceedings of the National Academy of Sciences USA* 99: 9527–32.
11. M.J. Tovëe, Is face processing special? *Neuron* **21**, 1239–42 (1998).
12. G.W. Leibniz, *La Monadologie* (1714), translated as *The Monadology* by R. Latta (Clarendon Press, Oxford, 1898).
13. S. Zeki and A. Bartels, Toward a theory of visual consciousness, *Consciousness and Cognition* **8**, 225–59 (1999).
14. K. Moutoussis and S. Zeki, A direct demonstration of perceptual asynchrony in vision, *Proceedings of the Royal Society of London B* **264**, 393–9 (1997).
15. K. Moutoussis and S. Zeki, Functional segregation and temporal hierarchy of the visual perceptive systems, *Proceedings of the Royal Society of London B* **264**, 1407–14 (1997).
16. D.H. Hubel and T.N. Wiesel, Receptive fields, binocular interaction and functional architecture in the cat's visual cortex, *Journal of Physiology* **160**, 106–154 (1962).

17. P. Gouras and J. Kruger, Responses of cells in foveal striate cortex of the monkey to pure color contrast, *Journal of Neurophysiology* **42**, 850–60 (1979).
18. D.H. Hubel and T.N. Wiesel, The Ferrier Lecture. Functional architecture of macaque monkey visual cortex, *Proceedings of the Royal Society (London) B* **198**, 1–59 (1977).
19. S.M. Zeki, Functional organization of a visual area in the posterior bank of the superior temporal sulcus of the rhesus monkey, *Journal of Physiology* **236**, 549–73 (1974).
20. J.H.R. Maunsell and D.C. Van Essen, Functional properties of neurons in middle temporal visual area of the macaque monkey. I. Selectivity for stimulus direction, speed, and orientation, *Journal of Neurophysiology* **49**, 1127–47 (1983).
21. T.D. Albright, Direction and orientation selectivity of neurons in visual area MT of the macaque, *Journal of Neurophysiology* **52**, 1106–30 (1984).
22. S. Zeki and L. Marini, Three cortical stages of colour processing in the human brain, *Brain* **121**, 1669–85 (1998).
23. A. Bartels and S. Zeki, The architecture of the colour centre in the human visual brain: new results and a review, *European Journal of Neuroscience* **12**, 172–93 (2000).
24. C. Galletti, P.P. Battaglini and P. Fattori, Parietal neurons encoding spatial locations in craniotopic coordinates, *Experimental Brain Research* **96**, 221–9 (1993).
25. E.H. Land, The retinex theory of colour vision, *Proceedings of The Royal Institution of Great Britain* **47**, 23–58 (1974).
26. E.H. Land and J.J. McCann, Lightness and retinex theory, *Journal of the Optical Society of America* **61**, 1–11 (1971).
27. N.K. Logothetis, J. Pauls and T. Poggio, Shape representation in the inferior temporal cortex of monkeys, *Current Biology* **5**, 552–63 (1995).
28. D.L. Sheinberg and N.K. Logothetis, Noticing familiar objects in real world scenes: the role of temporal cortical neurons in natural vision, *Journal of Neuroscience* **21**, 1340–50 (2001).
29. A. Bartels and S. Zeki, The neural basis of romantic love, *Neuroreport* **11**, 3829–84 (2000).
30. R. Penrose, *Shadows of the Mind* (Oxford University Press, Oxford, 1994).
31. P. Donke, *Dante's Second Love* (Society for Italian Studies, 1997).
32. L. Nelson, *The Poetry of Guido Cavalcanti* (Garland, New York, 1986).
33. J. Petrie and J. Salmons (eds.), *Vita Nuova*, by Dante Alighieri (Belefield Italian Library, 1994).
34. W.W. Jackson, *Convivio*, by Dante Alighieri (translation) (The Clarendon Press, Oxford, 1909).
35. M. Musa, *Vita Nuova*, by Dante Alighieri (translation) (Oxford University Press, Oxford, 1992).
36. J. Schulz, Michelangelo's unfinished works, *Art Bulletin* **58**, 366–73 (1975).

37. C. Tolnay, Michelangelo's Rondanini Pietà, *Burlington Magazine* **65**, 145–57 (1934).
38. J. Langerholc, *L'Accordo di Tristano come Immagine Ambigua: "Figure Vuote" nell'Opera di Wagner*, *Rivista di Psicologia dell'Arte* **VII**, 55–68 (1986).
39. E. Newman, *Wagner Nights* (Putnam & Co., London, 1949).
39. . Zeki and M. Lamb, The neurology of kinetic art, *Brain* **117**, 607–36 (1994).
40. W.L. Benzon, *Beethoven's Anvil* (Basic Books, New York, 2001).
41. I. Newton, *Opticks* (Dover, New York, 1704).
42. W. Furtwängler, *Gespräche uber Müsik* (Zurich, 1949), p. 115 (cited by Langerholc, 1986).
43. J. Langerholc, Sphinx und Janus: der Tristan-Akkord, *Richard Wagner Blatter* 7, 42–9 (1983).
44. N.K. Logothetis, D.A. Leopold and D.L. Sheinberg, What is rivalling during binocular rivalry? *Nature* **380**, 621–4 (1996).
45. N.K. Logothetis, Single units and conscious vision, *Philosophical Transactions of the Royal Society of London B* **353**, 1801–18 (1998).
46. E.D. Lumer, K.J. Friston, and G. Rees, Neural correlates of perceptual rivalry in the human brain, *Science* **280**, 1930–4 (1998).
47. A. Kleinschmidt, C. Buchel, S. Zeki and R.S.J. Frackowiak, Human brain activity during spontaneously reversing perception of ambiguous figures, *Proceedings of the Royal Society of London B* **265**, 2427–33 (1998).
48. D.H. Crosby, Beyond analysis: Richard Wagner's *Tristan und Isolde*; lecture delivered at the Washington Opera, 8 March 1999.

Chapter 3

The Neurology of Art: An Overview

F. Clifford Rose

Introduction: Science and Art

The Egyptologist Sir Flinders Petrie claimed that in all civilisations there is a regular sequence in the development of cultural activities: painting comes before sculpture, after which comes architecture, followed by literature, and only then by science. Although art and medicine have the same patron saint, Luke, who was both a doctor and a painter, their origins are separated by millennia. They share the purpose of improving the lot of man, the former chiefly on the physical side and the latter in mental well-being.[1] The practitioners of each are trained to see more than the average.[2] Art, like medicine, reflects society, and both are interwoven with history. We find that in those countries and periods where one flourished, so did the other.

The artist and the scientist were compared by William Harvey in "*De Generatione*": "Each has its origin in sense and experience, and it is impossible that there can rightly be either art or science without visible instance or example." Sigerist[3] has pointed out the distinction, "Art and medicine—they are both aspects of human civilisation . . .", but the former "is the creation of an imaginative mind . . ." while the latter "is the endeavour of man to succour his fellowmen . . .".

Whilst in ancient civilisations medicine and religion were closely associated, they began to separate in the Middle Ages in Europe, where the church became the chief patron of paintings with religious themes. Up until the 15th century, doctors were members of religious orders and were ordered to be celibate. With the Renaissance, art and medicine came together, largely because of anatomy and the works of da Vinci, Vesalius and Michelangelo, all of whom had been involved in human dissection.[a] The great importance that neuro-anatomy has played in the development of artists' portrayal of the human body has been extensively reviewed.

The title of this chapter suggests that it concerns neurological disorders of artists and how these may influence their work. There are several other meanings, such as paintings of neurologically sick patients, works of art by neurologists, e.g. Charcot, or portraits of famous neurologists which may be works of art. In addition, the neuroscience of painting deals with how special parts of the brain (magno, blob and parvo sub-systems) appreciate colour, form, depth and motion.[4] There is also the question of cerebral localisation of creativity (see previous chapters). Yet another fundamental problem is how brain perception produces aesthetic experience. Since these are huge topics, this chapter can only be an overview giving examples of a few of them. Attempts are made to follow a chronological order and to consider some challenging controversies.

Poliomyelitis

It has been claimed that the earliest example of neurological disease portrayed in art is the funeral stele of the priest Ruma, from the 19th Egyptian dynasty.[5] This work, in the Carlsberg Museum of Copenhagen, shows the priest, accompanied by his wife, approaching a small table on which are offerings to the god Astarta (Figure 3.1). Ruma's leg is clearly atrophied and shortened, so that he walks on his toes with the help of a cane. The suggestion that this was a representation of "what is probably the residue of poliomyelitis" was repeated more recently[6] but with the suggestion that the *bas relief* figure was that of a pharaoh's mummy of the 18th dynasty (1500 BC). The interpretation that it was a case of polio (acute anterior poliomyelitis) is not universally agreed on. Kinnier Wilson, the late eminent neurologist, thought that it might be a club foot (personal communication from his son, Kinnier Wilson Jr, a professor of Assyriology), a view also held by Denis Browne, the late famous orthopaedic surgeon at the Hospital for Sick Children, Great Ormond Street, London. I have pointed out that this is also my interpretation, because there has been no description of polio before the 18th century.[7]

a. Dissection had previously been banned, due to a papal decree excommunicating those who cut human flesh—the reason why surgeons were only aids and had to work as barbers.

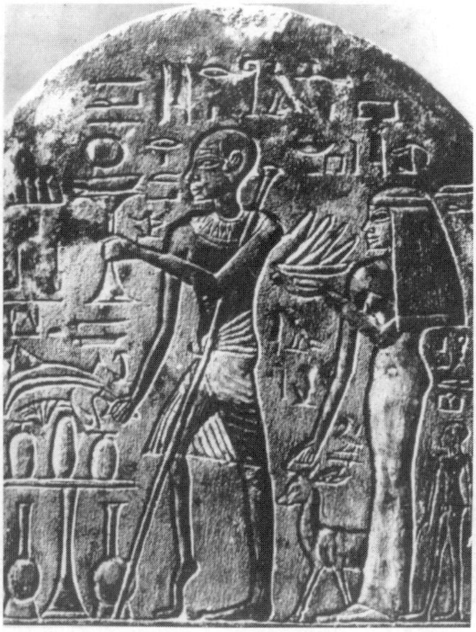

Fig. 3.1. Funeral stele of the priest of Ruma, in the Carlsberg Museum of Copenhagen.[5]

Masaccio

Masaccio (1401–1428)[b] was among the great Renaissance painters who inaugurated the modern painting era by new ideas of perspective and light. His innovations were taken up by such artists as Piero della Francesco, Filippo Lippi and Fra Angelico. This style may owe something to Giotto, who lived in the previous century, but he was more influenced by his friends, the sculptor Donatello and the architect Brunelleschi;[8] all three have been called the founders of the Renaissance. Since Florentine painters were buying their pigments from apothecaries, they had frequent contact with physicians; for example, Masaccio joined the League of Physicians and Apothecaries.

---

b. He was born Tommaso Cassai in San Giovanni Valdaino, in the Tuscan province of Arrezzo, 40 miles southeast of Florence. "Masaccio" was his nickname—translated, according to Vasari, as "Big Tom" or "Lazy Tom", as he was careless and absent-minded, albeit good-natured. Having trained in Florence, Masaccio joined the confraternity of St Luke, composed mainly of painters, at the age of 23. At the age of 26, greatly in debt, he moved to Rome, where he died the following year. He worked for only six years but his relatively small output had a profound effect on the history of art. Only four of Masaccio's works survive and all are in churches, as either altar pieces or frescoes.

(a) (b)

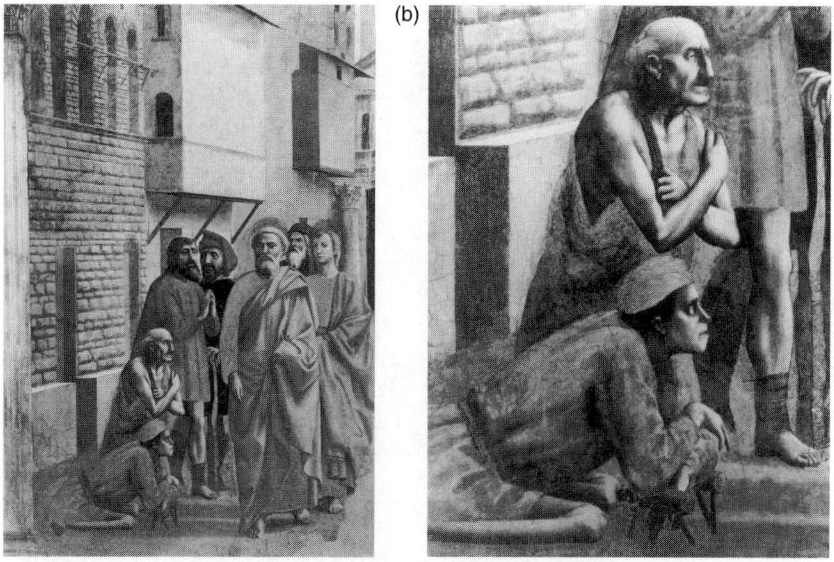

Fig. 3.2. (a) *St Peter Healing the Sick with His Shadow*, by Masaccio. (b) Focus on the wasted leg.

Masaccio's most famous works are the frescoes in the Brancacci Chapel of Santa Maria del Carmine, Florence, painted on wood (poplar) in 1426 as an altar piece for a Carmelite church. One of the six fresco paintings shows a beggar with crippled legs (Figure 3.2) from the painting *St Peter Healing the Sick with His Shadow*,[9] based on the episode recounted in the "Acts of the Apostles" (5:15–16). It has again been claimed that the disease portrayed is polio,[10] but this is highly unlikely since the first known epidemic of this condition was in the 18th century.[7]

Migraine

Whilst there is much writing about how visual acuity affects the artist,[11] there is evidence that Georgio de Chirico[c] and Picasso used their migrainous visual auras as a source of artistic invention.[12] Headache is an experience common to most of mankind and migraine is the commonest disorder of the brain,

c. Giorgio de Chirico was born in 1888 in Greece of Italian parents. Trained in Munich, he lived in Paris before settling in Rome. He founded his own school of metaphysical painting, homage being paid to him by the surrealists, but later became more of a classical painter.

affecting up to 1 in 3 women and 1 in 6 men at some time of their lives. Only about 10% of migraine attacks are associated with a visual aura, but one personality in medieval times whose visions were claimed to be due to the aura of migraine was Hildegard of Bingen.

Hildegard of Bingen

Many books have been written about Hildegard of Bingen (1098–1179), who was one of the first women to be accepted in a man's world. A polymath famous for her music composition, she was also writer, artist, theologian and poet, as well as being knowledgeable about science and herbalism. Born in the famous wine-growing region of Rheinhessen in Germany, she was the tenth (and last) child.[d] When she was eight years old, she was entrusted to Jutta von Spanheim at the monastery of Disibodenberg, and she took the veil at the age of 14.

Hildegard had frequent illnesses and, at the age of 12, a particularly serious but unspecified one. From the age of 3 she had experienced visions[13]: "I was only in my third year when I saw a heavenly light which made my soul tremble, but because I was a child I could not speak out." When she was 24 years old: "I saw an extremely strong, sparkling, fiery light coming from the open heavens. It pierced my brain, my heart and my breast through and through like a flame which did not burn; however, it warmed me.... And suddenly I had an insight into the meaning and interpretation [of the Holy Books]." Terms she used included "*lux vivens*", "perceptions", "illumination", "reflections of the living light" and "visionary insight". During the visions, she was always fully awake, neither in a trance nor in a state of ecstasy. "Hildegard may have been fully conscious when she had her visions, but she seems to have fallen into some sort of cataleptic[e] trance beforehand.... Her monk biographers describe her suddenly rising from her bed and pacing the anchorage from corner to corner, all the while unable to speak."[14]

In her 43rd year, in the midst of another prolonged and severe bout of illness, the call came; she was "... gazing with great fear and trembling attention at a heavenly vision. I saw a great splendour in which resounded a voice from Heaven saying to me." She was told by God in this vision to write and she began work on her book "*Scivias*", which included 26 visions. It took her over ten years to finish and she set the last vision to music. By that time she had

d. Her parents had promised her as a tithe to the church; known as oblation, it was not infrequent, as happened to the Venerable Bede and Thomas Aquinas *et al.*

e. See Chapter 24 for discussion of catalepsy.

moved to the convent at Rupertsberg, near Bingen on the Rhine.[f] She also wrote two non-visionary books: "*Physica*" (on nature) and "*Causae et Curae*" (on medicine). In the latter book, she identifies migraine as a headache affecting part of the head rather than being generalised. Although she admits that migraine is hard to cure, "...she did not connect the malady with her own catalogue of afflictions".

Charles Singer[15] was the first to attempt a connection between her visions and migraine: "Hildegard reportedly assures us that most of knowledge was revealed to her in waking visions. Some of them we shall seek to show had a pathological basis, probably of a migrainous character and she was a sufferer from a condition that would nowadays be classified as hystero-epilepsy... visions, it must be remembered, were 'The fashion' at the period and were a common literary device."[15] This latter view is supported by comparing a contemporary, Elizabeth of Schönau, and Hildegard's successors, e.g. Gertrude of Robersdorf. Singer continues: "From a very early age, she was the subject of trances and visions, and from time to time she was prostrated with protracted illness."[15] Hildegard writes: "In this affliction I lay thirty days while my body burned as with fever.... And throughout those days I watched a procession of angels innumerable who fought with Michael and against the dragon and won the victory... and thus I began to get back my strength."[15] The length of time of her illness is very much against migraine as the cause of her visions. "Three years were thus passed during which the Cherubim pursued me with a flaming sword... and at length any spirit revived within me and my body was restored again... and thus I was healed."[15] Again it is difficult to explain a continuous illness of three years based on migraine. "These visions which I saw," writes Hildegard, "I beheld neither in sleep, nor in dream, nor in madness... but wakeful, alert, with the eyes of the spirit.... I perceived them in open view and according to the will of God. And how this was compassed is hard indeed for human flesh to search out."[15]

Singer writes: "In all a prominent feature is a point or a group of points of light, which shimmer and move, usually in a wave-like manner, and are most often interpreted as stars or flaming eyes. In quite a number of cases one light, larger than the rest, exhibits a series of concentric circular figures of wavering forms; and often definite fortification figures are described, radiating in some cases from a coloured area. Often the lights gave that impression of *working*, boiling or fermenting, described by many visionaries from Ezekiel onwards."[15]

f. The "*Scivias*" is divided into three parts, the first containing 6 visions, the second 7, and the third 13, each of these parts having a varied number of chapters.

Singer claims that even though Hildegard "herself variously interpreted" the visions, " . . . the medical recorder or the sufferer from migraine will, we think, easily recognise the symptoms of scintillating scotoma". The description given is not typical of a scintillating scotoma.[16]

Singer states: "The condition from which she was suffering was clearly a functional nervous disorder; this significantly demonstrated by her repeated complete recoveries, her activity between the attacks, and the great age to which she lived." It is difficult to know to which particular "functional nervous disorder" Singer is referring, but it would not be unreasonable to point out that Singer, although a well-known historian, was not recognised as either a neurologist or a psychiatrist.

Hildegard writes: "I saw a great star most splendid and beautiful, and with it an exceeding multitude of falling sparks which, with the star, followed southward. And they examined Him upon the throne almost as something hostile, and turning from him, they sought rather the north. And suddenly they were all annihilated, being turned into black coals . . . and cast into the abyss that I could see them no more" (Figure 3.3). She interpreted this vision as the Fall of the Angels.

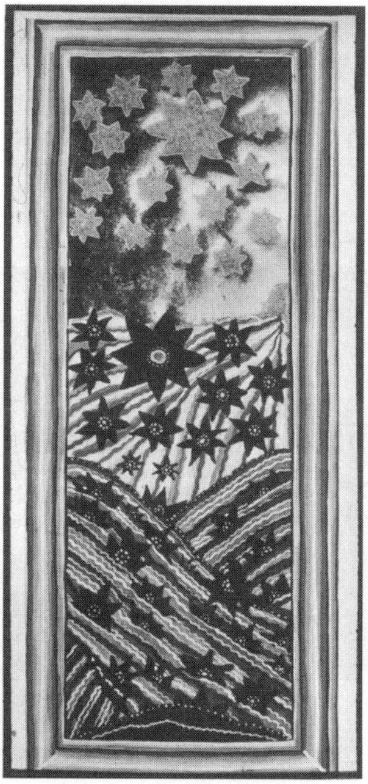

Fig. 3.3. *The Fallen Stars of Hildegard of Bingen.* Lucifer, the great dark star, and his followers are turned to cinders and tossed in a whirlwind towards the abyss.[14]

Oliver Sacks also thought that Hildegard's visions were due to migraine but acknowledged that they were rare, concluding: "Invested with this sense of ecstasy, burning with profound theophorous and philosophical significance, Hildegard's visions were instrumental in directing her towards a life of holiness and mysticism."[17] "Our literal interpretation of [Hildegard's visions] would be that she experienced a shower of phosphenes in transit across the visual field, their passage being succeeded by a negative scotoma." On no occasion does she mention headaches in relation to her vision; nor does she state how long the visual phenomena lasted. Hildegard had the imagination of a mystic, and although Sacks considers her visions "indisputably migrainous", I have grave doubts, for the reasons stated, that Hildegard's visions were migrainous in origin.

Ergotism

St Anthony's Fire

A case has been made regarding the fingers of St Anthony as painted on the altar in the Antonite monastery at Isenheim in southern Alsace but now in the museum Unterlinden, Colmar, France. The hands show bluish atrophy, considered a sign of peripheral vascular disease, which can lead to gangrene (Figure 3.4). The painting was done by Mathias Grünewald

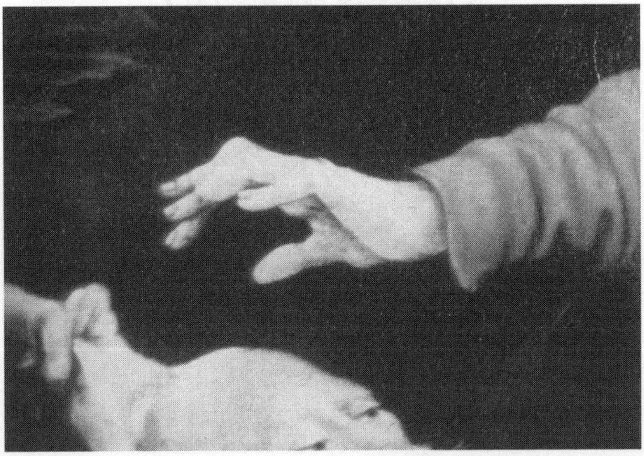

Fig. 3.4. The Isenheim Altar piece, now in the Musée Unterlinden, Colmar, France.

(Goxhardt-Neihardt) (1480–1524), who was also a sculptor, a contemporary of Albrecht Dürer. He was born in Würzburg, the date of birth being uncertain but between 1455 and 1480, and died in Halle in 1524. Grünewald had stayed at a monastery of St Anthony's order which had the privilege of looking after patients with St Anthony's Fire, later recognised as ergotism.[g] The monks of the order of Hospitallers of St Anthony had opened wards for patients whose fingers and toes burned like fire, and the walls were painted red. Pictures of this saint (Figure 3.5) show him with a bell, which indicated his hermit status, and a pig, since the monks of that order allowed their pigs to roam the streets. He was often depicted as being surrounded by vile creatures or tempted by gold or the Devil dressed as a woman. Known also as St Anthony of Thebes, or St Anthony the Great, he gave all of his money away and lived as a third century wandering hermit in the Egyptian desert, dying at the age of 99 years. Although frequently consulted, he disliked fame and asked that his burial site not be revealed.[h]

St Anthony's Fire probably included other diseases such as erysipelas. Ergotism is poisoning from the ergot fungus, *Claviceps purpurea*, which forms on cereal grains, especially ears of rye, and could poison any food, such as bread or porridge made from them. It could affect either the brain, causing convulsions, or constrict the arteries to the limbs, giving, in its extreme form, gangrene. In its less severe form, it causes redness and blistering of the extremities, which explains the appellation "St Anthony's Fire". Many of the epidemics occurred

---

g. Ergotism was so serious and widespread that it was no doubt felt that as much divine help as possible was needed. For 130 years from 591 AD, epidemics of ergotism were recorded on average every ten years (Kiple, 1997, p. 32). An outbreak could cause as many deaths as 40 000 in France (in 922 AD) or 14 000 in Paris alone (in 1128–1129 AD). The mortality of those affected could be over 40% (Kiple, 1997, p. 53). Epidemics occurred in Germany and Italy as well as in France, particularly in those areas where rye was eaten. Since this was often in the countryside, ergotism was often called *morbus ruralis*. It especially affected children (who needed more food per body unit) and involved urban orphanages and foundling hospitals. Ergot toxins can be secreted in the milk of nursing mothers and infant mortality in Russia was highest at the beginning of the 20th century. The ergot fungus grows best in wet conditions, so the epidemics tended to occur after a severe winter, or during a rainy spring or in newly cultivated marshy land. In Russia, for 250 years from the first recorded epidemic in 1785–1786, the disease was particularly common because the cold climate necessitated a hardy grass such as rye. It may be that the increasing production of the potato during the 17th century helped to lessen the effects of ergotism.

h. This request was kept for two centuries, until he was reburied in Alexandria. A century after this, his remains were taken to St Sophia Church in Constantinople when a French crusader obtained permission to relocate them home to the Dauphine region of France. A series of paintings of St Anthony's life was done by the 15th century Sienese artist known as the Osservanza Master, so called as the altar piece came from the church of the Osservanza in Siena. His contemporaries include Sassetta and Sano di Pietio and he may have been Vico di Luca, who worked with Sassetta.

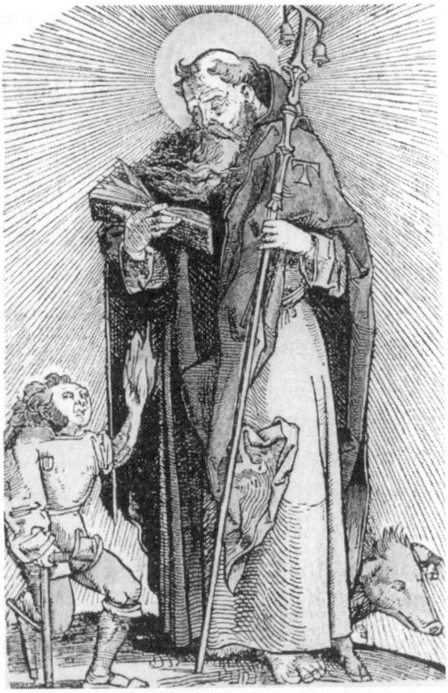

Fig. 3.5. St Anthony of Egypt (from Henry VII's Chapel, Westminster Abbey).

in France, where monastic hospices attending patients would name a patron saint for each disorder. The association of St Anthony with ergotism came about in the Middle Ages, before which the condition was known as *ignis sacer* — "holy fire". There are two medical St Anthonys: the one of the Fire is St Anthony of Egypt (*c.* 251) (Figure 3.5), possibly earning him fame since his shrine, which was visited by sufferers, was outside the area where the rye fungus flourished; the other St Anthony (1195–1231), of Padua, was born in, and is the patron saint of, Lisbon,[i] as well as of the poor, seamen and victims of traffic accidents. Other than hagiologists, it is inevitable that the average person confuses the two saints (Figure 3.6).

i. He was a Franciscan monk who preached in France and Italy, and was hence called St Anthony of Padua. His name was also invoked for help with infertility and as the finder of lost articles. The hospitals of his order tended to specialise in diseases of the skin and venereal diseases.

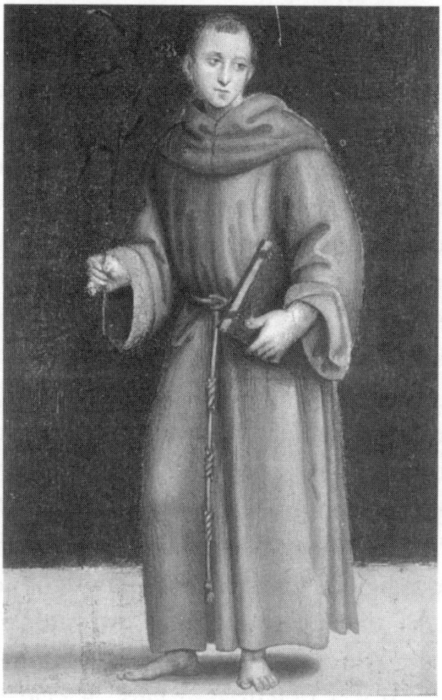

Fig. 3.6. St Anthony of Padua, from the Colonna Altar piece (oil on panel) by Raphael (1483–1520).[46]

The Stone of Folly

Hieronymus Bosch

Hieronymus Bosch (*c.* 1450–1516) was born Jerome van Aaken (Aachen), but his surname derives from the Dutch provincial town of s'Hertogenbosch, of which he was a respected citizen and where he worked from 1480 till his death in 1516, probably in his 60s. His father, grandfather and uncles were all painters; although he was married, it is unknown whether he had any offspring. He was no painter of portraits, and his 40 surviving paintings can be divided into the genres of religion and fantasy, the latter from earlier in his career. He drew cripples and lepers, painting the minutest details of their diseases. His art is mostly incomprehensible to modern generations, possibly because his ideas came from medieval religious tracts, astrology and folklore.[18] Not much was written about him by his contemporaries but a modern day psychiatrist might deduce from his paintings that he was schizophrenic.

Bosch was the first painter to illustrate the widespread belief that a stone in the head was responsible for brain illness which could be cured by operation. The Cure of Folly, also known as "The Operation for the Stone" or "The Stone of Insanity", involved an incision into the patient's scalp but trephination, i.e. penetration of the skull, was not done. Quacks who claimed to cure epilepsy may have held an object in the palm of their hand or hide a stone up their sleeves to produce during or after the operation. This "madness" stone, removed by sleight of hand, was occasionally dropped into a metal container, giving an impressive sound.[19] Contemporary Flemish literature suggested that the cause of madness was a stone ("rocks") in the head, a view supported by physicians who reputedly found at post-mortem examination stones in patients with similar disorders and migraine. Poems were written and plays performed regarding the manoeuvre.

In the following two centuries, Bosch was copied by many Flemish and Dutch painters, possibly because genre paintings were common in the low countries where religious pictures were less common than elsewhere in Europe. Painters of this operation include Peter Breughel the Elder, Jan Steen, Frans Hal the Younger, Jan Sanders van Hermessen, David Teniers and Adriaen Brower.[20] It was practised at fairs, as evidenced in the painting by Jan Steen.

Bosch's *The Cure of Folly* is circular in form, a 15th century symbol of creation, giving a sense of universality (Figure 3.7). In the 16th century the

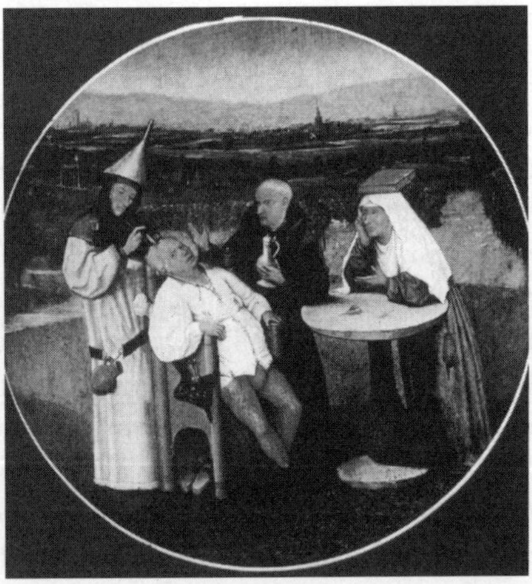

Fig. 3.7. *The Cure of Folly*, by Hieronymus Bosch, now in the Prado Museum, Madrid.

funnel hat was a symbol of deception, possibly because an inverted funnel cannot hold anything and was the precursor of a dunce's hat. Close to the head of the surgeon is a gallows with its ominous suggestibility; the empty jug hanging from the surgeon's belt may signify hollow vanity; the nurse balances a volume on her head symbolically, unable to see it. In Bosch's painting, the monk holds an alcoholic beverage which would have been the only anaesthetic used. The background includes a torture instrument, as well as gallows, presumably symbolising the pain of the world.[19] The object removed looks like flowers—at that time thieves' jargon for money—but may be a tulip, perhaps because the old Dutch words for "tulip" and "stupidity" were similar. "The nun's red, heart-shaped purse may be a depiction of the Flemish proverb 'His heart is where the money is'."[19,j] The inscription translated into English means "Master, cut the stone out, My name is Hubbert Das." One explanation is that the operation was performed on a cuckolded husband to relieve his suspicions of unfaithfulness; one such husband was called Hubbert, a name often given for duped husbands. An alternative explanation is that the name of the patient may have been Lubbert Das—hence the word "landlubber", i.e. "a stupid person".

Among the considerable literature on this theme, the most interesting interpretation[21] is that these paintings could be divided into three groups: the interpretation of the metaphor "rocks in the head"; a theatrical interpretation, where players act parts of patients and doctors; they were genre paintings. Schupbach concluded that there was no evidence that the operation was done at all and that these quacks never existed.[k]

Neuro-Anatomy

It was the Crusades that brought back the Arabic translations of Greek thought. During the Renaissance "the *leaders* of medicine were the artists, who made the greatest contribution to Anatomy"[22] and ". . . anatomy became the basis for the teaching of medicine".

j. The Bishop of Utrecht displayed this painting in 1524 but it is now in the Prado Museum, Madrid.

k. The Persian physician Rhazes (854–925 or 935) denounced those who attempted to cure epilepsy by incising the patient's scalp and pretending to extract an object with sleight of hand. Five hundred years later, the many paintings of this operation appeared, but it is now assumed that they showed quacks at work.

Leonardo da Vinci

Leonardo da Vinci (1452–1519) left more than 6000 pages of notebooks and closely written diary, of which 190 pages are devoted to anatomy. He dissected 30 bodies to help his art—an endeavour that provided the impetus for the development of systematic anatomy. In the late 15th and early 16th centuries (*c.* 1487–1509), he was particularly concerned with the nervous system, an interest not simply anatomical but because he wanted to explain "the function of man's mind as an instrument for logical revelation of natures laws".[23,1]

Leonardo's dissections were performed before fixatives were used, so they had to be done quickly as putrefaction would ruin the anatomical specimens, especially the brain, which deteriorated rapidly, "virtually dissolving into a soupy consistency within a few days."[23] It is thus not surprising that dissectors paid less attention to the brain than those organs which were less perishable. Between 1504 and 1507, Leonardo injected the cerebral ventricles with liquid wax, labelling each with a Galenic function; this work was not publicised until the 19th century and so had no effect on Leonardo's contemporaries. Leonardo was basically an engineer and did cross-sections in anatomy, but such drawings were not generally published until hundreds of years later. He studied various facial expressions, inducing the smile of Mona Lisa (the third wife of Francesco de Giocondo) by music and surrounding her with pleasant objects.[8]

---

1. Leonardo was born in 1452 in Vinci, a mountain village near Empoli, west of Monte Albano. His father, Ser Picio da Vinci, was the Notary of the Signoria of Florence; his mother, Caterina, a peasant girl. Since each of his parents married someone else in their own class, he was raised by his paternal grandparents. His father married three times and had 11 children from the second and third marriages, who, on the death of their father, disputed Leonardo's inheritance, a lawsuit that lasted two years (Rosenberg, 1903). At the age of 20, "... his name was entered in the red-letter book of the Florentine Guild of Painters". At the age of 24, when he was still at the workshop of Verocchio, he was "... accused of immoral conduct subject to severe penalties" but was acquitted. Leonardo entered the workshop, probably in 1468, of Andrea del Verocchio, who was a pupil of Donatello, and probably began his career as a sculptor, working on clay, bronze and marble; he was also a goldsmith. One of the first Renaissance painters to produce anatomical exactness in painting, Verrochio was a friend of Leonardo's father, but only a few of his paintings survive. Even before then, according to Vasari, Leonardo had drawn and made reliefs. It was at the age of 26 that he received his first great commission, viz. to paint a picture for the Chapel of St Bernard in the Palace of the Signoria of Florence; in spite of being advanced 25 gold ducats, he did not get beyond preliminary studies; he "never produced finished works" (Rosenberg, 1903). He undertook "deeper anatomical studies during his stay in Milan with the help of Marcantonio della Torre, a doctor who had become his friend. . . ." (Rosenberg, 1903).

Vesalius

It has been said that Leonardo was an artist with the mind of a physician, whereas Vesalius (1514–1564) was the reverse.[22]

The collaboration of artist and scientist reached its Renaissance peak in 1543, with the publication of "*De Humanis Corpora Fabrica*"[m] in Basel by Vesalius; "Andreas Vesalius Bruxellensis" was the name he preferred.[n] Written before he was 28 years old, this work consisted of two parts: the first and better-known consisted of seven chapters or books (*libri*) of woodcut illustrations of the human body, with a Latin text bound in one volume; the second was a thinner volume, called *Epitome*, which had the same format but showed arterial and venous structures and was intended for a less specialised audience, such as artists and students.

The fourth book of *Fabrica* deals with peripheral nerves, while the seventh and last concerns the central nervous system and sensory organs. The best-known plates of Vesalius are the full-figure dissections of the 12 "muscle men"

---

m. The term "*fabrica*" derived from "*fabes*", meaning an artisan who works his material ingeniously. It was used in classical Latin for trade, later for art, then the process of making a product and finally for the product, and he probably meant it to indicate the ingenious structure of the human body.[24] Henry VIII ordered an English translation of "*De Fabrica*" with its first important copperplate engravings in 1545 (Heirlinger, 1970).

n. His forebears came from the town of Wesel on the lower Rhine in Germany. There were several generations of distinguished doctors in his family before Andreas was born on the last day of 1514 in Brussels. He matriculated in 1530 at the University of Louvain, where he later studied the structures and functions of the human body as described by Albertus Magnus and Michael Scotus. From 1533 to 1536, he studied medicine at the University of Paris, the faculty being "a stronghold of Galenism". His teachers included Sylvius (1478–1555), Jean Fernel (1497–1558), and Jean Gunter (1505–1574), who was said to have translated the works of Galen directly from Greek to Latin.[24] Because of the outbreak of hostilities in 1536 between King Francis I of France and Emperor Charles V, Vesalius, the son of the imperial dispenser, had to leave Paris and was unable, to his eternal regret, to complete his studies and take his degree. He returned briefly to his home in Brussels and then back to Louvain. There he continued anatomical studies but, following arguments, left Louvain after a year, never to return. He headed for Italy, passing via Basel, where he met the printer Robert Winter, who published the second edition of his book on Rhazes. He then went to Venice for six months, where he heard of Titian (1477–1576), whose pupils included his fellow Fleming, Jan Stephen van Calcar (1499 – *c.* 1546), who would later prepare his anatomical drawings. Venice was the Italian centre for printing and there he published his works on dissection of nerves, veins and arteries. During this time he cooperated with John Kaye (1510–1573) (for whom Caius' College is named), who was a confirmed Galenist. He then went to Padua, where the university was governed by the Venetian Senate, and graduated as a doctor in December 1537. Almost immediately he was appointed to lecture on anatomy; his fame grew and he was asked to lecture in Bologna. Towards the end of 1542, he left Italy to get his major work—"*Fabrica*"—published in Basel. This was done by a relative of Winter, namely Johannes Herbst (1507–1568), better known as Oparinus, the son of a poor painter in Basel, and was until then a relatively unknown publisher.

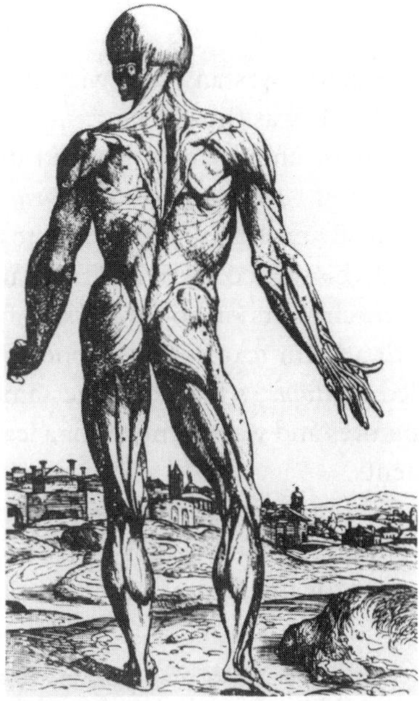

Fig. 3.8. Woodcut of a full-figure *ecorché* ("flayed") dissection from "*De Humanis Corpora Fabrica*" of Vesalius (1543).

revealing successive deeper layers of muscle (6 from the front and 6 from the back). When these plates are put in two rows, the background forms a complete picture[24] (Figure 3.8). They show a frontal view of a flayed (*écorché*) man at the first stages of dissection. These drawings are characterised by an illusion of life in what is clearly a dead body with slack and deteriorating musculature. Vesalius' muscle men had no arteries, veins or nerves.

These plates are probably the work of Jan Stephan van Calcar, a Flemish student of Titian. The background portrayal of ancient Rome with monuments, obelisks, rotundas and pyramids was probably added and may be the work of yet another of Titian's students, Domenico Campagnola (*c.* 1484 – *c.* 1563), who was well known for his landscapes.[o] Vesalius had produced an earlier work in 1538, *Tabular Sex*, in which there were drawings of skeletons by van Calcar, the pupil of Titian's from whom he had acquired his Italian method of painting. In this book there were three representations (back, front and side) of the same skeleton of a male teenager who had suffered from rickets. There

o. Harvey Cushing recognised the background as the Eugenian hills surrounding Padua between the town and Leguatro.

were several errors, such as the loss of spinal curves, exaggerated rounding of the thorax and a tilt of the pelvis, which had been twisted anti-clockwise from the side, and the clavicle was upside down. Some of these errors were removed in the *Fabrica* of 1543. Here, Vesalius showed the incus and malleus but not the stapes. He was not interested in the cerebral gyri and thought of them as coils of small intestine or clouds drawn by schoolboys without a fixed pattern.

It has been claimed that the work of Vesalius was the beginning of modern observational science. Expert as an anatomist, Vesalius was also keen on surgery, albeit not always a successful operator. Before Emperor Charles V died, he raised Vesalius to be a Count Palatine; following the Emperor's death, Vesalius passed into the service of his son Philip II, to whom *Epitome* had been dedicated.[p]

On a personal level, Vesalius had a protuberant forehead and a sandy beard. He was not an extroverted, amiable character but was occasionally depressed, surly, gruff, and aggressive in his opinions. It was on returning from the Holy Land in 1564 that he met his death following a shipwreck.

The Spanish School

José de Ribera

Born in Spain, José de Ribera (1591–1652) went to Italy as a young man. After working in Palma and Rome, he settled down in Naples, which was then

p. One of his more important consultations occurred with the celebrations of the marriage of Philip II to the sister of the King of France in 1558. Tournaments were held and on June 30th King Henry jousted with a 29-year-old captain, whose lance struck the metal neck plate of the King so hard that the point broke off and was pushed into the opening visor, striking the left orbit and upper part of the right orbit. The King tottered from his saddle, tried to walk, collapsed twice and vomited. Vesalius, who was in Flanders, was sent for and arrived in Paris on July 5th. The King had become drowsy and developed a left hemiparesis, with the right side showing occasional twitches. On arrival, Vesalius inserted a handkerchief into the King's mouth for him to bite on and removed the lance, whereupon the King put his hand on his head, complaining of severe head pain. Vesalius was then heard to mutter "*Chironium Vulnus*" ("an incurable wound"), an opinion confirmed five days later when the King died. The following year, in 1559, Phillip II went to Spain accompanied by Vesalius, who could do little anatomy there. He had another important consultation on the Infante Don Carlos, the King's mentally abnormal son, who, in a nocturnal sexual escapade, fell down a staircase, sustaining a severe head injury. Vesalius found his pulse to be weak and the diagnosis of a depressed skull fracture was made, indicating that trepanation should be undertaken. Others thought that the more likely diagnosis was osteitis without fracture. A local incision to expose the skull bone was made, which confirmed severe inflammation; there was some, but incomplete, recovery. At Vesalius' recommendation both orbits were cut and drained, after which recovery was rapid, and complete within weeks.

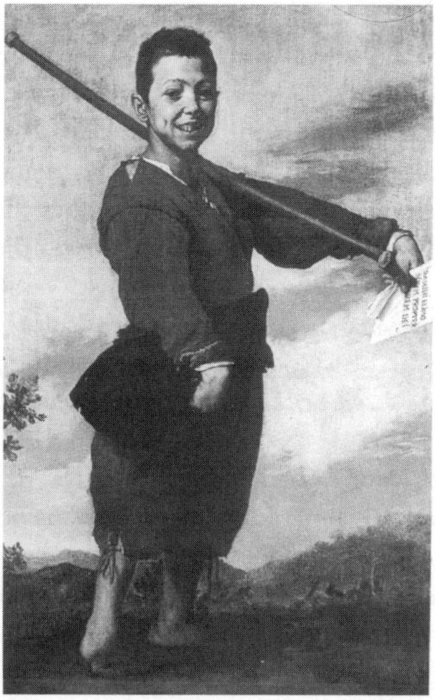

Fig. 3.9. *The Clubfoot* of José de Ribera (1593–1632), in the Musée de Louvre, Paris (oil on canvas, 164 × 93 cm).

under Spanish rule, and married at the age of 25. Although his paintings were mainly of religious subjects, a few were of a popular genre, e.g. *The Clubfoot*, now in the Louvre (Figure 3.9). The note that the boy holds in his left hand reads "Give me alms for the love of God" and suggests that he is unable to speak. As evidenced by his bright face, he does not appear to be an idiot. From the title we can assume that he has difficulty with his right leg. Of particular significance is the posture of the right arm, with the appearance of flexion of the right wrist and the fingers of the right hand. One explanation is that he has a right infantile hemiparesis[5] and the suggestion is made that "The painting also most likely represents the first and only graphic portrayal of aphasia."[5] If the causative lesion was confined to the left cerebral hemisphere to explain his right infantile hemiparesis, then he would not be aphasic because, with right infantile hemiparesis, the surviving right hemisphere takes on the capacity for language. Either the right hemisphere was also affected or the note may be a ploy to obtain sympathy and "alms".

Francisco Goya

Francisco Goya (1746–1828) (Figure 3.10) was born at Fuendetodos, near Saragossa, the capital of Aragon, halfway between Madrid and the French border. The son of a small landed proprietor, he became at the age of 14, having already painted frescoes in his local church, an apprentice in Saragossa.[q] After further art training in Italy, he returned to Spain to design tapestries and became a pupil of the Court painter, Francisco Bayeu, whose sister he married in 1772. His early Baroque paintings were influenced by the Venetian painter Tiepolo, who spent the last years (1762–1780) of his life in Madrid, where he painted ceilings in the royal palace. Goya studied and copied the paintings of Velásquez, who, like the Spanish school in general, had a tendency to portray humble models and often invalids. Popular with the ladies, Goya painted over 200 portraits. A member of the San Fernando Academy in 1780 and Court Painter in 1786, he became Director of the Madrid Academy in 1795 but resigned two years later for health reasons.[25]

His Illness

Goya fell ill after delivering his report on teaching to the Academy and went to recover in Seville. Whilst there in January 1793, at the age of 46 years, he sustained the "... devastating illness that nearly killed him. He survived, but lost his hearing, and remained deaf to the end of his life."[26]

Goya convalesced in Cadiz from March 1793, when his friend wrote: "Goya is slightly better but progress is sadly slow. The noises in his head and his deafness have not passed away; however, his sight has improved and he no longer has fits of dizziness and can walk up and down stairs without difficulty."[27] The sudden illness had caused, besides deafness and giddiness, partial blindness. Goya's sudden deafness has been explained by the diagnosis of the Vogt–Koyanagi syndrome,[27] where in addition there is uveitis (inflammation of the eye); there may also be loss of pigmentation of the skin and hair.[28] The eye problem tends to clear up but the deafness is permanent. Unknown in his day, this disease is now recognised as an auto-immune disorder affecting melanin, the black pigment found in the inner ear (to give

q. Goya was considered to be the best swordsman in Spain. Sought by the Inquisition, because of a duel, he left Madrid at the age of 20 for Italy, where he continued duelling, both wounding and being wounded (Symmons, 1998). From his letters and those of his friends, Goya had a warm but quick-tempered personality, enjoyed good food and wine, as well as hunting with dogs and hearing the latest popular songs. He was concerned when his children fell ill. His peasant background and matador bull-neck appearance made him stand out from others at Court.

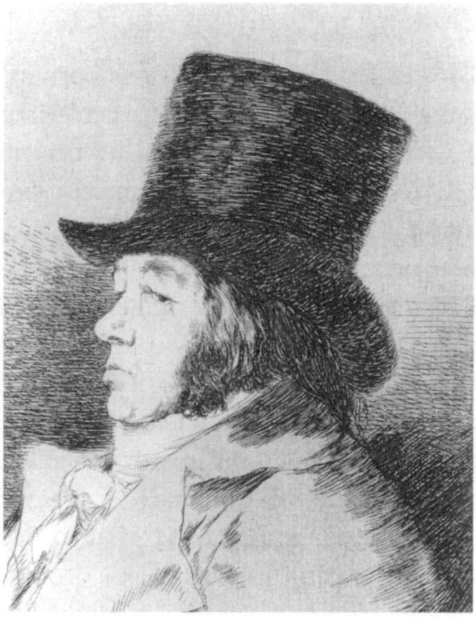

Fig. 3.10. Self-portrait of Francisco Goya.

dizziness, tinnitus and permanent deafness), the uveal tract (to give blurred vision) and sometimes the skin (to give vitiligo or depigmentation) and hair (to give poliosis or whitening). Each of these can be affected alone or in combination.[29] The trigger in Goya's case may have been coldness and over-exertion when he was trying to mend the axle of a coach in which he and the Duchess of Alba were travelling. His illness lasted nearly a year, and the fact that he survived 35 years after this is against the diagnosis of syphilis, which has been suggested.

After this illness, his paintings changed from establishment portraits to such pictures as a shipwreck, prison, lunatic asylum or a fire at night—"a microcosm of the darker side of human experience. . . ."[26]

Six years after his illness, in 1799, he published "*Los Capricos*", a set of 80 prints featuring weird and colourless cartoons, with "Satirical representations of popular superstition, bitter, mordant attacks on the aristocracy, the government and all social conditions, unprecedented assaults on the Crown, on religion and its doctrines. . . ."[30,r]

r. These 80 paintings in etching and aquatint were advertised in 1799 but withdrawn two days later and handed back to the royal painter under threat of the Inquisition in 1803. The reasons were that 12 attacked the aristocracy and even more the church. In the ten years after the

Goya painted "*Los desastres de la guerra*" between 1810 and 1814. These included scenes of terror from the Napoleonic invasion; he added 17 plates in 1814 on the restoration of Ferdinand VII. Hating tyranny, social injustice and human stupidity, he went into exile in France towards the end of his life and died in Bordeaux in 1828, from a stroke.

El Greco

Although El Greco (Domenikos Theotokoponolos) was born in Greece (hence his popular name), his paintings were done in Spain. He painted the in-patients of St James Hospital, Toledo, which may explain why the so-called distortions in his paintings were not due to artistic licence but to revealing neuromuscular disorders. Examples given are the dystrophic facial muscles of San Sebastian, the hand wasting of Santiago el Mayor, the *pes cavus* of the angel in *The Crucifixion*, the peroneal muscular atrophy of St John in *The Baptism of Christ* and the facioscapulohumeral dystrophy in *Adoration of the Shepherds.*[31]

France

Théodore Géricault

An example of portrayal of a neurological disorder is given by (Jean-Louis-André) Théodore Géricault[s] (1791–1824), who was born at Rouen, Normandy. His first exhibit was of a "Mounted Officer" at the age of 21 and he was best known for his bravura paintings of cavalrymen. He was a close friend of several Parisian physicians and, in seeking the truth, to study the sick and dying, he moved into a studio closer to a hospital in order to study corpses in the hospital mortuary. He was thus able also to paint the dead victims of a shipwreck in *The Raft of Medusa*, at the same time as he commissioned a ship's carpenter to make a model of the raft for his painting. This hangs in the Louvre,[2] and shows the 15 survivors of a ship's complement of 150.

Géricault spent a year in Italy from autumn 1816, because he was aware of the need for a change of scene from the stagnant art of contemporary Paris, as

---

age of 62 he produced over 700 paintings; his entire oeuvre comprised almost 2000 paintings, drawings, engravings and lithographs.[25]

s. Sturdily built and with a serious manner, he was a depressive who preferred the darker aspects of life. Hasty, unruly, bold and passionate, he "was a fashionable dandy and an avid horseman whose dramatic paintings reflect his colourful, energetic and somewhat morbid personality".

well as the need for the usual Grand Tour, specially for artists.[t] He had lived through the exciting Napoleonic period, when his paintings were noted for the portrayal of valiant cavalrymen, such as *Charging Chasseur* of 1812. But, after the retreat from Moscow, he suffered from the same disillusionment as his compatriots and his artistic style changed—for example, *Wounded Cuirassier* of 1815. His final paintings include five portraits of the criminally insane, illustrating varieties of mental illness, which are now in the Musée des Beaux Arts, Lyon.

Géricault's lithograph entitled "A Paralytic [*sic*] Woman" (from *Various Subjects Drawn from Life and on Stone*, Rodwell and Martin, London, 1821) was drawn while in England in 1820–1821, when he recorded his impressions of England in lithographs, drawn from the streets of early 19th century London. This paralysed woman has a hopeless expression and is slumped in a heavy wooden wheelchair with large wheels. The unkempt porter is resting from his task, as evidenced by the slack harness and leaning against the chair. This is in sharp contrast with the young girl, who appears to be recoiling, and the passing elegant carriage. In 1821, this lithograph was not a commercial success and the stone was erased.

Géricault's trip to London in 1820 was the last major event of his life. Following a fall from a horse, he lingered for two years with spinal paralysis, from which he died at the age of 32.

The Low Countries

Rembrandt van Rijn

Anatomy Lesson of Dr Nicolaes Tulp, painted in 1632 by Rembrandt van Rijn (1606–1669), shows the eminent surgeon surrounded by pupils of the Amsterdam Guild of Surgeons. Dr Tulp was not only an alderman but also a member of the Amsterdam town council (Figure 3.11). Many such paintings were done because anatomy was no longer forbidden. Now in The Hague, this picture was Rembrandt's first group painting. It has been suggested there is an anatomical error which shows the long finger flexors coming off the lateral, rather than the medial, epicondyle. A more important error is that dissection in those days would start with the abdomen because putrefaction took place there earlier; for the same reason, dissections were in winter and annual events

t. Another reason why he went was that he had a scandalous affair with the wife of his maternal uncle, Alexandine-Modeste Camel (1785–1875), who was six years older than him (Whitney, 1997).

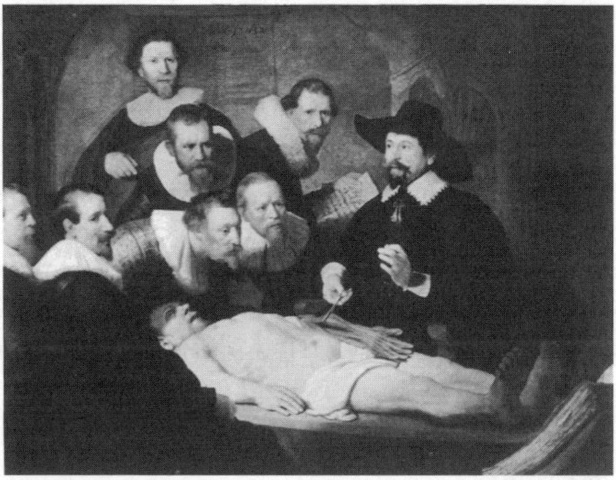

Fig. 3.11. Rembrandt's *Anatomy Lesson of Dr Nicholaes Culp*, now in The Hague, Holland.

for which entrance tickets had to be bought. It is the asymmetrical grouping that makes us feel that we are looking at the cadaver. Although some in the painting are looking at the dissection, others are looking at an anatomical atlas, probably that of Vesalius. Schupbach[32] has written a learned monograph on this one painting, showing that the original has been markedly altered, *viz.* there is a traditional doctor on the left, a hat has been removed from the apex of watchers, and there is a list of the doctors' names instead of an anatomical diagram.

Vincent van Gogh

Vincent van Gogh (1853–1890), a vicar's son and deeply religious, was a self-taught artist. A quiet boy, he showed high spirits alternating with depression; he was obstinate, secretive and not a good mixer. "Red-headed, self-willed, temperamental and inclined to wander off. . . ." His life was full of self-mutilatory acts: putting his hand in a flame when frustrated in love, drinking turpentine and speaking of joint suicide.[33] He stayed in London from the age of 22 for two years, during which time he fell in love with his landlady's daughter, who was in love with someone else.[34] Although zealous as a missionary, he failed, and it was after this that his parents thought that he first began "to go to the bad", and of putting him in a lunatic asylum ("*en curatelle*"). At that time he fell in love with his widowed cousin, and when her father refused to let him see her he held his hand over a lamp flame. It was after this rejection that he began to concentrate more on painting.

Family History

He was the eldest of six surviving children and was born when his mother was aged 35; labour was prolonged and he was born with craniofacial asymmetry. One of his sisters was confined to an asylum for 38 years, having become schizophrenic in the latter part of her life. On his mother's side there were several with epilepsy, a maternal aunt reputedly dying from this condition.

His Art

In the years 1882–1883, van Gogh made many mixed-media drawings in The Hague, teaching himself to paint from a manual and from books illustrating the old masters. "Based in Paris during the years 1886–1888, van Gogh, after a unique 5-year apprenticeship, works with colour."[35]

A review of his work[36] reported: "Van Gogh was 27 when he became an artist, having failed as an art dealer, teacher, and minister. A thoughtful, well-educated man who was a fervent religious scholar and champion of the downtrodden, he sought to evoke the humanity and emotions in everyday existence. His subjects were nature, peasants at work, and other ordinary people. Carefully and methodically following his vision, he produced over 2000 works in ten years. Van Gogh was a heavy smoker. He moved to Paris in 1886, discovering Japanese prints and the Impressionists' bright colours. Travelling south to Arles in 1888, van Gogh, deriving inspiration from the bright sun and colour, painted with speed and intensity, determined to capture fleeting effects and emotions."

His Illnesses

In the winter of 1886 van Gogh was short of money, eating only bread and smoking heavily. He developed dizzy spells and abdominal pain, and consulted a doctor as he feared "that I was not long for this world". He was living with an English painter, and they had the idea of a joint suicide. He found relief in painting, writing to his sister that "... it is a relief to paint a picture and, without it, I should be more miserable than I am".

Van Gogh left Paris for Arles in February 1888, and there he produced his first Fauve painting, with broad strokes and crushed paint. He felt he was "... now bereft of control, or at the mercy of blind or mechanical forces ...".

He was often tired and hungry and, in a letter to his brother, wrote: "The more ugly, old, vicious, ill and poor I get, the more I want to take my revenge by painting in brilliant colours, well arranged, resplendent." In October 1888, the month that Gauguin arrived in Arles, he wrote to his brother, Theo: "I suffer from vertigo."[37]

The Ear Amputation

Gauguin lived with him for only a few weeks but they often argued, and Gauguin left after van Gogh threw a glass of absinthe at him. This happened on December 23rd, 1888, after which van Gogh, according to Gauguin, followed him into the street with an open razor but turned back when Gauguin fixedly stared at him. Gauguin refused to return to their house and stayed that night in a hotel. Van Gogh went home and cut off the lobe of his ear (Figure 3.12) by a diagonal incision beginning "posteriorly towards the top of the ear and cut anteriorly through the tragus (the prominence in front of the external opening)".[38] He then went to the local brothel, and presented the ear to the prostitute Rachel, who had apparently slept with Gauguin. The day following his ear amputation, having lost a good deal of blood, he was taken to hospital, where he was delirious with visual and auditory hallucinations. This was diagnosed as acute mental derangement accompanied by generalised delirium, and Theo was not allowed to see him. His illness cleared within three days and he was discharged on January 7th, 1889.

There have been various explanations of the ear amputation, from being a phallic symbol to the influence of bullfighting at Arles, where the bullfighter was presented with the dead bull's ears.[38] As it occurred before Christmas day, it may have been done in a fit of religious despair; even more far-fetched is that at about the same time, Jack the Ripper was removing ears from Whitechapel prostitutes. A more recent suggestion is that Gauguin, who has been considered a poor witness, was the only observer of the incident, and was responsible for the ear amputation as he was a fencer.[42] Whatever the explanation, the ear amputation was perhaps the first unequivocal evidence of definite "madness".

His Attacks

On January 7th, 1889, van Gogh wrote: "I hope I have just had simply an artist's fit, and a lot of fever after *very* considerable loss of blood, as an artery was severed...." Later that month he wrote: "...the unbearable hallucinations have ceased, and are now getting reduced to a simple nightmare, in consequence of my taking Bromide of potassium, I think...."[37] In April 1889 he

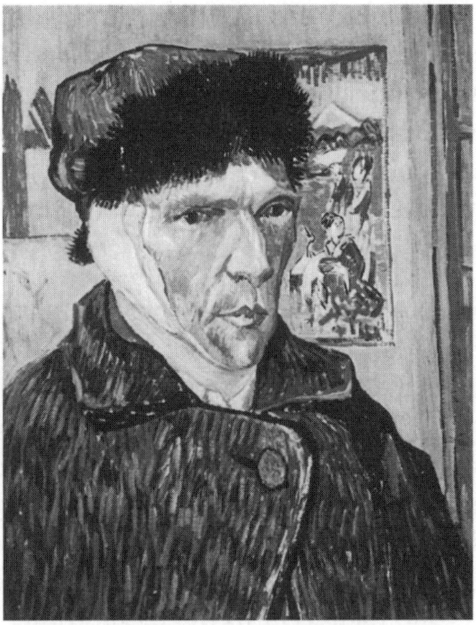

Fig. 3.12. Van Gogh's self-portrait.

wrote: "I have had in all four great attacks, during which I didn't in the least know what I said, what I wanted and what I did. Not taking into account that I had previously three fainting fits without any plausible reason, and without retaining the slightest remembrance of what I felt."[37] In the same letter (April 30th, 1889) he wrote: "Every day I take the remedy which the incomparable Dickens prescribes against suicide. It consists of a glass of wine, a piece of bread with cheese and a pipe of tobacco."

As van Gogh's mental infirmities (diagnosed at the time as epilepsy) had increasingly incapacitated him after 1888, he committed himself to St Rémy asylum, where he alternated between healthy outdoor painting and incoherent spells.

Van Gogh wrote: "... there is quite definitely something or other deranged in my brain...." In July 1889, while settling down to paint, his orderly by his side, his eyes "suddenly became wild, his hand began to move convulsively, his body arched backwards". For three weeks he suffered attacks of dementia and prostration. Afterwards he was remorseful and depressed. In September 1889 he noticed that attacks came every three months. In December 1889, another attack occurred but was less severe and lasted one week.

The year 1890 is important in his disease progression. On January 23rd he had an attack after visiting Arles. On February 1st his nephew was born, and this may have affected him as he would be a rival for Theo's financial interests. On February 24th, 1890, he had visited a brothel and had another severe attack; he escaped from a cell to sprawl on a heap of coal, snatched lamp oil to drink, sank into a dazed state, and only in April did he begin to improve. During convalescence he suddenly kicked his orderly in the stomach and said: "Forgive me, I'm not very clear what I've done. I thought I was at Arles being hunted by the police." During this time he was erratic and moody and again began to drink. He lost his temper with boys who teased him by putting salt in his coffee.

In all, van Gogh had seven attacks at Arles and St Rémy. Four were "*grandes crises*" and three fainting spells, but he was amnestic for all of them. They were all sudden in onset and slow in resolution. He recovered from most within one to two weeks but two lasted two months. Whilst he was at St Rémy, three of four episodes occurred after he had gone to Arles.[38] The attacks were initiated by an "acute state of delirium and disorientation", accompanied by visual and auditory hallucinations and paranoia. He was suicidal, drinking turpentine, kerosene and oil colours, so that his tubes of colour paints had to be removed. During these episodes he was unable to paint, did not always recognise people and "complained of dizziness which was provoked by heights and he disliked climbing stairs".[39]

In the year that Vincent was in St Rémy-de-Provence, he produced 150 oils, 100 drawings and 10 watercolours. He was in a private asylum from May 1889 and left in May 1890. While in the Saint Pare de Mausole asylum, he wrote 750 letters, which were all lucid. Dr Peynon, director of the asylum, diagnosed epilepsy, but others thought he had schizophrenia.

On "one bright, hot July day in 1890 in Auvers-sur-Oise, 20 miles to the northwest of Paris, he mounted two flights of steps to his windowless attic room and shot himself."[35] He died at the age of 37 years, the same age as artists like Toulouse-Lautrec, Watteau, Caravaggio and Raphael, and composers like Mozart.

Differential Diagnosis

There is no consensus as to the diagnosis of van Gogh's illness.

Pennemen,[40] a surgeon in Washington, gave as the differential diagnosis:

1. Epilepsy
2. Schizophrenia
3. Neurosyphilis
4. Bipolar disorder

5. Substance abuse
6. Absinthe
7. Delirium tremens
8. Meniere's disease
9. Lead poisoning
10. Acute intermittent porphyria

Epilepsy

At Arles, the house surgeon, Dr Rey, talked of epileptic crises and Dr Peyron, director of the St Rémy asylum, considered attacks of epilepsy, although there was no evidence of convulsions. An ex-ophthalmologist, Dr Peyron may have given weight to the family history of epilepsy and concluded that the cause of van Gogh's illness was some form of epilepsy, "whether exacerbated by absinthe, glaucoma, digitalis poisoning or syphilis . . .".[39] "Between his breakdowns in the asylum he had long periods of absolute lucidity. . . ." He had three blackouts without warning in April 1889. On other occasions, there was "prolonged loss of consciousness, often preceded by irrational behaviour".[41] "A tuberculous abscess, in particular, is a distinct possibility."[41] The diagnosis of epilepsy would fit in with his complete recovery between attacks. Professor Gastaut of Marseilles, a famous epileptologist, diagnosed temporal lobe epilepsy. Van Gogh's attacks were controlled by bromides, then the only anti-epileptic drug known. But this diagnosis would not explain his prolonged attacks lasting weeks, with hallucinations.

Schizophrenia

Van Gogh's sister was diagnosed as schizophrenic, and some of his early behaviour, such as burning his hand deliberately, would support this diagnosis, as would his later self-mutilation, paranoia and suicide; but it does not fit in with complete recovery in between episodes. Schizophrenia is considered the most likely diagnosis by Karl Jaspers and the German school of neuropsychiatrists. Van Gogh's violent attacks were initially rare; the interludes were good except for suicide gestures by attempting to swallow turpentine.

Neurosyphilis

In 1882 van Gogh had an attack of gonorrhoea in Antwerp when he may have contracted syphilis. The following year he developed eye trouble, and generalised weakness. Later he may have contracted syphilis from his mistress, who was a prostitute. In either case the time intervals were too short for the development of GPI (general paralysis of the insane), although not for meningo-vascular syphilis, the other type of tertiary neurosyphilis.

Bipolar disorder

Bipolar disorder has been diagnosed because of confusional episodes, from which van Gogh made a rapid recovery, with prolonged periods of normal mentation. Also in favour of this diagnosis is that his illness developed in his third, and lasted into his fourth, decade. When he was admitted to hospital at Arles, the diagnosis of the director, Dr Uspur, was acute mania with generalised delirium. There were periods where he would gesticulate and talk wildly; at other times he had great agitation, followed by prostration and calm. These sudden attacks could be provoked by trifling incidents and he had no recollection of his attacks of hallucinations, during which he had uncontrollable aggression with threatening behaviour. He also had nocturnal fantasies. But he was constantly plagued by abdominal symptoms; he had auditory and visual hallucinations and epileptic attacks, and these features could not be explained by manic-depressive psychosis.

Substance abuse

Alcohol

Van Gogh's health was not the best due to excessive smoking and drinking. During the winter of 1887–1888 in Paris, he had problems with his "blood", variously described as poor circulation or anaemia, as well as indigestion, nerves and melancholy; the latter was made worse by attempts to reduce his alcohol intake and smoking. In Paris he had a "tired brain" and "tired eyes" after painting and referred to a "stroke" and "breakdown". He talked of "bad wine" in Paris and brandy in Arles but did not mention absinthe, possibly because this was noted specifically as a toxin at that time.[u]

A toxic psychosis consists of disorientation, hallucinations, delusions, feelings of terror and violent behaviour. Following withdrawal of alcohol, delirium tremens ensues, which includes visual rather than auditory hallucinations. Tremor is almost invariable (hence the name) but there are usually no fainting

u. Another example of substance abuse, in the case of another artist, was Toulouse-Lautrec, who was an alcoholic; it was while being "dried out" in a clinic that he drew his famous circus scenes. He had many medical connections; for example, he spent Saturday mornings visiting hospitals with his cousin, who was a doctor. He also shared a flat with a doctor and often said that would have been his chosen profession if he had not become a painter, and his last paintings often had a medical association. He was said to have died of a stroke at the age of 37 (his friend van Gogh died at the same age).

spells, and it would be strange if this was not diagnosed at that time, when it was a well-recognised condition.

Absinthe

Van Gogh was said to have drunk absinthe excessively in Paris, the suggestion being that he was "a manic-depressive who developed confusional periods and fits due to his addiction to the liqueur called absinthe" (Hemphill, 1961). The absinthe drinker painted by Edgar Dégas (1834–1917) indicated that this drug addiction was not uncommon.[v]

Unlike the hallucinations of schizophrenia, which are usually auditory, absinthe can also cause visual hallucinations.[w] The symptoms may present after drinking ceases. There was a high consumption of absinthe in Bouches-du-Rhône, where Arles is situated. In excess, it gave seizures, vertigo, hallucinations and delirium. Its constituent, thujone, is a brain toxin, which is also found in cannabis. Complete recovery in between attacks is against the diagnosis in van Gogh. Toulouse-Lautrec and Modigliani also drunk absinthe, as did the poets Baudelaire and Verlaine.

Digitalis

Used now in cardiac conditions, in the 19th century it was used to treat epilepsy. Van Gogh's propensity for yellow and halo effects may have been due to digitalis. On two occasions in 1890 he painted Dr Paul-Ferdenand Gachet; in both pictures there is a "a foxglove flower of dark purple", i.e. *Digitalis pupurea*, the purple foxglove.[x]

The Czech Jan Evangelista Purkinje experimented in 1825 with digitalis, which produced circular concentric light and dark waves.

---

v. It was unusual for Dégas to use models; he knew the portrayed couple well and asked them to pose in the Café de la Nouvelle-Athénes on Place Pigalle. Painted in 1876, the man was Marcellin Desbontin, a painter and engraver, who introduced Dégas to the café, and the woman, Ellen Andrée, an actress. While she is portrayed as innocent and youthful and fashionably dressed, he is mature and worldly. They both sit with sad eyes starting distractedly, being reduced to a state of apathy.

w. Absinthe was popular in 19th century France and was obtained from wormwood (*Artemisia absinthium*). It was thought to be a cure-all and was used by French soldiers in Algeria to reduce fevers. The first commercial producer was Henré Louis Pernod (in 1797), who obtained the recipe from a Swiss GP. "The extract was prepared by steeping the pungent herb in alcohol and distilling the spirit" (Bell, 1984). Other herbs such as fennel and licorice, were added to lessen the bitter taste. Its production was prohibited in France in 1915, since absinthe was found to be addictive. Modern Pernod is an aniseed-flavoured beverage. The ban has recently been lifted and a less powerful absinthe is available, known as the "Green Fairy".

x. Digitalis intoxication causes confusion, delirium and hazy yellow vision.

Delirium tremens

Van Gogh's attacks seemed to be provoked after alcohol intake rather than its withdrawal, as would be the case in delirium tremens.

Meniere's disease

Although he complained of dizziness (presumably vertigo), there was no suggestion of episodic attacks or accompanying nausea or tinnitus, nor would Meniere's disease explain all the other symptoms of his disorder.

Lead poisoning

He could have inhaled lead from his paints but his symptoms were not suggestive of lead poisoning, which more likely could have acted as a trigger.

Porphyria

Van Gogh's attacks were precipitated by going without food and alcohol. He was better when the last two triggers were obviated and also by bromide therapy. A single explanation for all these features would be acute intermittent porphyria.[43] Low protein and low carbohydrate diets are especially detrimental. The first diagnosis of this condition was reported in Dutch medical literature just before his death, so his attending doctors would not have been aware of this diagnosis. The condition is transmitted by an autosomal dominant gene and this would fit in with the fact that van Gogh had several relatives with neuropsychiatric disorders.[44,y] The main country for variegate porphyria is South

y. The word "porphyrin" is derived from the Greek word meaning reddish-purple. The porphyrias are so called because the urine of sufferers turns reddish-purple on standing; they are inherited as autosomal dominant traits (except for congenital erythropoietic porphyria). They are due to abnormalities in the synthesis of haem and associated with excessive secretion of porphyrins (Green, 1976). Although *porphyria variegata* and *acute intermittent porphyria* are both genetically determined, they are two distinct unborn errors of metabolism. Both types occur in Holland. Patients may complain of abdominal pain, made worse by barbiturates; they may be unstable, neurotic or mentally disorientated.[44] The skin may be sensitive and easily upraided. The red pigment that gives a reddish urine does not contain iron. In the 1963 classification, porphyrias are broadly divided into hepatic and erythropoietic. The first group includes:

(1) acute intermittent porphyria

(2) porphyria variegata

(3) coproporphyria

(4) porphyria cutanea tarda

Africa, where 10 000 cases have been reported, nearly all of whom could be traced to two Dutch settlers who married in the Cape in 1688. The disease became more evident with the introduction of barbiturates at the beginning of the 20th century. Triggers included overwork and a proclivity for camphor and other terpenes. The reason why there has been no report of coloured urine in van Gogh may be: "Freshly voided urine is colourless, but on exposure to air and light it becomes dark or a wine red colour after several hours."[43] Since van Gogh did much of his painting out of doors, the urine would have been colourless.

Not only the central nervous system but also the peripheral nervous system can be involved, as well as the liver and skin. The cerebral features include anxiety, agitation and seizures, all of which van Gogh had. The psychiatric symptoms may be diagnosed as schizophrenia, psychoneurosis, hysteria or paranoia.[45] Behavioural disturbances, e.g. irritability, confusion, mania or depression, occur in 30% of cases, and epilepsy in 25%. The attacks are precipitated by drugs, especially including alcohol, and this may be the reason why van Gogh often developed attacks after visiting Arles. As in his case, there may be no symptoms in between attacks.

Conclusion

While, in this chapter, the case histories of Goya and van Gogh have been elaborated, because of the rarity of their neurological diagnoses I hope to have indicated the wide and fascinating topics falling within the ambit of the chapter's title. This also points to many more research areas for investigation.

References

1. F.C. Rose, The medicine of art. Presidential Address, *Trans. Med. Soc. London* (1985).
2. D.R. Karps (ed.), *Ars Medica: Art, Medicine and the Human Condition* (Philadelphia Museum of Art, 1985), pp. vii, x, 191.
3. H.E. Sigerist, The historical aspects of art and medicine, *Bull. Inst. Hist. Med. II* Vol. 271–97 (1936).

The second group is divided into:

(1) congenital porphyria

(2) erythropoietic protoporphyria

4. C.H. Espinel, Art and neuroscience: how the brain sees Vermeer's *Woman Holding a Balance*, *Lancet* **352**, 2099 (1998).
5. L. McHenry, Neurology and art. In *Historical Aspects of the Neurosciences*, eds. F. Clifford Rose and W.H. Bynum (Raven, New York, 1982), pp. 481–519.
6. F. Loschiovo, Masaccio's cripple, *Lancet* **347**, 628 (1996).
7. F.C. Rose, Masaccio's cripple, *Lancet* **347**, 628 (1996).
8. J. Beck, *Italian Renaissance Painting* (Harper and Row, London, 1981), pp. 285–304.
9. O. Casazza, *Masaccio and the Brancacci Chapel* (Scara, Florence, 1990).
10. C.H. Espinel, Masaccio's cripple: a neurological syndrome. Its art, medicine and values, *Lancet* **346**, 1684–86 (1995).
11. P. Trevor-Roper, *The World Through Blunted Sight* (Thomas and Hudson, London, 1970).
12. K. Podell and D. Robinson, Migraine experiences as artistic inspiration in a contemporary artist, *J. R. Soc. Med.* **93**, 263–5 (2000).
13. B. Hozeski, *Hildegard von Bingen's Mystical Visions* (Bear, Santa Fe, 1995).
14. F. Maddocks, Hildegard of Bingen; The Woman of Her Age. Headline, London, 2001, p. 62.
15. C. Singer, The scientific views and visions of Saint Hildegard (1098–1180). In *Studies in the History and Methods of Science*, ed. C. Singer (Oxford University Press, London, 1917), pp. 21, 51–3.
16. F.C. Rose, Transient blindness, *Br. Med. J.* **3**, 763–4 (1969).
17. O. Sacks, *Migraine* (University of California Press, 1992).
18. F. Jowell, The paintings of Hieronymus Bosch. *J. R. Soc. Med.* **58**, 131–6 (1965).
19. J.G. Ravin, G.P. Hodge and J.J. Hartman, *Stones of Madness* (Michigan Medicine, 1974), pp. 185–8.
20. N.H. McAlister, The cure of folly, *Can. Med. Assoc. J.* **110**, 1380, 1383 (1974).
21. W. Schupbach, A new look at *the cure of folly*, *Med. Hist.*, **22**, 267–81 (1978).
22. F. Martí-Ibáñez, The artist as physician: medical philosophy in the Renaissance, *Ins. Rec. Med. G.P. Clinics*, **167**, 221–42 (1954).
23. E.W. Todd, *The Neuroanatomy of Leonardo da Vinci* (American Association of Neurosurgeons, Park Ridge, 1991), pp. 26, 59.
24. G.A. Lindebloom, *Andreas Vesalius and His Opus Magnus* (De Fanel, Nieuwendyk, 1975), p. 12.
25. J. Tomlinson, *Painting in Spain: El Greco to Goya* (Weidenfeld and Nicolson, London, 1997), pp. 139–61.
26. J. Wilson-Bareau, *The Daily Telegraph*, 3 Feb. 2001.
27. T. Cawthorne, Goya's illness, *Proc. R. Soc. Med.* **55**, 213–17 (1962).
28. R.S. Manor, Vogt-Koyanagi-Harada syndrome and related diseases. In *Handbook of Clinical Neurology*, eds. P.J. Vinken and G.W. Bruyn (North-Holland, Oxford, 1978), Vol. 34, pp. 513–44.

29. A.F. Ryan, E.M. Keithley and J.P. Harris, Autoimmune inner ear disorders, *Current Opinion in Neurology* **14**, 35–40 (2001).
30. R. Muther, *The History of Modern Painting* (J.M. Dent & Co, New York, 1907), pp. 222–51.
31. J.R. Heron, El Greco and muscular dystrophy? *Br. Med. J. II*, **256** (1979).
32. W. Schupbach, *The Paradox of Rembrandt's Anatomy of Dr Tulp* (Wellcome Institute of the History of Medicine, London, 1982).
33. P. Cabanne, *Van Gogh* (Thames and Hudson, London, 1963).
34. I. Dunlop, *Van Gogh* (Wiedenfeld and Nicolson, London, 1974).
35. P. Tuchman, Facing Van Gogh at the PMA, *Lancet* **356**, 1529–30 (2000).
36. W.J. Reif, Van Gogh's Van Goghs, *Lancet* **352**, 1478 (1979).
37. R. Pickvance, *Van Gogh in Arles* (Harry N. Abrams, New York, 1984), pp. 28–30.
38. A.J. Lubin, *Strangers on the Earth: The Life of Vincent Van Gogh* (Parladin, St Albans, 1975), pp. 184, 186, 187, 217.
39. R. Pickvance, *Van Gogh in St Rémy and Auvers* (Harry N. Abrams, New York, 1986), p. 15.
40. M.F. Penneman, Vincent van Gogh: what do his letters suggest about the diagnosis? *J. Med. Biog.* **3**, 43–9 (1995).
41. E.M.R. Critchley, *Hallucinations and Their Impact on Art* (Carnegie Press, Preston, 1981) pp. 157, 158.
42. P. Conradi, Gauguin cut off van Gogh's ear, *Sunday Times*, London, 22 July 2001, pp. 1–4.
43. L.S. Loftus and W.N. Arnold, Vincent van Gogh's illness: acute intermittent porphyria, *Br. Med. J.* **303**, 1589–91 (1991).
44. G. Dean, *The Porphyrias* (Pitman, London, 1971), p. 1.
45. A. Goldberg, *Porphyria: A Royal Malady* (British Medical Association, London, 1968), pp. 66–8.
46. K.F. Kiple, *Ergotism and Erysipelas: St Anthony's Fire in Plague, Pox and Pestilence*, ed. K. F. Kiple (Weidenfeld and Nicolson, London, 1997), pp. 32–7.
47. M.H. Bell, The cover, *JAMA* **252** 14, 1838 (1984).
48. W. Bosing, Hieronymus Bosch (c. 1450–1516). Between Heaven and Hell (Taschen, London, 2000).
49. F. Garin, *Murillo* (Aldlasa, Sevillé, 1995).
50. M. Green, Porphyria, in *Handbook of Clinical Neurology*, eds. P.J. Vinker and G.W. Bruyn (North-Holland, Oxford, 1976), Vol. 27, pp. 429–48.
51. R. Heirlinger, *History of Medical Illustration from Antiquity to AD 1600* (Pitman, London, 1970).
52. A. Rosenberg, *Leonardo da Vinci* (M.J. Lohse) (H Grevel & Co., London, 1903).
53. S. Symmons, *Goya* (Phairon, London, 1998).
54. W. Whitney, *Géricault in Italy* (Yale University Press, London, 1997).

Chapter 4

Galen and the Artful Symmetry of the Brain

Julius Rocca

A mainstream tenet of Greek philosophy is that human beings possess a rational soul. Its actions, according to the most famous physician of antiquity, Galen of Pergamum (129–*c*. 216 AD),[a] are possible only because of a set of communicating cavities deep within the brain substance known as the ventricles of the brain. The anatomical descriptions and physiological functions given for the ventricles and their interconnecting passages arguably represent one of Galen's chief contributions to the history of anatomical science. The account he provides of the ventricular system is eloquent testimony of a precise and detailed knowledge of the subject.[b] Galen based his decision to accord the ventricles their role on strict empirical grounds, determined by his knowledge of anatomy, his vivisectional experiments, and, in part, by

a. On Galen's life, career and achievements see: Moraux, 1985; Nutton, 1995; Singer, 1997.

b. For a survey see: Rocca, 1997. Galen records his anatomical demonstrations on the ventricles chiefly in *De usu partium* (*UP*) I.481–87, 489–96; *Anatomicis administrationibus* (*AA*) IIK, 717–31; *Anatomical Procedures*, IX.7ff. Although the 15 anatomical books which constitute the last two mentioned works were revised and expanded some 25 years after *UP*, which may partly account for some of the differences in anatomical descriptions between the two works, this has no direct bearing on the internal consistency of Galen's anatomy of the brain. In citing Galen, most references are given according to the edition of C.G. Kühn, *Claudii Galeni Opera omnia*, Vols. 1–20, Lipsiae, 1821–33 (hereafter, K). Kühn's text is, however, not a critical edition. Citations from the critical series *Corpus Medicorum Graecorum* are given by the pagination of the editor concerned. References to Galen's *De usu partium* are from the critical edition of G. Helmreich, *Galeni de usu partium libri xvii*, Teubner, Leipzig, I: 1907; II: 1909. Quotations from *Anatomical Procedures*, which constitute the latter six-and-one-half books (IX, 6–XV) of *Anatomicis administrationibus*, and which exist only in Arabic translation, are cited according to the edition of Duckworth, Lyons and Towers (= Duckworth).

his observations of brain-injured patients.[c] Although the importance of the ventricles was first formally stated by the pioneering anatomists Herophilus and Erasistratus in Alexandria in the third century BC, it was Galen who provided for the first time a comprehensive account of ventricular anatomy.[d] This anatomy is a complex record which is not easy to comprehend at first reading. In that part of *Anatomical Procedures* which has survived only in Arabic translation, Galen asks his readers to carefully study the "reciprocal symmetry" or "reciprocal harmony" of the four ventricles in the brain.[e] Although the ultimate elucidation of Galenic ventricular anatomy is only possible as the result of a highly refined methodology of painstaking and repeated dissection, an idea of the ventricles as three-dimensional, symmetrical structures is crucial for understanding their anatomical and topographical relationships.

I

As is well known, Galen elaborated his anatomy of the brain using, for the most part, the ox. It is striking that anything constructive in an anatomical sense can be made using a fresh brain.[f] Its cavities, in particular, represent a considerable anatomical challenge. Their intercommunications are delicate passages readily obliterated unless extreme care is taken.[g] Outside the skull the brain will collapse under its own weight.[h] It is this loss of structural integrity which Galen was well aware of, and forms one of the reasons why, for example, he stresses the importance of the structural support of the dural folds which make up the tentoria and falx.[i] It is also why Galen emphasises that a large amount of detailed dissection work should take place whilst the brain remains *in situ*.

---

c. Cf. Rocca, *Galen on the Brain: Anatomical Knowledge and Physiological Speculation in the Second Century AD* (E.J. Brill, Leiden, 2003).

d. The extant testimonia and fragments of Herophilus and Erasistratus do not allow the conclusion that the focus and direction of their work parallelled that of Galen in all respects.

e. IX.7; 2, Duckworth. Cf. Simon, 1906, II, 3.

f. Woollam (1958, 14) correctly notes that the brain is, in its unpreserved state, "an amorphous gruel". Nevertheless, what he calls the "distinguishing features", represented by the ventricles, are in fact remarkably featureless in a fresh brain.

g. The corollary is of course that false passages may easily be created.

h. It has been well compared to a blancmange (King, 1987, 22). A brain retains the shape it has due to the cushioning effect of the cerebrospinal fluid. It is highly likely that what Galen described as "residues" (*περιττώματα*) in the ventricles were traces of cerebrospinal fluid (cf. *UP*, II.2–3). Siegel (1968, 124) states that Galen "did not recognise that cerebrospinal fluid was lost by his faulty autopsy technique". This is best interpreted in light of most of Siegel's interpretations of Galen's physiology.

i. Cf. *UP*, II.20–21, where the dural foldings, the veins and the surrounding structures they support are presented as parts of a contiguous and logical whole that are critically important for the structural and functional integrity of the ventricles.

This will not of course prevent the brain from partly collapsing, but it does provide stability in a dissection. But more is needed to complete the picture, and Galen asks the dissector to envisage the ventricles as a set of symmetrical structures. The ventricular system consists of two lateral ventricles, which are Galen's anterior (or first) ventricles (there is no "second ventricle" because of the twin lateral ventricles), located deep within each cerebral hemisphere and communicating with each other and with the third (or middle) ventricle across the midline of the brain through the interventricular foramen (of Monro).[j] The third ventricle communicates with the fourth (or posterior) ventricle by the cerebral or mesencephalic aqueduct (of Sylvius).[k] The roof of the fourth ventricle is dominated by the mass of the cerebellum. The floor of the fourth ventricle narrows at its caudal end into the central canal of the spinal cord.[l] This canal is interpreted by Galen as a passage through psychic pneuma, which, elaborated and refined in the anterior ventricles, thereby has access to the nerves of the body. The most important features of the ventricular anatomy of the brain of higher mammals can best be appreciated by casts.[m] Galen's ventricular system is a continuous series of symmetrical chambers, linked by passages or canals, communicating with the brain substance, the cranial nerves and the spinal cord.

II

Arguably one of the greatest of Galen's achievements in the history of anatomical science is that of constructing a coherent description of a set of cavities that are not immediately discernible on first inspection of a fresh brain. The following from *Anatomical Procedures* perfectly encapsulates the Galenic notion of a series of communicating, symmetrical chambers deep within the brain:

> What you should carefully study is the reciprocal symmetry of the four ventricles in the brain. For if you proceed carefully, you find that the part which the anatomists have compared to the sharpened end of the writing reed is

j. Alexander Monro *Secundus* (1733–1817). Monro, however, is not the "discoverer" of this passage, and was mistaken on the actual site of the communication. Cf. Sharp, 1961; Last and Tompsett, 1953, 535. The third ventricle in the bovine brain is noticeably smaller than the lateral ventricles, and is "only a ring-like space" (Fitzgerald, 1961, 41).

k. This aqueduct is relatively large and quite long in the bovine brain, and it progressively widens as it approaches the fourth ventricle.

l. Here the anatomy is distinctive: "In large ruminants the fourth ventricle is an elongated almost quadrangular cavity. . .(it) communicates through the mesencephalic aqueduct with the third ventricle" (Sisson and Grossman, 1975, 1073).

m. Cf. Fitzgerald, 1961; Sharp, 1961, 88. Leonardo Da Vinci first performed castings (in wax). Cf. O'Malley and Saunders, 1952. Leonardo's cast work is all the more impressive as casting is a difficult technical procedure. Cf. Kier, 1977, 2788; Last and Tompsett, 1953, 525.

> fashioned similarly to an outflow which discharges into the spinal marrow. Further you see how, above this part, a passage opens out from the posterior ventricle, which extends itself to the middle ventricle. Then you see how the two anterior [*R. and L. lateral*] ventricles open themselves, discharging into the middle ventricle, as I have described above [Book IX, chap. 4].[n] And you see how the anterior end of each of the two anterior ventricles [*rostral horn*][o] goes to each one of the two nasal cavities like a hollow horn, wide at its commencement from its upper part and then steadily narrowing itself. You must now detach and remove all that surrounds these two horns, and go on uninterruptedly along them until you arrive at their termination... Previously also, if you will, inspect thoroughly the discharging effluents on the two sides [*R. and L.*] of the anterior ventricles, and remove completely all the parts lying around them, so as to get a fair view of the duct which comes out from the end of each of the two ventricles, noticing how for a wide stretch it descends in the same way as the commencement of the spinal marrow [*central canal*]. However, the top of that duct does not resemble the point of the calamus scriptorius. For it has in this spot no sort of vaulting; on the contrary each of the two ventricles steadily narrows and diminishes, so that the duct comes into being thereout.[p]

The whole thrust of this description is to visualise the ventricular system as an unbroken set of intercommunicating passages extending from the anterior part of the brain to the spinal cord. This is an absolute necessity for the passage of psychic pneuma. In view of the wide-ranging physiological claims Galen makes on each of the ventricles, the need to comprehend their individual anatomical characteristics within the paradigm of a symmetrical order becomes a high priority. Therefore, Galen prefaces his grand tour of ventricular anatomy by commending to the dissector their "reciprocal symmetry".

In the concluding chapter of his physiological masterwork, *On the Use of the Parts of the Body* ("*De usu partium*"), the importance of symmetry is placed in a teleological perspective. It is here that Galen cites Polykleitos:

> Here is something to marvel at in these men who say that Nature has no skill; namely, that they praise sculptors for making the parts on the right side precisely like those on the left but fail to praise Nature, who in addition to making

---

n. That is, at the interventricular foramen.

o. Duckworth glosses this as the "inferior horn". But Galen is providing a description of that part of the anterior ventricle which terminates at the olfactory tract. This is the superior or rostral horn. However, this interpretation depends on how Galen has oriented the brain in regard to this dissection. Thus, if Galen has turned the brain over and is examining it from its base, then the anterior horn becomes "inferior". However, Galen nowhere in the above description cites this particular orientation, and it should be assumed that he is proceeding from the surface of the brain downwards. It seems best to regard this part of the anterior ventricle described above as the anterior (rostral) and not inferior (caudal) horn. See Rocca, 2003, 118.

p. IX.7; 2–3. Square brackets Duckworth.

> the parts equal also supplies them with actions and, more than this, with usefulness that is taught to the animal right at the beginning, at birth. Or is it correct to admire Polykleitos for the symmetry of the parts in his statue known as *The Canon*, and yet necessary to deprive Nature not only of praise but of all skill—Nature, who exhibits the symmetry of the parts both externally, as sculptors do, but also deep below the surface? Or was it not Polykleitos himself who was her imitator, at least in that which he was able to imitate?[q]

According to Galen, Polykleitos successfully exhibited the correct symmetry of the surface of the body.[r] He is praised by Galen as someone who stresses the "precise symmetry" (ἀκριβῆ συμμετρία) of each part with the other.[s] Together with his rival Phidias, Polykleitos was one of the most famous of the Greek sculptors, active in the second half of the fifth century BC. Among his works, familiar to the Romans as copies of the Greek original, the most famous is the *Doryphorus* ("spear-carrier"), which formed a template for other artisans.[t] Indeed, Polykleitos also used this statue to promulgate his writings on symmetry and form.[u] Other works include the *Cyniscus*, in the Westmacott Youth in the British Museum, the *Amazon* of Ephesus, and the gigantic statue of Hera of Argos, said to have rivalled Phidias' *Olympian Zeus* in its execution.[v] Clearly, the reputation and skill of Polykleitos would have been familiar to Galen's audience. Galen usefully exploits this analogy with sculpture in the following way. Properly conveying the external symmetry of the body, says Galen, is a difficult skill for sculptors.[w] By implication, only a careful *anatomy* by a well-trained anatomist can reveal useful information about the more difficult internal structures of the body forever beyond a sculptor's ken. There is also a philosophical component to Galen's thinking. Plato noted that if the component proportions of a structure are incorrect, then that which is constituted from such elements, as well as the elements themselves, will be destroyed.[x] According to Plato, "the qualities of measure and proportion invariably . . . constitute beauty and excellence".[y] Symmetry is associated quantitatively with καιρός, *right proportion* or *correct measure*, and it is this sense

q. *UP*, II.441; tr. May 1968, 726–7, slightly modified. See also: Borbein, 1996, 66–90; Gourevitch, 1987, 275ff; Pollitt, 1972, 105–10; *idem.*, 1990, 75–9.

r. *De placitis Hippocratis et Platonis* (*PHP*), 308.21–25, De Lacy.

s. *De temperamentis*, I. 566 K.

t. The Roman copy is not an altogether exact one. The original lacked the prominent tree trunk, was of bronze, and was over seven feet in height. The spear rested on the left shoulder and was carried in the left hand. Cf. Cook, 1976, 125–6.

u. Cf. Pliny, *Naturalis Historia*, XXXIV.55. Polykleitos' text on this subject has not survived.

v. Strabo, *Geographica*, VIII.372.

w. Cf. *UP*, II.442.

x. *Philebus*, 64E; Cf. *Republic*, 530A, *Sophist*, 228C.

y. *Philebus*, 64E. Cf. Beardsley, 1966, 43f.

of the correct proportion of a structural component that operates in Galen's description of ventricular symmetry.[z]

Yet Galen's concept of symmetry is not simply a proportional set of parts but reflects an ordered pattern imposed by Nature which is the key to the proper function of the part of the body concerned. Examples from the plastic arts are important to Galen precisely because the symmetry of the various components of the body is neither easy to grasp nor to defend. An example is the topographic relationship of certain abdominal organs. For example, each kidney may be considered as reciprocally symmetrical with the other. Nevertheless, Galen holds that the right kidney lies higher than the left.[aa] However, this seeming imbalance is deemed necessary in order for all the abdominal organs to be in correct equilibrium with each other, for only this allows their proper function.[bb] In *On the Doctrines of Hippocrates and Plato* ("*De Placitis Hippocratis et Platonis*"), a work in which philosophy is pressed into the service of physiology, and where Galen seeks to establish that the brain alone is responsible for sensation and voluntary motion, he nevertheless states that all internal organs are said to be symmetrical. But here the context is that even single structures are symmetrical from the point of view of their constituent parts.[cc] A symmetrical relationship is fundamental in Galen's eyes in order to begin to comprehend the proper function of each constituent part of the body. The idea of the ventricles as symmetrical structures is thus a deliberate construct designed to allow better systematisation and comprehension of their complex anatomy. This is well brought out in the following from *Anatomical Procedures*:

> When you have cut away these bones (sc. of the top of the skull), then pay particular attention to that spot where the two meninges alone lie over the end of the posterior ventricle, since this is one of the most useful points for you in connection with the dissection which you intend to carry out in the living animal body. Pay attention also to the middle ventricle which the cupola or vault-like structure roofs over (sc. the *fornix*). This ventricle is situated in the upper regions of the head. Observe further, very thoroughly and carefully, the two anterior ventricles at the sides of the longitudinal (sc. *sagittal*) suture, and search out and remember well the position of each of the two as you see it. Then, when you have also seen quite clearly how the two optic nerves mount upwards towards the two anterior ventricles, and

z. Cf. Pigeuad, 1993, 92 n.18; Wilson, 1980, 202–3. For Aristotle, symmetry is commensurability. *Metaphysics*, 1004b.11, 1061b1. Cf. Lloyd, 1966, 342–5.

aa. *AA*, II. 579 K. Cf. *UP*, I.245, 266, 269–71; II.305. Cf. Scarborough, 1976, 173ff; Triolo, 1966, 113–4, 119.

bb. Cf. *Anatomical Procedures*, IX.1; 70–1.

cc. *PHP*, 594.30–596.4. The correct constitution of our bodies arises from the right proportion of the elements which constitute them, as stressed in *PHP*, 584.38–586.5.

> how this takes place at each side of them, preserve this also in your recollection. For in the course of this operation which I have described for you, you will have to investigate what takes place in the body of the living animal when one compresses or severs all these single structures.[dd]

Galen is asking for the ventricles to be considered in their entirety as three-dimensional entities, which, in their description and their relation to other structures in the brain, also possess a symmetric order. The above citation invites the dissector to reflect on both the internal anatomy of the ventricles and their physiological role. In the case of the anterior ventricles, their bilateral symmetry represents for Galen a useful way in which he can interpret their function as well as their importance compared to the other ventricles. Thus, when Galen discusses a case of head injury, which is interpreted in ventricular terms, the fact that the person in question survived is ascribed to damage of only one of the two, symmetrical, anterior ventricles. Were both to be effected, says Galen, the result would be fatal.[ee] The symmetry of the third ventricle might easily be elucidated from its midline position, but this ventricle's importance lies more in its symmetrical relationship with the fornix and corpus callosum, which will next be considered. The fourth ventricle's symmetry is demonstrated when it has been exposed by dissection. The symmetrical arrangement of the *calamus scriptorius*, in particular, invites one to reflect on the harmonious pattern of a well-ordered Nature.[ff]

III

The ventricles are not the only symmetrical structures for which an analogy with the plastic arts is sought. The *fornix* is compared to fundamental architectural forms. It, together with the *corpus callosum*, is one of several well-defined components which to Galen are of crucial importance for the protection and support of the ventricles.[gg] For Galen, all the deeper parts of the brain have a purpose and collectively represent a comprehensive functional entity on which the ventricular system depends for its identification, support

dd. IX.10; 14. Glosses in round brackets mine.

ee. Cf. *UP*, I.481–2.

ff. The description of the *calamus scriptorius* is given in *AA*, II. 731 K. Cf. *Anatomical Procedures*, IX.7; 2–3.

gg. Another deep structure, the *pineal body* (σῶμα κωνοειδές or κωνάριον), which, in spite of the importance it later assumed in some quarters as the locus of the soul, is for Galen a supporting structure for certain blood vessels in that area. It also acts as a landmark for the third ventricle. For its later elevation, the *locus classicus* is Descartes, *Les Passions de L'Ame*, 1649, § 31 and 32. Cf. Gaukroger, 1995, 272–4, 369–70, 401–2.

and integrity. The structure described by Galen as "in substance like a callus"[hh] lies between the two parts of the cerebrum in the sagittal plane and is known as the *corpus callosum*.[ii] It is only once the roof of the corpus callosum has been incised that it is seen to partly overlie—and support—each anterior ventricle. The next important structure for Galen has an even more critically important supportive function. It is described as a *vault* (καμάρα), an *arch* (ψαλίς), or an "arch-like body" (σῶμα ψαλιδοειδές). This is the *fornix*. If the role of the corpus callosum is to support the overlying brain and to anchor the *septum pellucidum*, providing it with the necessary tension to separate each anterior ventricle, then the task of the fornix is to give more immediate structural support to the anterior ventricles and the middle ventricle. The fornix lies below the corpus callosum, extending like a broad arch from the region of the interventricular foramen to roof over the middle ventricle.[jj] It is deliberately compared to the vault or arch of a roof, with the same load-bearing and protective function.[kk] Architects, according to Galen, are well aware of this.[ll] Although this reference to architects is a general one, Galen may well have been aware of the structural principles of the arch expressed in Vitruvius' *De Architectura*, although Galen nowhere uses the Latin expression for "arch" or "vault"—*fornix*—itself.[mm] Vitruvius, architect and military engineer in the early part of the reign of Augustus, was the author of a ten-volume work on architectural theory and practice. Not all his principles were acknowledged as such, but there can be no doubt of his influence in Imperial Rome as well as in the Renaissance.[nn] Leonardo's famous male figure, the *Vitruvian Man*,

---

hh. *AA*, II. 718 K.

ii. *AA*, II. 719 K. Clarke and O'Malley (1968, 577) correctly note that Galen's concept of the corpus callosum referred to "a more extensive structure than is implied today… It could include not only the midline connection of the white matter but also the white matter in the cerebral hemispheres that it connects."

jj. *AA*, II. 724 K.

kk. *AA*, II. 724–5 K. Cf. Hyrtl, 1880, §51. Willis (1681) decribes the "*Fornix* so called, or arched Vault, as it were a string or ligament, which arising before, where the brain is hanging to it, is carried to its hinder border, to which it is united as it were with two stretched out arms, and so it holds together the whole frame of the brain" (Tr. Pordage, 60).

ll. *UP*, I.484.

mm. Cf. *De Architectura*, VI.C.VIII.3. The Latin *fornix* is a direct translation of the Greek ψαλίς. Although Willis (cf. footnote kk) gave the term a more general currency, reinforcing both the anatomical accuracy and the appropriateness of its name, the fornix remains, in all probability, Galen's discovery. Cf. Rocca, 1998.

nn. "Vitruvius was very keen to lay down rules, and it must be emphasized that many of them were not universally acknowledged, even at the time and place of his writing. More important, however, are the principles behind the rules, and in that respect he is a faithful representative of Roman architecture" (Blagg, 1983, 52). Donato Bramante's *Tempietto*, Church of San Pietro in Montorio, Rome, 1502, is based on Vitruvian principles.

is based on Vitruvius' third volume, which is devoted to symmetry (III.I.2). For Galen, the curved shape of the fornix has the correct configuration to bear loads evenly, without harm to any part of the brain at the expense of another.[oo] Galen even states that some (unnamed) anatomists deny that the fornix exists, or else (more reasonably, one might interpolate here) they conflate it with the corpus callosum.[pp] It is likely that the fornix is Galen's discovery.[qq] The description of the fornix resembling the arch in a domed building vividly and accurately conveys its essential nature. Moreover, the appropriateness of its curved shape fulfils an important, didactic role. For Galen, the fornix describes part of the curvature of a sphere, and Galen, doubtless in common with Vitruvius, regarded the sphere as the best geometric form for any organ or structural component that has a load-bearing capacity.[rr] A sphere allows a load to be evenly distributed, and Galen extends this analogy to account for the shape of all vessels in the body—whether passages, canals, blood vessels or ventricles—that contain or receive any substance.[ss] For Galen, the ventricles—considered as a whole—can conceptually be regarded as "precisely sphere-like" (σφαιροειδὲς ἀκριβῶς).[tt] In this way, Galen deliberately invites the comparison of these anatomical structures not only with the aesthetic perfection of the sphere, but with the axiomatic properties of spherical geometry as seen in architecture. The deeper structures of the brain provide Galen with another example of how geometric demonstration may be extrapolated to an empirical methodology of dissection.[uu]

---

oo. *UP*, I.484.

pp. Cf. *AA*, II. 725 K. Whether this is also an allusion to Herophilus cannot be determined (see footnote qq). The description of the fornix in *AA* complements that of *UP*. In the latter description, however, Galen also uses the term καμάριον, the diminutive of καμάρα, a vaulted chamber, and a more general term, according to Galen, than ψαλιδοειδές (cf. *AA*, II. 725 K). The fornix has the same consistency as the corpus callosum, which might well account for some confusion regarding knowledge of its existence.

qq. Galen mentions the fornix together with Herophilus' contribution to the importance of the ventricles. However, there is no indication from Galen that Herophilus either cited or employed the fornix in a way similar to his own. Cf. *UP*, I.484 (see also: Von Staden, 1989, T138, pp. 315–6). There is no extant evidence that Herophilus himself employs the term καμάριον or otherwise cites the fornix. Galen fully credits Herophilus with discovering other parts of the brain: the *torcular Herophili* and *retiform plexus* are two such examples. Although this priority dispute cannot be completely resolved, it would seem unusual for Galen to appropriate the anatomy and function of the fornix without citing Herophilus as its discoverer, if that were indeed the case. See Rocca, 2003, 96–103.

rr. *UP*, I.485.

ss. *UP*, I.485.

tt. *UP*, I.486.

uu. On this topic see: Lloyd, 1987, 192–4, 231ff; *idem.*, 1996.

IV

For Galen, as the dural foldings are seen in the living animal to elevate the underlying brain substance (thereby maintaining its integrity), so too the fornix and corpus callosum maintain the structural integrity of the anterior and middle ventricles.[vv] If this support fails for any reason, their physiological role is extinguished, as a building ceases to function if its roof collapses. This structural integrity is necessarily destroyed in a dissection.[ww] In Galen's teleological *Weltbild*, no structural component of the body is without purpose. Galen's anatomical demonstrations are, in part, deliberately designed to draw attention to nature's Grand Design, to highlight an entity which, as Galen so often famously states, not only "does nothing in vain", but performs it *skilfully* (τεχνικῶς).[xx] Galen's own proficiency in elucidating the architecture of the ventricles of the brain, whilst obviously not on the same order of magnitude as that of Nature, is framed from a similar perspective and is designed to be equally as incontrovertible and to elicit as great a sense of wonder as the contemplation of a well-executed sculpture or a building. In his discussion of the parts of the brain, Galen informs his audience that:

> . . . those who perform a dissection badly not only make such mistakes in anatomy itself, but introduce those mistakes into their physiological explanations. For it is inevitable that, just as the uses of those things properly observed in anatomy provoke amazement, so too the account of the use of things mis-observed is impossible.[yy]

Galen here implicitly stresses that his own anatomical discourse is correct precisely because his observations have been made in an appropriate, and, one might say, artful way. An anatomy performed in the correct manner must evoke a sense of wonder similar to that experienced in contemplating a great work of sculpture or of architecture. Inviting us to consider what for him is the most important part of the brain, Galen—a technically proficient anatomist of the first water—exploits the artistic and philosophical nuances of symmetry to excellent effect. He reminds us that, on occasion, the plastic arts can bridge the gap between scientific conceptualisation and achievement.

---

vv. *AA*, II. 725–6 K. Daremberg (1841, 27) finds it difficult to reconcile the description of the role of the fornix description here with that in *UP* I. 485f. But Daremberg perhaps has failed to fully appreciate the analogous role Galen gives here to the dural foldings.

ww. *AA*, II. 726–7 K.

xx. *UP*, II. 438.

yy. *AA*, II. 727–8 K.

Bibliography

M.C. Beardsley, *Aesthetics from Classical Greece to the Present* (University of Alabama Press, 1966).

T. Blagg, Architecture. In: Henig (ed.) (1983), pp. 26–65.

A.H. Borbein, Polykleitos, *Yale Classical Studies* **30**, 66–90 (1996).

E. Clarke and C.D. O'Malley, *The Human Brain and Spinal Cord* (California, 1968).

L.I. Conrad, M. Neve, V. Nutton, R. Porter and A. Wear (eds.) *The Western Medical Tradition* (Cambridge, 1995).

R.M. Cook, *Greek Art: Its Development, Character and Influence* (Pelican, 1976), pp. 125–6.

C. Daremberg, *Exposition des Connaissances de Galien sur L'Anatomie, La Physiologie et La Pathologie, du Système Nerveux* (Paris, 1841).

W.L.H. Duckworth, M.C. Lyons and B. Towers, *Galen: On Anatomical Procedures, The Later Books* (Cambridge, 1962).

W. Feindel (ed.), *The Anatomy of the Brain and the Description and Use of the Nerves in the Remaining Medical Works of That Famous and Renowned Physician Dr. Thomas Willis*, Englished in 1681 by Samuel Pordage, Tercentenary Edition, 1664–1964, two volumes (McGill University Press, 1965).

T.C. Fitzgerald, Anatomy of cerebral ventricles of domestic animals, *Vet. Med.* **56**, (1961), pp. 38–45.

M. Frede and G. Striker (eds.), *Rationality in Greek Thought* (Clarendon, Oxford, 1996).

S. Gaukroger, *Descartes: An Intellectual Biography* (Oxford, 1995).

D. Gourevitch, *L'esthetique Médicale de Galien, Les Études Classiques*, LV (1987), pp. 267–89.

M. Henig (ed.), *A Handbook of Roman Art* (Phaidon, 1983).

J. Hyrtl, *Onomatologia Anatomica* (1880). Reprinted, George Olms, Hildesheim, 1970.

E.L. Kier, The cerebral ventricles: a phylogenetic and ontogenetic study. In: Newton and Potts (eds.) (1977), pp. 2787–914.

A.S. King, *Physiological and Clinical Anatomy of the Domestic Mammals, Vol. I: Central Nervous System* (Oxford, 1987).

J. Kollesch and D. Nickel (eds.), *Galen und das hellenistische Erbe*. Verhandlungen des IV. Internationalen Galen-Symposiums, Sudhoffs Archiv Beihefte 32, Franz Steiner Verlag, Stuttgart, 1993.

P. De Lacy, *De Placitis Hippocratis et Platonis*, CMG V, 4, 1, 2. Parts 1–3 (Berlin, 1978, 1980, 1984).

R.J. Last and D.H. Tompsett, Casts of the cerebral ventricles, *Br. J. Surg.* **40**, 525–43 (1953).

G.E.R. Lloyd, *Polarity and Analogy. Two Types of Argumentation in Early Greek Thought* (Cambridge, 1966); *The Revolutions of Wisdom: Studies in the Claims *and Practice of Ancient Greek Science* (University of California Press, 1987); Theories and practices of demonstration in Galen, in: Frede and Striker (eds.) (Oxford, 1996), pp. 255–77.

M.T. May, *Galen: On the Usefulness of the Parts of the Body,* 2 vols. (Cornell University Press, 1968).

P. Moraux, *Galien De Pergame. Souvenirs d'un médecin* (Les Belles Lettres, Paris, 1985).

T.H. Newton and D.G. Potts (eds.), *Radiology of the Skull and Brain. Volume III: Anatomy and Pathology* (C.V. Mosby, St. Louis, 1977).

V. Nutton, Medicine in the Greek world, 800–50 BC, in: Conrad, Neve, Nutton, Porter and Wear (eds.) (1995), pp. 11–38; Roman medicine, 250 BC to AD 200, in: Conrad, Neve, Nutton, Porter and Wear (eds.) (1995b), pp. 39–70.

C.D. O'Malley and J.B. Saunders, de C.M., *Leonardo da Vinci on the Human Body* (Henry Schumann, New York, 1952).

J. Pigeaud, *Les problèmes de la création chez Galien.* In: Kollesch and Nickel (eds.) (1993), pp. 87–103.

J.J. Pollitt, *Art and Experience in Classical Greece* (Cambridge, 1972); *The Art of Ancient Greece: Sources and Documents* (Cambridge, 1990).

F.L.N. Poynter (ed.), *The History and Philosophy of Knowledge of the Brain and Its Function* (Blackwell, Oxford, 1958).

J. Rocca, Galen and the ventricular system, *J. Hist. Neurosci.* **6**(3), 227–39 (1997); A Note on the term Fornix, *J. Hist. Neurosci.* 7(3), 243 (1998); *Galen and the Brain: Anatomical Knowledge and Physiological Speculation in the Second Century AD,* forthcoming.

J. Scarborough, Galen's investigations of the kidney, *Clio Medica* **11**, 171–7 (1976).

J.A. Sharp, Alexander Monro Secundus and the interventricular foramen, *Med. Hist.* **5**, 83–9 (1961).

R.E. Siegel, *Galen's System of Physiology and Medicine: An Analysis of His Doctrines and Observations on Bloodflow, Respiration, Humors and Internal Disease* (S. Karger, Basel, 1968).

M. Simon, *Sieben Bücher Anatomie des Galen,* 2 vols. (Leipzig, 1906).

P.N. Singer, *Galen: Selected Works* (The World's Classics, Oxford, 1997).

S. Sisson and J.D. Grossman, *The Anatomy of the Domestic Animals,* 5th edition, two vols. (W.B. Saunders, Philadelphia, 1975).

H. Von Staden, *Herophilus: The Art of Medicine in Early Alexandria* (Cambridge University Press, 1989).

V. Triolo, An Interpretative analysis of Galenic renal physiology, *Clio Medica* **1**, 113–28 (1966).

D.H.M. Woollam, Concepts of the brain and its functions in classical antiquity. In: Poynter (ed.) (1958), pp. 5–18.

maternal transmission of congenital cases DM1. However, the intergenerational differences of CTG repeats have been measured by comparing progenitor allele sizes in the blood DNA of parent and child. Our data correlated with the data of other investigators in that most transmissions result in a true germline increase in allele size. However, the actual germline contractions are relatively rare, at least during passage through the male germline (Monckton *et al.*, 1995). Some investigators suggested that expanded alleles are limited in size to less than 1000 repeats in the sperm of the affected DM1 males (Jansen *et al.*, 1994). Out of 20 parent–child pairs, we found contraction in size of the CTG repeats only in one father–child pair. This contraction may be a true germline reduction, but it may actually represent true germline expansions masked by age-dependent somatic expansion. As reported previously, the number of CTG repeats was related with muscular disability and intelligence quotient ($P < 0.05$). However, the presence and severity of cardiac abnormalities, respiratory insufficiency, cataracts, gastrointestinal and endocrinological disturbances was not related to the number of CTG repeats (Rakocevic-Stojanovic *et al.*, 2000, 2003). This suggests that pathogenetic mechanisms of DM1 may differ in various tissues.

References

Ashizawa T, Dubel JR, Harati Y (1993). Somatic instability of CTG repeat in myotonic dystrophy. *Neurology* **143:**2674–2678.

Brook JD, McCurrach ME, Harley HG *et al.* (1992). Molecular basis of myotonic dystrophy: expansion of a trinucleotide (CTG) repeat at the 3′end of a transcript encoding a protein kinase family member. *Cell* **68:**799–808.

Harley HG, Brook JD, Rundle SA, Crow S. *et al.* (1992). Expansion of an unstable DNA region and phenotypic variation in myotonic dystrophy. *Nature* **355:**545–546.

Jansen G, Willems P, Coerwinkel M, Nillesen W, Smeets H. *et al.* (1994). Gonosomal mosaicism in myotonic dystrophy patients: involvement of mitotic events in (CTG)n variation and selection against extreme expansion in sperm. *Am J Hum Genet* **54:**575–585.

Martorell L, Monckton DG, Gamez J, Beiget M (2000). Complex patterns of male germline instability and somatic mosaicism in myotonic dystrophy type 1. *Eur J Hum Genet* **8:**423–430.

Monckton GD, Wong LJ, Ashizawa T, Caskey T (1995). Somatic mosaicism, germline expansions, germline reversions and intergenerational reductions in myotonic dystrophy males: small pool PCR analyses. *Hum Mol Genet* **4:**1–8.

O'Hoy KL, Tsilfidis C, Mahadevan MS, Neville CE *et al.* (1993). Reduction in size of the myotonic dystrophy trinucleotide repeat mutation during transmission. *Science* **259:**809–812.

Rakocevic-Stojanovic V, Grujic M, Savic D, Romac S, Lavrnic D *et al.* (2000). Myotonic dystrophy and cardiac disorders. *Panminerva Med* **42:**257–261.

Rakocevic-Stojanovic V, Savic D, Lavrnic D, Vujic A, Pavlovic S *et al.* (2003). Genotype-phenotype correlation in myotonic dystrophy type 1. *Eur J Neurol* **10:**40.

Chapter 5

Leonardo da Vinci's Mechanical Art and the Origin of Modern Neurology

David A. Steinberg

This chapter identifies a commonality in the thought processes of Leonardo da Vinci in his theory of machines, as illustrated in his mechanical art, and John Hughlings Jackson in the formation of a science of neurology. Though there is no evidence of any influence of one on the other, the common features suggest a general historiographic principle that may be applicable to the history of any science.

Introduction

In this chapter, I will discuss a similarity between Leonardo da Vinci's mechanical art and John Hughlings Jackson's idea of brain function that is the foundation of modern clinical neurology. There is no evidence of any direct influence of Leonardo on Hughlings Jackson, but this commonality is a curiosity in its own right, and also sheds light on general characteristics of a productive science.

I want to emphasize that though I will briefly describe Leonardo's views of the brain and mind for completeness, the topic of this chapter is not a comparison of the neurologies of Leonardo da Vinci and John Hughlings Jackson. I will explore a similarity in thought processes that, for Leonardo, resulted in a complete theory of mechanical devices, and that, for Hughlings Jackson, resulted in a scientific theory of neurology.

Leonardo da Vinci and His Mechanical Art

Leonardo da Vinci needs little, if any, introduction. As one of humanity's transcendent geniuses, his accomplishments in art, science, and engineering are recognized by all. Nevertheless, the details of his life are worth briefly reviewing.

Leonardo was born on April 15, 1452 in the Italian village of Vinci, about 20 miles from Florence. He was the illegitimate son of Ser Piero d'Antonio and a peasant woman named Caterina from Anchiano, a nearby village.[a] Though little is known of Leonardo's early life, he probably had a rudimentary formal education consisting of reading, writing, and basic mathematics. Later in his life he regretted the lack of additional education as he struggled with Latin and geometry. There is a story, of uncertain authenticity, explaining why Ser Piero agreed to let him study painting—a vocation far below the social station of his family's traditional employment as notaries. According to this story, a local peasant brought Ser Piero a wooden shield to take to Florence for decoration. Instead, he gave it to his son, who created a design consisting of a marvelous and fearsome mythic creature. Ser Piero bought another shield for the peasant and sold Leonardo's for a large sum. This supposedly convinced him of Leonardo's talent and earning potential, and as a consequence he apprenticed Leonardo to the studio of the noted Florentine artist Andrea del Verrocchio.[b]

Verrocchio's workshop was one of several in Florence competing for large public projects and commissions from wealthy individuals. A workshop's final products were collaborative efforts, yet even in the company of such great artists as Verrocchio, Botticelli, and Lorenzo di Credi, Leonardo's contributions can often be identified by their quality and grasp of subtle physical principles of optics and engineering.

Leonardo's earliest-known work is a pen-and-ink drawing of the Arno valley dated August 5, 1473. A significant event for historians of Leonardo's life, if not for Leonardo himself, occurred in 1476, when the entire staff at Verrocchio's workshop was anonymously accused of sodomy. All charges were dismissed, but in conjunction with Leonardo's solitary nature, this incident may have contributed to the prevalent notion of his homosexuality. From 1491 until 1505 Leonardo created the various documents that are collected in what is now known as the *Codex Madrid*. This codex contains references to *Elementi macchinali*, or "elements of machines," which must therefore have been written earlier. At the end of this period, i.e. 1504–05, Leonardo painted the portrait of Mona Lisa del Giocondo.

---

a. There are numerous sources for biographical information on Leonardo da Vinci, e.g. Santi (1990).

b. This story is related in Reti (1974), p. 12.

In 1517 Leonardo moved to Amboise in France with a commission from Francis I to design a palace for the Queen Mother. Leonardo da Vinci received the full sacraments of the Church and died on May 2, 1519 at the age of 67 years. He was buried at Amboise, but during later religious wars his grave was desecrated and his bones were lost.

Though over 5000 folio pages of Leonardo da Vinci's notebooks are known, most estimates suggest that this represents only 20–35% of his actual written work.[c] In addition to the known manuscripts, there is a class of Leonardo's investigations that have survived only as references in extant codices. One such manuscript is a four-volume work known as *Elementi macchinali*, referred to earlier.[d] In these four volumes, Leonardo lists a universal directory of components from which all mechanical devices can be constructed. In *Codex Madrid I*, which was lost until 1967,[e] Leonardo states that "[o]nce the instrument is created, its operational requirements shape the form of its members. They may be of infinite variety but will still be subject to the rules of the four volumes."[f]

Prior to the discovery of the *Codex Madrid*, the theory of elemental construction of machines was thought to originate with the work of early 19th century French scholars from the École Polytechnique. In the late 19th century, Franz Reuleaux enumerated 22 constructive elements of machines.[g] Of these, all but one are explicitly presented in Leonardo's mechanical drawings. The one element that is missing is the rivet, which was well known to Leonardo but was excluded because he chose to examine the machines "without their armatures or other structures that might hinder the view of those who will study them."[h]

The small set of elements of all mechanical devices has been described in biological analogy as the "organs" of machines.[i] A machine for any particular task is constructed out of the apposite combination of these organs. The operation of any organ of a machine is invariant and is regulated by the input and output connections. Thus, for example, the organs that connect to the two ends of a rope of a simple pulley, regulate its action. If one considers

---

c. These figures are found in Reti (1968), p. 22.

d. This four-volume work is referred to in several of Leonardo's extant writings. It is possible that some of the original is present in the *Codex Madrid*, but definitely not all of it. See Reti (1974), p. 275.

e. Publication of an analysis of the *Codex Madrid* can be found in Reti (1968), p. 10.

f. This quotation is found in *Codex Madrid I*, folio 96V, and reproduced in Reti (1974), p. 275.

g. Elaboration of the elemental concept of machines is in Reuleaux (1963), pp. 437 and 580.

h. In Galluzzi (1996), p. 192.

i. This analogy is expanded in Galluzzi (1996), p. 192.

a whole machine to consist of a collection of subunits that are each harnessed to perform some particular function, then the output of each subunit is regulated by every subunit to which it is connected. In this manner, any organ of a machine is controlled by all organs to which it is harnessed.

In summary, according to Leonardo, every machine is composed of a particular selection of elemental machines that perform a single and invariant function. In the construction of a machine, the appropriate elements are combined, and the output of each one is regulated, or controlled, by the other elements to which it is attached.

I again would like to emphasize that it is Leonardo's views of machines that I will be comparing to modern neurology. However, because of the general interest, I will briefly review his ideas of neurophysiology and neuroanatomy. Though Leonardo extended his axiomatic and mechanical ideas about machines to nature as a whole, he did not completely do so concerning the brain and mind. Nonetheless, his theory of neurophysiology is predictably sophisticated.

Leonardo located the soul in the third ventricle of the brain on the basis of geometric arguments and believed that it was the nexus of all sensory and motor function.[j] He was careful to point out that, though the soul resided in the third ventricle, it did not occupy any physical space. He believed that sensory and motor functions were the result of the action of four "powers"—movement, weight, force, and percussion—and he saw the soul as the source that animates these powers. The soul, as this animating force, was transmitted through what Leonardo called the "tree of nerves." A rigor and perspicacity that is remarkable informed even his philosophical musings about the nature of the soul and of man. "The soul," he said, "finding itself enclosed in the human body is ever longing to return to its author. And you must know that this same longing is that quintessence which is inseparable from nature; and that man is a model of the world."[k] This sophisticated perspective is much closer to Aristotle or some modern scientific views than to Renaissance Christianity and is manifestly heretical. However, it appears that Leonardo was spared the consequences of his ideas by the simple fact that no one in a position to object was aware of, or understood, them.

---

j. The following summary of Leonardo's neuroanatomy and neurophysiology is from Todd (1983).

k. This quote is from the foreword to Todd (1983), p. 13, by Kenneth Keele.

John Hughlings Jackson and Scientific Neurology

John Hughlings Jackson was born on April 4, 1835 in the village of Green Hammerton in Yorkshire. His mother and father died during his early life, and his sole formal education was at a boarding school. Hughlings Jackson was then apprenticed to William Anderson at the York Hospital Medical School. Here, one of his teachers was Thomas Laycock, who later became Professor of Medicine at Edinburgh. Laycock had a profound influence on Hughlings Jackson's developing ideas concerning the nature of the brain in health and disease. In 1855, he was a student at St. Bartholomew's Hospital in London, attending the lectures of Sir James Paget. He received the diplomas of M.R.C.S and L.S.A. in 1856 and took the position of House Surgeon at the York Dispensary shortly thereafter. After two years, Hughlings Jackson decided to return to London. This move was at least partially influenced by Sir Jonathan Hutchinson, who had preceded Hughlings Jackson as a student at the York School and was at that time working in London as a medical journalist and physician at the London Hospital. In London, Hughlings Jackson took the degree of M.D. (St. Andrews) in 1860 and M.R.C.P. (London) in 1861. He was appointed Assistant Physician to the National Hospital for the Paralyzed and Epileptic in 1862, and promoted to Physician in 1867. He retained this position until 1906, when he was appointed Consulting Physician. He also held appointments at the London Hospital from 1863 until 1894, when he retired. He was elected the first president of the London Neurological Society in 1885 and was president at one time or another of every medical society of which he was an active member. Hughlings Jackson died in his home on Manchester Square in London on October 7, 1911.[1]

Hughlings Jackson's greatest accomplishment is the creation of a scientific neurology. By this I mean a theoretical framework of reproducible and predictive neurological diagnosis based solely on observable symptoms. There are three aspects of Hughlings Jackson's theory that I will highlight. These three elements are necessary for his theory of neurology but are not quite sufficient. First, the brain is a sensorimotor machine. That is, the entire operation of the nervous system can be explained in terms of observable sensorimotor events. Second, the nervous system is composed of anatomically localized centers, and each center performs a single function. Finally, nervous system centers

---

1. This summary of the life of Hughlings Jackson is taken from his obituary in the *British Medical Journal.*

are organized hierarchically, with higher centers inhibiting the action of lower centers.

The realization that the entire nervous system, including the most complex functions of the brain, is a manifestation of the sensorimotor reflex was the culmination of an evolving idea known as the law of reflex action. This law states that sensation and movement are anatomically separate, connected at each spinal segment and to segments above and below on the neuraxis.[m] In 1845, Thomas Laycock extended the law of reflex action to the cerebral cortex and, thereby, to the entire nervous system.[n] However, Laycock did not exclude the possibility that metaphysical functions may coexist with sensorimotor physiology within the brain. In particular, he did not exclude the soul as a possible resident of the neocortex. Hughlings Jackson realized that the key to a science of neurology is a consideration of purely sensorimotor physiology. He thus completed the evolution of the law of reflex action by claiming that not only is the nervous system a sensorimotor machine, but it is exclusively so.[o]

Modern diagnostic neurology depends on the reliable localization of observable symptoms to specific lesions in the central nervous system. The implicit assumption underlying this diagnostic process is that there are separate organs within the nervous system, each with a particular function and each occupying a delineated anatomic region. However, each aspect of this assumption is ambiguous. The definition of a function, the anatomic delineation of an organ, and the nature of a symptom reveal profound difficulties when analyzed in detail. Nonetheless, the efficacy of this diagnostic principle is obvious to any clinician who takes the time to consider it.

The origin of the belief that separate functions of the brain are localized within the central nervous system can first be found in the discredited pseudoscience of phrenology. The idea that nebulous functions such as "aptness to receive an education" or "friendly attachment or fidelity" could be consistently reflected in calvarial irregularities now seems absurd. But the novel concept that particular functions of the mind or brain could be localized to particular regions of neuroanatomy was essential for the creation of a science of neurology.[p]

---

m. This topic is discussed in detail in York and Steinberg (1994), p. 4.

n. Laycock (1845) describes reflex action and the cortex.

o. Hughlings Jackson (1958), p. 15.

p. The phrenological functions are widely variable in their number and description. The two cited above are from an English translation of Gall's original list of 27 and can be found in van Wyhe (2001).

The third principle of Hughlings Jackson's neurology is that the anatomically delineated sensorimotor centers of the nervous system are hierarchical in organization. He identified four key characteristics of these centers:

> ...[T]here is from lowest to highest centers: (1) increasing complexity (differentiation), representation of a greater number of different movements; (2) increasing definiteness (specialization), representation of movements for more particular duties; (3) increasing integration, representation of movements of wider ranges of the body in each part of the centres; (4) the higher the centres the more numerous the interconnections of their units (cooperation).[q]

An origin of these principles can be traced to *Naturphilosphie*, the ideas of Karl von Baer, and Herbert Spencer's application of evolution to the nervous system.[r] However, Hughlings Jackson's interpretation of these ideas derived from his unique perspective as a careful physician who understood the clinical symptoms of neurology. He found that viewing the nervous system as discrete evolutionary levels best fit his observations in the clinic.

Any evolutionary explanation must include a process or force of evolution. In the Darwinian sense this is natural selection. Because Hughlings Jackson believed the nervous system to be completely sensorimotor, a natural assumption was that the process of nervous system evolution was representation of the body. Thus, the lowest level represents the body directly, the next level re-represents the body, and the highest level re-re-represents it. The nature of this ordinal representation of the body implies that higher levels control, or inhibit, lower levels.[s]

Discussion

It is interesting to speculate on the essential characteristics of science, though any consensus would be difficult to obtain. However, the scientific thinking of Leonardo da Vinci in mechanical theory, as expressed in his mechanical art, and John Hughlings Jackson's formation of a science of neurology do provide evidence for a generally productive approach to the natural world. This similarity occurs in three areas. First, both systems reduce the scope of a particular science to observable events. In the case of Leonardo this is tautological, since his investigation is limited to physical machines. Hughlings Jackson, on the

q. Hughlings Jackson (1958), p. 80.
r. See York and Steinberg (1994), p. 6.
s. See, e.g., Steinberg and York (1994).

other hand, had to explicitly limit the purview of neurology to observable events of sensation and movement, a significant change from previous analyses. Second, both Leonardo and Hughlings Jackson explicitly reduced a wide range of observed output behavior to the operation of a relatively small set of fundamental organs, each of which is endowed with a single simple function. For Leonardo, this significantly simplified the design of machines by combining the "organs" necessary for the particular task at hand. Hughlings Jackson developed a reproducible and predictive cerebral localization by recognizing that the nervous system was organized as a collection of functional units localized consistently within the nervous system. Finally, both scientists recognized that there is a hierarchical ordering of elements such that more deeply nested organs are controlled by those to which their output is harnessed.

Though it is clear that the discoveries of Leonardo and Hughlings Jackson were independent, their contraposition does support the historiographic notion that similar ideas in science tend to recur at various times and in different eras. To indicate that this is not a completely isolated occurrence, I would like to briefly, and without detail, identify the same guiding principles in what is probably the 20th century's archetypal science, quantum mechanics.

Werner Heisenberg explicitly stated, in his 1925 formulation of quantum mechanics, that his conceptual breakthrough was to realize that a physical theory could contain only variables pertaining to observable events.[t] This corresponds exactly to the implicit recognition by Leonardo da Vinci and the explicit one of Hughlings Jackson. All analytic science, including quantum mechanics, is an attempt at unification and simplification and, as such, has as its goal the reduction of complex descriptions to the interaction of a small number of fundamental elements. Again, this is explicitly the case in Leonardo's mechanical art and Hughlings Jackson's science of neurology. Finally, the hierarchical organization in quantum mechanics takes the form of a reduction in the degrees of freedom in an interacting system, conceptually identical to the hierarchical arrangement in Leonardo's machines and Hughlings Jackson's nervous system.

In conclusion, the correspondence of scientific analyses by Leonardo da Vinci and John Hughlings Jackson is fortuitous, in the sense that no direct influence is present. Even as general principles of scientific discovery, it is possible that the three identified similarities are so general that they are of little prospective utility in ordering scientific hypotheses and experimentation.

---

t. This insight of Heisenberg is well documented and can be found in his own words in Heisenberg (1989), pp. 26, 113.

On the other hand, the common principles of scientific inquiry identified by Hughlings Jackson and Leonardo da Vinci suggest some validity for the historiographic principle that aspects of scientific thinking are continuous through different eras and contexts.

References

Editors; Obituary, *Br. Med. J.* **2**, 950 (1911).

Galluzzi, P., *Renaissance Engineers from Brunelleschi to Leonardo da Vinci* (Florence, Instituto Museo della Scienza, 1996).

Heisenberg, W., *Encounters with Einstein and Other Essays on People, Places and Particles* (Princeton University Press, 1989).

Hughlings Jackson, J., *Selected Writings of John Hughlings Jackson*, ed. J. Taylor (Basic Books, New York, 1958).

Laycock, T., On the reflex function of the brain, *British and Foreign Medical Review* **19**, 298–310 (1845).

Reuleaux, F., *The Kinematics of Machinery* (Dover, New York, 1963).

Reti, L., The two unpublished manuscripts of Leonardo da Vinci in the Biblioteca Nacional od Madrid—I, *The Burlington Magazine* **110**, 10–22 (1968).

Reti, L., *The Unknown Leonardo* (McGraw-Hill, San Francisco, 1974).

Santi, B., *Leonardo da Vinci* (Riverside, New York, 1990).

Steinberg, D.A. and York, G.K., Hughlings Jackson, concomitance and mental evolution, *J. Hist. Neurosci.* **3**, 169–176 (1994).

Todd, E., *The Neuroanatomy of Leonardo da Vinci* (Capra, Santa Barbara, 1983).

van Wyhe, J., The history of phrenology on the Web (http://www.jmvanwyhe.freeserve.co.uk, 2001).

York, G.K. and Steinberg, D.A., Hughlings Jackson's theory of cerebral localization. *J. Hist. Neurosci.* **3**, 1–16 (1994).

Chapter 6

The Art of Sir Charles Bell[1]

Christopher Gardner-Thorpe[2]

There's no art to find the mind's construction in the face.[3]

The name of Charles Bell (1774–1842) is commemorated in the long thoracic or external respiratory nerve, in a variety of lower motor neurone facial palsy, and in Bell's sign, where the eyeball rolls upwards on attempted closure of the eye. Well known too is his description of the difference between the fifth and seventh cranial nerves, and between the anterior and posterior roots of the spinal cord, which is named Bell's law. The first description of a patient with muscular dystrophy has also been attributed to Charles Bell.

Charles Bell and His Family

Charles Bell's father was the Reverend William Bell (1704–1779), who was ordained into the Episcopal Church of Scotland. He had come with his father, John Bell (1676–1708), to the Counties bordering the River Forth. His second wife was Margaret Morice, daughter of Bishop White, later Primus of Scotland, who was a good artist. John Bell preached the Sermon in Edinburgh Cathedral on the death of William III and is buried in an ornate tomb at Gladsmuir Church. He was the son of Sir John Bell of Hamilton (1640–?), who was the son of Patrick Bell, who was the son of John Bell (1580–1646), who was the son of James Bell of Kirkconnel and Blackett House. William and Margaret had four sons (some records suggest six). Their oldest son, Robert (1757–1816), became Professor of Conveyancing to *The Society of Writers to The Signet*. George (1759–1759) was the second and William (1763–1763) the third. Their fourth son, John (1763–1820), was the outstanding surgeon in Edinburgh at the close of the 18th century and trained Charles in anatomy and surgery. James (1767–1830) was the fifth. George Joseph (1770–1843) was the sixth and he held the Chair of Scots Law in Edinburgh University.

On 8 November 1774 Charles, the youngest, was born in Fountainbridge, a straggling suburb of Edinburgh.[4] In 1778 the family moved into Edinburgh due to the infirmity of Charles' father, who had died about 1779, when Charles was five years old. To this has been attributed Charles' tendency to depression and lack of self-confidence, and thus he leaned upon George for advice in many areas. Charles' mother struggled to look after the family. The family moved to the upper part of a house in George Street, a road 115 feet wide. Charles attended Edinburgh High School (from 1784 to 1788), where Walter Scott was a contemporary.

As a boy Charles assisted his brother John, 11 years older, in his extra-mural school and attended lectures in the university. He listened to Dugale Stewart, the philosopher whose influence was to be seen later in Bell's *Treatise on the Hand* and in his commentary on Paley's *Natural Theology*. Charles was taught to paint by his mother and by David Allan (1744–1796), whose self-portrait hangs in the National Gallery of Scotland and who is well known for his portrait of Robert Burns.[5] David Allan, the Scottish Hogarth, was a kind and facetious old gentleman. Allan gave Bell drawings to copy and called him "Brother Brush". Artists of this time included Reynolds, Gainsborough, Constable, Zoffany, Turner, Corot, Opie, Millais, Fragonard, Goya, Canaletto, Guardi, Landseer and others. Later Mrs Head, wife of the neurologist Henry Head, was to discuss some of these artists.[6,7]

Medical Education in Edinburgh

John Monro, a surgeon in the army of William of Orange, wished that a medical school existed in Edinburgh, as at Leyden, where he had studied. His enthusiasm led to the Edinburgh Medical School. The Edinburgh Faculty of Medicine was established in 1726. His son, Alexander Monro *Primus*, was the first of three generations of Alexander Monro[8–10] who held the Chair of Medicine and Anatomy in Edinburgh, in total for 126 years. They were Alexander Monro *Primus* (1697–1767), Alexander Monro *Secundus* (1733–1817) and Alexander Monro *Tertius* (1773–1859).

Bell attended lectures of Monro *Secundus*, who, in turn, had attended the lectures of William Hunter (1718–1783) in London and then studied at Leyden. One of his works, *Observations on the Structure and Functions of the Nervous System Illustrated with Tables*, was published in Edinburgh in 1783.[11] He described the communications between the lateral ventricles and the third ventricle—the Foramina of Monro. He also wrote *Of the Termination of the Nerves in the Muscular Organs; and Whether Muscles Possess a Vis Insita Different from the Vis Nervea*. Monro believed that all the spinal nerves passing through ganglia were motor nerves. He commented:

> "When a person examines an object brought near to the eye, the pupil is contracted, although the object be of a black colour, so as not to affect the eye by an increase of light. With this observation let us connect another, to wit, that, when a small printed book is brought so near the eye, that its letters begin to seem confused and intermixed, if we interpose a card, with a very small hole in it, the letters are again seen distinctly."

Monro *Primus* and Monro *Secundus* were not practising surgeons and John Bell felt that the needs of surgeons were not met by the teaching of classical anatomy. John introduced the subject of surgical anatomy.[12] In 1793 he published *The Anatomy and Physiology of the Human Body*, which by 1829 became a two-author volume by John and Charles Bell in three volumes.[13] Charles wrote[14]:

> "And here we are led to observe a fact of great consequence to the Pathologist; the muscles are not equally under the influence of the sensorium; some are prompt and exact, under the guidance of the will, whilst over others we have no command at all; and there are not a few which we command indirectly, that is, we put a certain class of muscles into operation, which are followed by the combination of others, over which we have no direct power."

In 1797 John published *The Anatomy of the Human Body* in four volumes,[15] which was described as "the first great textbook contributed by the British school to modern anatomy".[16]

In 1798 John looked after casualties from the Battle of Camperdown, fought off the south-east coast of Scotland between Napoleon's Dutch fleet and the English Navy. John Bell ceased teaching anatomy in 1799 and for 13 years became the leading surgeon in Edinburgh. He is remembered for the Muscles of Bell—slight thickenings, not always present, in the trigonal muscle sheet passing between the openings of the ureters and the internal urethral orifice.

Regarded as a founder of surgical anatomy, John published in 1801–1808 *The Principles of Surgery* in three volumes.[17] Like Charles, his illustrations were his own work and of a high standard. He was said to be the first to ligate the gluteal, common carotid and internal iliac arteries.

Charles Bell's Early Career in Surgery

At around that time other Bells were in medicine in Edinburgh who do not seem related to Charles. They include Benjamin Bell (1749–1806), who was President of the Physico-Chemical Society of Edinburgh (1819–1822) and a founder member of the Edinburgh Medico-Chirurgical Society, set up in May 1821. He wrote *A Treatise on the Diseases of the Bone*,[18] *A System of Surgery*, an important textbook in six volumes, and treatises on ulcers and on gonorrhoea. Joseph Bell, FRCS, FRCS Ed (1837–1911), worked at the Royal Infirmary in Edinburgh. He is depicted in a painting of 1888 in the Royal College of Surgeons of Edinburgh, where he was President. He emphasized that observation was an all-important quality in a doctor and he is recognized as the model for Sherlock Holmes.[19,20] Bell wrote on "Paraffin epithelioma of the scrotum"[21] and showed shale oil to be a cause of skin cancer.

From 1798 to 1799, and while still a student, Charles Bell embarked upon his first independent venture as an author and published *A System of Dissections*.[22] He described his injection methods in the preparation of specimens that may still be seen in the Museum of The Royal College of Surgeons of Edinburgh. On 1 August 1799 Charles was admitted as a Member of the College and operated in the Edinburgh Infirmary. However, both John and Charles were excluded from the Infirmary from 1800. Charles also contributed the description of the nervous system to John's *Anatomy of the Human Body*. By the age of 25 Bell was an authority on anatomy. The anatomical work of Charles Bell and his brother John became the most important in the British Isles during the early part of the 19th century.

In 1801 and 1802 Charles illustrated and published *Engravings of the Arteries, of the Nerves and of the Brain*. Later this was published in sections, such as the third edition of *Engravings of the Arteries; Illustrating the Second Volume of the Anatomy of the Human Body, and Serving as an Introduction to the Surgery of the Arteries*, in 1811.[23]

In Edinburgh John was unpopular and there was jealousy of Charles. The Faculty did not accept Charles' offer of his Museum of Anatomy and 100 guineas on the basis that he should attend hospital autopsies and make drawings of every remarkable autopsy case. Charles Bell left Edinburgh on 23 November 1804 and went to London.

London (1804–1836)

On arrival in London, Bell's carriage delivered him to the London Coffee House on Ludgate Hill. London was not all to his liking. Chimney boys still cleaned the flue, press gangs were around the neighbourhoods, and the Gas Light and Coke Company was yet to be formed in 1810. He wrote: "If this be the season that John Bull selects for cutting his throat, Sunday must be the day, for then London is in all its ugliness, all its naked deformity; the houses are like ruins, the streets deserted."

There was competition for surgery. Within two days of arriving in London he had called on Matthew Baillie (1761–1823), who was a nephew of John Hunter (1728–1793) and William Hunter (1718–1783);[24] James Wilson (1765–1821), who was successor to the Hunters in the Great Windmill Street School of Anatomy; John Abernethy (1764–1831);[25] and Sir Astley Cooper (1768–1841), who invited him to make drawings and to live in his house. From the London Coffee House Bell moved to 22 Fludyer Street in Westminster, from where he walked through St James's and Green Park to Piccadilly.

With total assets of £12 after settling down in Fludyer Street, Charles bought a dilapidated house in Leicester Street and moved there in October 1805. It was said to be haunted by a beautiful young woman whose body had been dissected. The house had been used by a magician in depicting the disappearing woman, which probably explained the hole in the floor into which Bell nearly fell. This might account for Thomas Hood's (1799–1845) comic poem "Mary's Ghost: A Pathetic Ballad":

> I vow'd that you should have my hand,
> But fate gave us denial;
> You'll find it there, at Dr. Bell's,
> In spirits and a phial.

One house pupil was John Shaw (1792–1827), second brother of Barbara, whom George had married in 1806, and of Marion,[26] whom Charles was to marry five years later.

The source of Charles' bodies for dissection was not clear before the 1832 Anatomy Act but appears to have been not without help from the Resurrectionists.[27] Charles set about studying the nerves.

Essays on the Anatomy of Expression in Painting, 1806

During his first year in London, Bell completed the plates for his work *Essays on the Anatomy of Expression in Painting*,[28] which he had brought from Edinburgh and which appeared in 1806 in quarto. Bell's artistic and literary skills combined with his knowledge of anatomy and physiology make this work a tour de force of art history and the anatomical and physiological basis of facial expression. It was read by Queen Charlotte, Consort of King George III (1738–1820) and grandmother of Queen Victoria (1819–1901), who drew and painted. Charles was not much pleased, however.

Artists were exhorted to have a good knowledge of the muscles. Bell visited art galleries and the theatre. He examined facial expression in the Royal Bethlem Hospital (now the Imperial War Museum). He watched Pitt and Fox in the House of Commons and Mrs Siddons in the theatre. He noted how the painter could depict his feelings and not just produce a facsimile of the subject.

Bell commented on the changes from infancy to old age and how the skull protects the brain, with a great increase in the size of the upper jaw and development of the maxillary sinuses. Expression in the human cannot be explained by direct influence of the mind upon the features. The muscles around the eye provide the most lively feature in the countenance and a large eye is essential to beauty. Passion is expressed in man by those muscles peculiar to him, those involved in facial expression. Laughter is not confined to the face but also involves much of the human frame. Bell considered how controlling the expression can modify the emotions. The tenth essay notes anatomy and its value to the painter.

Bell was a keen and accurate observer and he compared the facial muscles in man with those in animals and the limits of emotional display in animals. In Paris he was provided with a donkey rather than a horse to undertake his work on the stimulation of nerves—he had difficulty since the anatomy of the donkey and of the horse are different.

He felt that some muscles of facial expression had been created specifically to enrich man's expressive powers. Charles Darwin (1809–1882) disagreed but nevertheless thought highly of Bell's depiction of emotional expression and mentioned him in his *Expression of the Emotions in Man and Animals*, published in 1873.

Bell noted that the facial expression of joy is really anticipation and the immediate assurance of gratification. He advised artists to gain a perfect knowledge of the muscles, indicated a group action of muscles and condemned giving animals human expressions which they cannot produce. He indicated that the artist should not just copy but must communicate his thoughts—"The face: the index of a feeling mind".[29]

Famous as anatomist, physiologist and neurologist, Charles Bell was also, like his brother John, an eminent surgeon and his artistic talent was even greater than that of John.[30] Charles lectured on anatomy and surgery for medical men and on anatomy for painters. The first volume *A System of Operative Surgery* appeared in 1807, in two volumes.[31]

112

are not raised as in grief. The characters of such opposite passions are so distinct, that they cannot be combined where there is true and genuine emotion. When we see them united by those who have a ludicrous control over their muscles, the expression is farcical and ridiculous. It never is by the affection of an individual feature that emotion is truly expressed; there must be a consent and accordance of expression in the whole countenance systematized (if the expression be allowable) and united by the general tone of tension or relaxation.

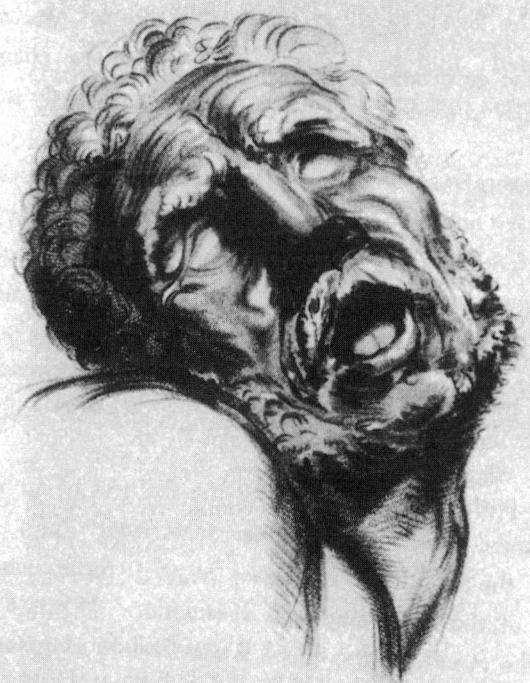

Fig. 1. A cartoon of facial expression.

La Coruña (1809)

The Peninsular War (1807–1814) was fought in Spain from 1808 to 1809. At La Coruña, on the north-west tip of Spain, Sir John Moore opposed the Duke of Dalmatia on 16 January 1809. One thousand were killed or wounded, but 14 000 British defeated 20 000 French under Soult. Moore was killed and lies in a granite tomb, commemorated by the Irish poet Charles Wolfe in the poem "The Burial of Sir John Moore".[32] In 1811 and 1812 Napoleon was to turn his attention to Russia.

By the end of January the wounded British from Corunna landed at Portsmouth. Bell offered to help at the nearby naval hospital at Haslar. He sketched in oil three soldiers wounded in the head at the Battle of Corunna, dying successively from gunshot fracture of the skull. He collected bones from the injured for the Museum of The Royal College of Surgeons of Edinburgh and painted his patients. The 15 oils (see Appendix 1) hang at the College and perhaps the most famous illustrates opisthotonos in tetanus, sometimes described as devil possession. The facial expression, *risus sardonicus*, is the "smile of death".

Later, in illustrations for his books, Bell described fear, terror, jealousy, rage and madness, and considered death as depicted by the great masters.

Marriage to Marion Shaw in 1811

In 1811 Bell married Marion Shaw (1788–1876) of Ayr and they honeymooned in Scotland, Oxford and the Lake District, about which Bell wrote: "Here is England in her most august and venerable aspect."

Bell gave up house pupils and the couple lived at 34 Soho Square, close to the private anatomical schools of Soho (Brooke's, Carpue's, Dermot's, Tuson's and Grainger's) and the Great Windmill Street School, as well as the home of Sir Joseph Banks, later President of The Royal Society. This was a good area of London, with Matthew Baillie in Grosvenor Street and John Shaw in Berners Street next to the Middlesex Hospital. Artists lived nearby.

Alexander Walker wrote in 1809 *New Anatomy and Physiology of the Brain in Particular and of the Nervous System in General*,[33] two years before Bell's idea and 13 years before the work of François Magendie (1783–1855). Walker got the concept right but the details wrong, because he described the anterior roots as sensory and the posterior roots as motor.

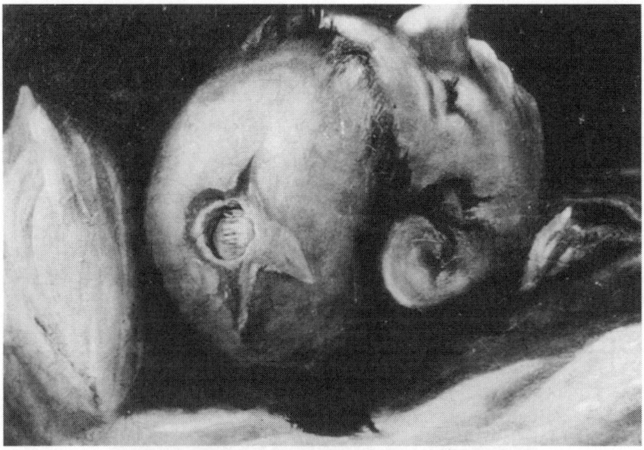

Fig. 2. Musket ball wound of the skull. Corunna oil (1809).

Idea of a New Anatomy of the Brain, 1811

In 1811 Bell published *Idea of a New Anatomy of the Brain*[34] a pamphlet printed privately in 100 copies and presented by Bell to friends and colleagues. [35] The work contains the first reference to experimental observations on the motor functions of the ventral spinal nerve roots but without establishing the sensory function of the dorsal roots.[36] In 1811 Bell enunciated Bell's Law.

Bell distinguished the sensory nerves and motor nerves by differences in texture rather than by the stimuli transmitted by them. Galen had pointed out that a limb could be weak yet with feeling. Bell contributed to the physiology of the nervous system rather than to anatomy, but he went astray in pressing the analogy too far when he attempted to link the hemispheres with the anterior columns of the cord and the cerebellum with the posterior columns. He believed the anterior roots were both sensory and motor and the cerebellum autonomic.

The Great Windmill Street School of Anatomy in 1812

In 1746 William Hunter established the Great Windmill Street School of Anatomy in Covent Garden and in 1748 his brother John joined him. In 1766 William bought a house in Great Windmill Street and rebuilt it to his

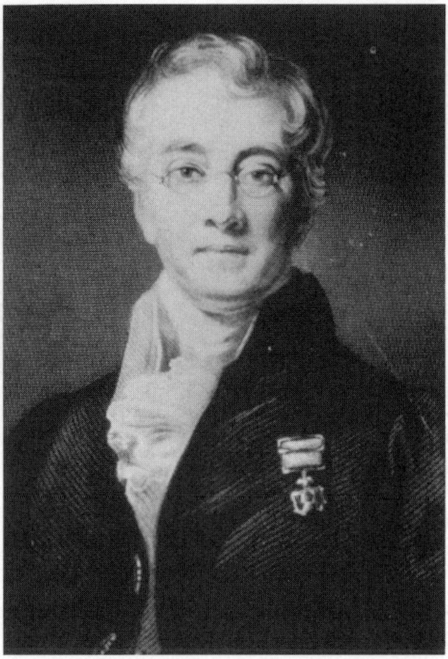

Fig. 3. Sir Charles Bell.

own specifications. Early in 1812, Bell became Proprietor of the School, which continued teaching until the late 1830s.[37]

The Hunterian School was better than many private or hospital schools as it had a library, a reading room and a museum, and was at the cheaper end of the scale at 34 guineas for attendance at all lectures. In 1834 the apprenticeship system for medical training came under heavy criticism in the *Report of the Select Committee on Medical Education*.

Surgeon to the Middlesex Hospital (1814–1836)

Early in March 1814, the year of the Great Frost, Henry Witham, Surgeon to the Middlesex Hospital, died and next morning the hospital staff asked Bell to take his place. Bell was voted in.

In 1814 Bell wrote *A Dissertation on Gunshot Wounds*. In May of 1812 the Russian Emperor sent General Baron Driessen to Bell with a musket ball from the Battle of Borodino lodged in the lower head of the femur. Bell used conservative measures that stopped the wound discharging until March

1816. The discharge resulted from the instillation of mercury into the joint at the suggestion of the German surgeon M. Kretowsky to "dissolve the lead ball". The limb was amputated in 1817 on the advice of Henry Cline (1781–1841).[38] A musket ball retriever, probably from the Crimean War (1854–1856), is exhibited at the Royal College of Surgeons of Edinburgh.

The Battle of Waterloo (1815)

Wellington and Napoleon (each was born in 1769) fought on Sunday, 18 June 1815. About 15,100 of the Anglo-Netherlands army were killed or wounded. News of victory reached London four days later, and Bell and John Shaw set out on 26 June. Bell operated and made copious notes while working continually for eight days, and he sent a moving account of the battlefield to his brother George, which was then passed to Sir Walter Scott, who remarked: "It sets me on fire when I read it." Scott himself set off for the Continent. Wellington's prize money amounted to £61,000 and the corporals, drummers and privates were each awarded £2, 11s, 4d.[39]

Bell wrote:[40]

> "All the decencies of performing surgical operations were soon neglected. While I amputated one man's thigh there lay at one time thirteen all beseeching to be taken next, one full of entreaty, one calling upon me to remember my promise to take him, another execrating. It was a strange thing to feel my clothes stiff with blood and my arms powerless with the exertion of using the knife! And more extraordinary still, to find my mind calm amid such variety of suffering; but to give one of these objects access to your feelings was to allow yourself to be unmanned for the performance of a duty. It was less painful to look upon the whole than to contemplate one object."

On 13 August 1815, H.H. Blackadder wrote noting how on 5 July Bell had removed a musket ball from the right hemisphere of the brain of a 27-year-old soldier who survived. This may be one of the earliest cases of operation on the brain and is probably represented in one of Bell's watercolour drawings. Forty-five sketches in watercolour were included in a notebook that survived to 1866, when it was donated to the Army by Bell's widow. In 1836 Bell was to prepare 17 watercolours based on the book as teaching aids in Edinburgh.

Professor Philbert Joseph Roux (1780–1854), Surgeon from the Hôpital de la Charité, visited Bell in London and later said to his students: "*C'est assez, messieurs, vous avez vu Charles Bell.*"[41]

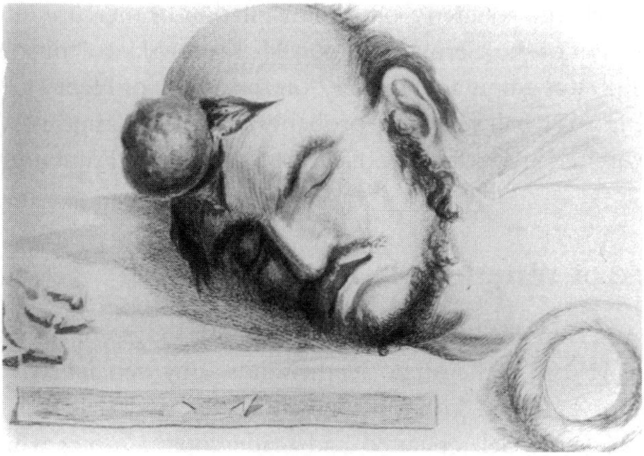

Fig. 4. Head wound. Sketchbook.

In 1819 a description[42] of the Anatomical Museum of the School of Great Windmill Street included an entry for "scapular, ulna, etc., with the triceps muscle preserved as a specimen of a triceps muscle".

In 1820–1821 Bell published in fascicles *Illustrations of the Great Operations of Surgery, Trepan, Hernia, Amputation, Aneurysm and Lithotomy*,[43] one of the most dramatically and beautifully illustrated works in the entire literature of surgery. Hand-coloured copies show more blood than is usual for surgical treatises of this period.

On 12 July 1821, Bell read his first paper to The Royal Society, entitled *On the Nerves, Giving an Account of Some Experiments on Their Structure and Functions, Which Lead to a New Arrangement of the System.*[44] Bell's nerve, the long thoracic, is described here,[45] as is, for the first time, Bell's palsy, the facial paralysis ensuing from a lesion of the motor nerve of the face.[46] Nobody else seemed very interested in the nerves. Bell described how he cut the first division of the trigeminal nerve in a man with tic douloureux and noted the absence of facial weakness. He designated the facial nerve as the respiratory nerve of the face. He wrote of angina pectoris and sudden death. In July John Shaw published the first and second editions of his *Manual for the Student of Anatomy.*

In 1822 François Magendie (1783–1855) published "*Experiences sur les fonctions des racines des nerfs rachidiens*"[47] and would probably not have entered the fray had it not been for Bell's 1811 essay. Magendie described the anterior root as motor and the dorsal root as sensory, although Romberg, Flourens, Sherrington and others credited the discovery to Charles Bell. In

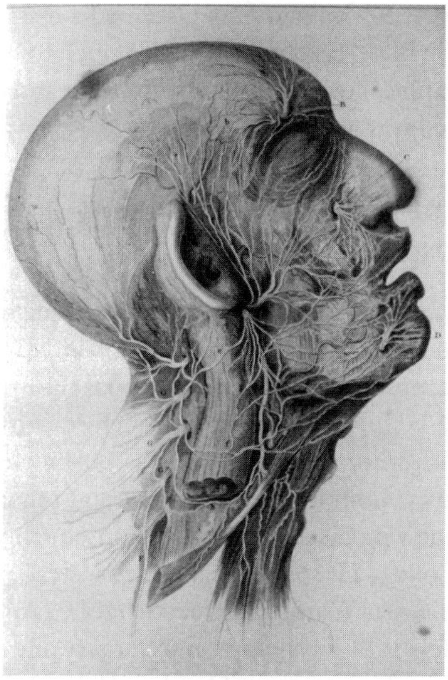

Fig. 5. Nerves of the face. Illustration.

this paper Magendie announced that "section of the dorsal root abolishes sensation, section of the ventral roots abolishes motor activity, and section of both roots abolishes both sensation and motor activity",[48] an observation called "the most momentous *single* discovery in physiology after Harvey". However, Bell and Magendie had rather less to go on, in contrast to Harvey, who discovered the circulation.

Bell made alterations to his papers in the light of Magendie's publication on nerve root function in June of 1822, and also on Herbert Mayo's (1796–1852) statements in 1822 on the trigeminal and facial nerves. Magendie cut the roots of the spinal nerves in pups—a classic of scientific literature.

In 1823 a printed catalogue[49] was made of Bell's Museum.[50] He continued to teach for 12 years at the Great Windmill Street School of Anatomy, and in 1825 he offered most of his Museum to The Royal College of Surgeons of Edinburgh for a consideration of £3000, and that is where it may be seen now.

Anatomy and Philosophy of Expression as Connected with the Fine Arts, minimally amended, was published in 1824. On his return from the Continent in 1840, Bell prepared a new edition, the third.[51] The later editions described the function of nerves and, in particular, the separate functions of the fifth and seventh cranial nerves.[52] Before Bell's time the nerves, pervading even the minutest portion of the human frame, seemed a mass of inextricable confusion and a subject of hopeless obscurity. Bell helped to sort this out. In those days before photography, illustration was by drawing and engraving, coloured by hand. In 1826 Bell was appointed FRS.

The University of London in 1828 and a University Hospital

Lord Brougham, afterwards Lord Chief Justice, was a lifelong friend of Charles Bell. Brougham founded the University of London in 1828 and hoped that the Middlesex would become the University Hospital. However, the University, known as the Godless University, advertised before consulting the hospital, and the Hospital Governors refused. This lesson in the destructive effects apparently of petulance and pique could be a good reminder today to those about to embark on new medical schools. As a consequence the Middlesex lost out and University College Hospital was founded instead, and this contributed to the closure of the Great Windmill Street School of Anatomy.

Bell became Professor of Physiology and Surgery and delivered the Introductory Address at the University in October 1828.[53] The Middlesex Hospital was linked to the University as a Centre of Clinical Study in the Faculty of Medicine. In 1829 the Royal Society of London awarded Bell its Gold Medal for his discoveries in science, and in 1830 he resigned from the University because everyone seemed to be teaching anatomy. He had already been elected a fellow of the Royal Society of Edinburgh in 1811. An entry dated 19 February 1830 in a notebook at the Middlesex provides perhaps the original example of the misconception that a draught on the face leads to Bell's palsy: "This is a case of paralysis of the face, coming on after exposure by falling asleep with the face at the open window of the carriage. Pain of the ear, erysipelous tumefaction of the outward ear and closing of the tube, puffiness of the side of the face."

In 1831 Bell was knighted by William IV (1765–1837), son of Queen Charlotte. In 1833 the University of Göttingen conferred an MD on Bell, and on Astley Cooper likewise. The men held each other in high esteem and Cooper recommended Bell as Queen's Surgeon in Scotland.

Bridgewater Treatise (1833)

From 1832 to 1833 Bell was Professor of Comparative Anatomy at The Royal College of Surgeons of England, and he accepted an invitation from the

President of The Royal Society, the Archbishop of Canterbury and the Bishop of London to prepare the Fourth Bridgewater Treatise. The Right Honourable and Reverend Francis Henry, Earl of Bridgewater, died in February 1829. By his will dated 25 February 1825 he left £8,000 for trustees to place at the disposal of the President of the Royal Society of London to fund tracts to counter the dissent from the traditional concepts of Creation. The Treatises, of which there were eight, were to "illustrate the power, wisdom and goodness of God, as manifested in the creation"—in other words, to advance arguments in favour of Natural Religion. Bell's contribution was entitled *On the Hand: Its Mechanism and Vital Endowments as Evincing Design*.[54]

In 1802 Archdeacon William Paley (1743–1805)[55] published *Natural Theology; or, Evidences of the Existence and Attributes of the Deity, Collected from the Appearances of Nature*.[56] He sought to argue the existence of God from a principle of design in nature and stated: "Suppose I had found a watch upon the ground, then it would be enquired how the watch happened to be in that place."

In 1815, at the age of 71, Lamarck (1744–1829) published his views on evolution in *Philosophie Zoologique*. In 1827 *The Library of Useful Knowledge*[57] included a "Section on Animal Mechanics", which refers to Paley, who "has composed a work of high interest, by taking the common anatomical demonstrations, and presenting them in an elegant and popular form". A diagram shows the tendons to the toes held down by a sheath to avoid bowing and loss of function.

In the preface Bell explains that he wrote *Animal Mechanics* at the request of the Lord Chancellor and later joined him in illustrating Paley's *Natural Theology*, believing that all in the world implies design. When the eye turns from the white paper to the painting, the reds and yellows must be deeper and the muscles which move the eyeball are powerfully affected in certain conditions of the mind: independently altogether of the will, the eyes are rolled upwards during mental agony, and whilst strong emotions of reverence and piety are felt. He includes a chapter on muscular sensation.

Bell's work shows many of Paley's ideas and was a suitable introduction to Darwin's *On the Origin of Species*. It advanced comparative anatomy. Bell notes the geological strata and the difference in the animals embedded therein. He notes the comparative anatomy of the shoulder in different animals or brutes and that the relationship between animals and the elements around them implies that one has been formed to correspond with the other, or vice versa. He notes the chain of animal creation. Bell contrasted the hand with other animals, emphasizing the delicacy of the hand: "Yet it is very remarkable that the muscles of the arm and hand should resemble so closely the muscles of the fore extremity of the lion, for example."[58]

He designated consciousness of muscular exertion as a sixth sense, needed for precision in the use of the hand. This led him to investigate the nerves. He notes how we are sensible of the position of our limbs, how after amputation pain and heat and cold can still be felt in the limb, and how the position of the phantom limb changes with the posture of the body. He did not seem aware of the posterior columns, spinocerebellar tracts or end organs.[59]

More Surgery in London (1834–1836)

In April 1835 six members of the staff, including Bell, wrote to the Board of the Middlesex Hospital pointing out the need to found a medical school, and on 1 October 1835 the Middlesex Hospital Medical School was opened with 60 students. Bell gave the Introductory Address on 1 October 1835.[60] One month later he was invited to take the Chair of Systematic Surgery (founded in 1831) at Edinburgh University, the medical school pre-eminent in Europe. The staff presented Bell with a silver urn when he resigned in 1836, and at that time John Shaw was appointed Surgeon and he continued to serve the Hospital for a total of 33 years.

In August 1836 Charles, now aged 58 years, with Lady Bell left their home at 82 Brook Street, to which they had moved in 1832 from Soho Square, and departed for Edinburgh.

Back to Edinburgh (1836–1842)

Charles Bell and his wife settled at Ainslie Place in Edinburgh, a city that had extended its boundaries since 1804, when they were last there. Bell was paid £400 a year as Professor of Systematic Surgery in Edinburgh.

In 1836, ten years before the invention of photography, Bell prepared 17 life-size watercolours from his 1815 notebook of Waterloo to use for teaching.[61–63]

James Syme (1799–1870) occupied the senior Chair (founded in 1803), the Regius Chair of Clinical Surgery. In Edinburgh nearly all the Surgery Chairs were Regius as they were technically supported by the Crown; that is to say, the Government, as the Town Council did not feel able to go against the wishes of the Monros. He was Bell's great rival and he refused Bell the use of surgical beds. Syme was also a rival of Robert Knox (1791–1862), a very determined man and a keen walker. In 1826 Syme went to Dublin to try to

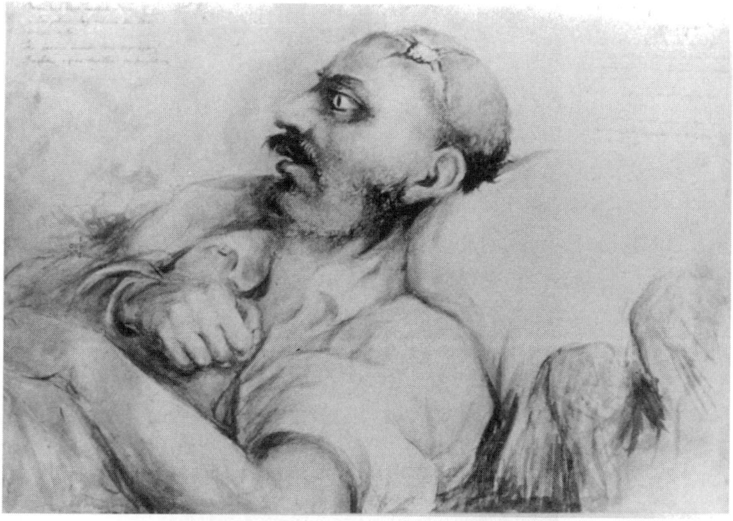

Fig. 6. A soldier suffering from head wounds and shock. Waterloo watercolour, 1836.

obtain bodies but was unsuccessful. When he returned to Edinburgh he had already made up his mind to give up teaching anatomy. Burke and Hare only offered bodies in 1827 but none was offered to Syme. Later, in 1852, Robert Knox's brief *Manual*[64] showed the relationship between anatomy and art. The volume contains illustrations of osteology and muscle structure.

In the first chapter Knox indicates that Charles Bell wholly misunderstood the true relationship of anatomy and art but that Leonardo da Vinci understood it perfectly. Knox states: "Suffice it to say, that in England, utilitarian England, the coping-stone of folly was placed by Sir Charles Bell and Mr. Haydon." Knox's thesis is that the hand bears little relation to its skeleton. The skeleton does not indicate where the soft tissues should lie, for "Do you find in the skeleton of the hand the taper form, the pulpy extremities of the fingers; the prominences of the skeleton's articulations turned into beautiful depressions or dimples, the soft elastic palm, the smooth and glossy elevated dorsum, the fleshy mass of the thumb, the beauteous curve of the antithenar eminence or base of the little finger?"

Knox then embarks on a description of the bones and joints. He asserts that Bell totally misunderstood the attitude and the force required to maintain the position of *standing at ease*, Bell stating that the patella was held tense though Knox said not.

Knox even criticises Bell, who measured the statue of Venus incorrectly on account of the stoop in the statue. Bell could have looked round London and

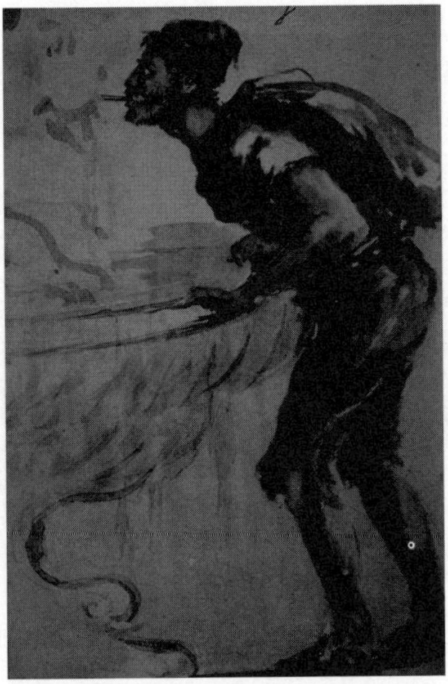

Fig. 7. *Thus a Roman Drinks.* "Italian Sketch", watercolour.

elsewhere to see hundreds and hundreds of persons whose profile equalled the finest models of antiquities, and Bell's assertion that the facial angle now rarely if ever equalled the antique was frankly not true.

All this competition prevented Bell from doing much surgery. He was a very sensitive person, recording the emotions of his patients. Often he vomited before operating.

While in Edinburgh Bell published a new edition of *The Anatomy and Philosophy of Painting*.

On 30 December 1837 William Whewell, polymath and alleged bully, and Professor of Mineralogy at Cambridge,[65] wrote in the *London Medical Gazette*[66] that Mayo (1796–1852) and Magendie had corrected the work of Bell and that the description of the dual function of the nerves should be attributed to all three.

In the spring of 1840 Bell started a three-month tour of Paris, Nice, Genoa and Rome, sketching and commenting on the art. He spent a month in Rome and visited the grave of his brother John, who had died there in 1820. He felt the strain of the angina that affected his stomach. His heart was not mentioned, though in all probability it was a warning of his impending demise.

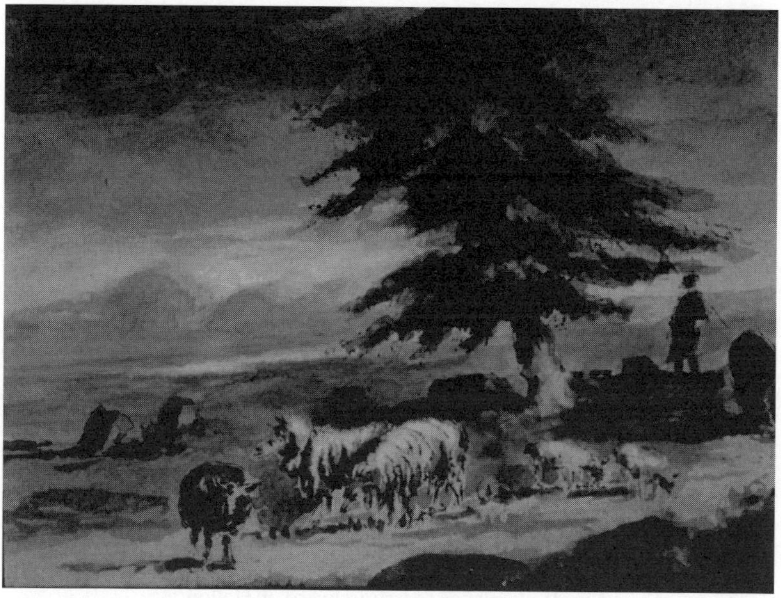

Fig. 8. *Pastoral Scene with the Malvern Hills in the Background*. Watercolour.

Bell's watercolours may be seen in the Royal College of Surgeons of Edinburgh and include the "Italian Sketches": *Man*, *Beggar*, *Peasant Girl*, *Taken Before St Peter's Rome*; *Old Man and a Girl*; *Thus a Roman Drinks*; *Italian Lake Scene*. Others include *Old Nanny*, *The Mad Bull*, *The Palsied Beggar of Richmond Hill*, *Loch Earn*, *The Derelict Ship*, *Fishing Sketch*, *Heart of Midlothian*, *Rejected*, *Take Care My Dears*, *Boys Are So Rash*, *Rural Sketch*, and *Man and Woman with Child*. The style of *Lowland Scot in Kilmarnock Bonnet* is different and the attribution to Bell less secure.

The Final Illness in 1842

On Wednesday 27 April 1842 Charles and Lady Bell arrived to visit their friend Mrs Holland at her beautiful home, Hallow Park, near Worcester. They had been frequent visitors to this area, originally given by the Bishop of Worcester to the monks to cultivate and develop.

While dining at Hallow Park Bell was uncomfortable, and the next day he sketched probably his last picture, *Pastoral Scene with the Malvern Hills in the Background*. At dinner that evening he felt cold and lacked appetite

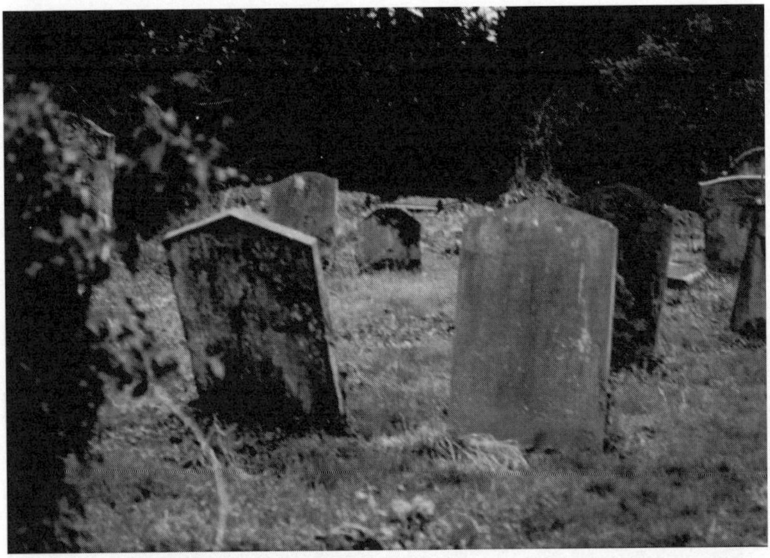

Fig. 9. Grave in old churchyard at Hallow.

and at one stage became deadly pale. A Worcester physician attended him and administered laudanum. After going to bed Bell had severe pain, and he awoke the next day in pain.

On 29 April 1842 Bell, a poor man, died from ossification of the heart—that is to say, coronary atheroma—and the verdict of the Coroner for Worcester was given as "Visitation of God".

Charles Bell was buried in the churchyard[67] of the old parish church at Hallow, which has since been demolished. The grave, at the far end of the churchyard on the right when entered from Church Lane, is a horizontal slab of sandstone, inscribed, surrounded by an iron railing and in some disarray.

A memorial of white marble was transferred from the old church to the north aisle of the new Hallow Church and the inscription reads:

SACRED TO THE MEMORY
OF
SIR CHARLES BELL
WHO AFTER UNFOLDING
WITH UNRIVALLED SAGACITY, PATIENCE AND SUCCESS
THE WONDERFUL STRUCTURE OF OUR MORTAL BODIES
ESTEEMED HIGHLY OF HIS GREATEST DISCOVERIES
EXCEPT ONLY

AS THEY TENDED TO IMPRESS HIMSELF AND OTHERS
WITH A DEEPER SENSE
OF
THE INFINITE WISDOM AND INEFFABLE GOODNESS
OF
THE ALMIGHTY CREATOR.
HE WAS BORN AT EDINBURGH
1774
DIED WHILE ON A VISIT OF FRIENDSHIP
AT HALLOW PARK IN THIS PARISH
1842
AND HE IS BURIED
IN THE ADJOINING CHURCHYARD

Thomas Hood in his *Silence* sums up the atmosphere:

> There is a silence where hath been no sound,
> There is a silence where no sound may be,
> In the cold grave—under the deep deep sea,
> Or in wide desert where no life is found,
> Which hath been mute, and still must sleep profound.

Lady Bell was awarded a pension of £100 a year from the Civil List. She returned to London soon after Charles died and lived with her brother, Mr Alexander Shaw. She died of bronchitis and pneumonia at the age of 89 at her residence in London, 47 Albany Street, Regents Park, on 9 November 1876 and was buried[68] in Brompton Cemetery.[69] Others of interest buried in Brompton Cemetery include the suffragette Emmeline Pankhurst (1858–1928) and the opera singer Richard Tauber (1891–1948). Of medical interest are John Snow (1813–1858),[70] and Edward Meryon (1807–1880),[71] who described the variety of muscular dystrophy later attributed to Guillaume Duchenne de Boulogne (1806–1875).[72] In 1862 Duchenne published work on the mechanics of human facial expression which he based on electrical stimulation studies and photographs.

Memories and Legacies

The Great Windmill School failed and the building was used as a surgery, a printing office, a Catholic school, and a French dining and billiard establishment later known as the Café de l'Étoile. In 1890 an entertainment company bought it. In 1958 it formed part of the Lyric Theatre in Shaftesbury Avenue and the entrance for the subjects for dissection became the stage door.

Hallow Park was demolished and rebuilt in 1914, only the cellars of the old house remaining. The last private resident was a clothing manufacturer from Chester, after whose death the house was sold to Dr Barnardo's as a children's home until about 1970. The house, still owned by Dr Barnardo's, is leased to Foley Park Estates, which has converted it to offices.

Despite the undoing of much of what surrounded Bell in life, his name should be known to every medical student and doctor by virtue of the five eponyms: Bell's law, the long nerve of Bell, Bell's palsy,[73] Bell's phenomenon and Bell's sign. His papers are classics and have been reprinted with biography and bibliography.[74] Biographies appear in modern works on the history of the neurosciences.[75] Neurological texts still describe the eponymous Bell disorders and Bell is still quoted in contemporary papers.[76] The study of ancient faces may give insight into neurological problems. Mummy portraits painted in colour from the beginning of the first millennium suggest facial hemiatrophy, deviation of the visual axes, and oval pupils. This, the study of palaeoneurology,[77] complements the study of neurohistory.

Elegy Written in a Country Churchyard[78]

Thomas Gray (1716–1771) could have the last words:

1

The *Curfeu* tolls the Knell of parting Day,
The lowing Herd winds slowly o'er the Lea,
The Plow-man homeward plods his weary Way
And leaves the World to Darkness, and to me.

⋮

4

Beneath whose rugged Elms, that Yew-Tree's Shade,
Where heaves the Turf in many a mould'ring Heap,
Each in his narrow Cell for ever laid,
The rude Forefathers of the Hamlet sleep

⋮

9

The Boast of Heraldry, the Pomp of Pow'r,
And all that Beauty, all that Wealth e'er gave,
Awaits alike th'inevitable House.
The Paths of Glory lead but to the Grave.

Acknowledgments

An unsurpassed biography of Charles Bell is that of Gordon Taylor and Walls.[79]

I am greatly indebted to Professor D.L. Gardner, who has kindly given me sight of his papers "Charles Bell: Surgeon and Artist" and "Charles Bell and the Faces of the Wounded". I have also enjoyed sight of the watercolours and oils in the Royal College of Surgeons of Edinburgh, and Mrs Jones from the Museum has been most helpful.[80] I am grateful to the College for permission to reproduce Figs. 2, 7 and 8. Other Bell paintings are held at the Wellcome Museum on behalf of the British Army and I am grateful to staff there for help and permission to reproduce Fig. 6. Mr M.F. Sturridge at The Middlesex Hospital has kindly given permission to reproduce Fig. 3, and the Royal College of Surgeons of England permission to reproduce Fig. 4. The Reverend Robert Latham at Hallow Vicarage has helped with details of the grave and memorial. Professor Matthew Kaufman has made many helpful suggestions, for which I am very grateful.

Appendix 1

Fifteen Sketches in Oil (the Corunna Oil Colours) at the Royal College of Surgeons of Edinburgh

Gunshot wound of the humerus (GC 13834)
Old standing gunshot fracture of the shaft of the humerus (GC 13830)
Bullet wound of the skull (GC 13832)
Sketch of a gunshot wound of the thigh (GC 13846)
Gunshot entry and exit wounds of the chest (GC 13829)
Old standing gunshot fracture of the fibula (GC 13828)
Gunshot wound of the testes (GC 13836)
Gunshot wound of the head (GC 13831)
Gunshot wound of the elbow (GC 13833)
Gunshot wound of the clavicle and scapula (GC 13845)
Tetanus following gunshot wounds (GC 13842)
Gunshot wound of the humerus (GC 13835)
Sketch in oil of a man wounded in the chest (GC 13844)
Bullet wound of the skull (GC 13837)
Sketch of a wound of the abdomen (GC 13843)

Appendix 2

Sixteen Waterloo Watercolours at the Wellcome Institute in London

Soldier with missing arm, lying on his side, grasping a rope, dated "11 Aug." (1815). Inscribed "XIII, Waterloo...". (L22539B)

Soldier suffering from head and facial injuries, head and shoulders. Inscribed "Waterloo". (L 22540)

Soldier with right arm missing, head and torso. Inscribed "XV". (L 22541)
Soldier suffering from head and facial injuries, profile. Inscribed "Waterloo". (L 22542)

Soldier suffering from neck wound, lying on his back. Inscribed "Waterloo". (L 22543)

Soldier suffering from open chest wound, head and right arm bandaged. Inscribed "VIII". (L 22544)

Arm wound. Inscribed "XII Waterloo". (L 22545)

Soldier with right arm missing. (L22546C)

Soldier suffering from stomach wound; sabre wound to abdomen. Peltier. Belgian Hospital, 2 July 1815. (L22547C)

Soldier suffering from head wounds and shock. (L22548)

Two examples of eye wounds, with inscriptions. (L 22549)

Leg wound. Inscribed "XVII". (L2250B)

Soldier with bandaged head. (L22551)

Soldier with left arm missing, bandaged head, with quill in right arm. (L22552)

Soldier suffering from a wound to left shoulder and bandaged head. Inscribed "XI". Gunshot wound to arm, James Ellard, York Hospital, September 1815. (L22553C)

Soldier with bandaged head, and arm in a sling. Inscribed "X Waterloo". (L22554)

Soldier suffering from head wound; part of scalp shaved. (L22555)

Notes and References

1. Based on a paper read at The Mansell Bequest Symposium on the Neurology of the Arts, held at The Medical Society of London from 30 April to 1 May 2001.
2. MD, FRCP, FACP, Consultant Neurologist. Exeter Neurosciences and Peninsula Medical School, Royal Devon and Exeter Hospital, Barrack Road, Exeter, EX2 5DW, UK. E-mail: cgardnerthorpe@doctors.org.uk
3. William Shakespeare (1606), *Macbeth*, Act 1, Scene 4, lines 12–13. Duncan.
4. Charles' gravestone gives the date of birth as 1775.
5. L. Stephen and S. Lee, *The Dictionary of National Biography* (Oxford University Press, 1921–2), pp. 293–4.
6. Mrs (Ruth) Head, *A Simple Guide to Pictures by Mrs Henry Head* (Chatto and Windus, 1914).
7. C. Gardner-Thorpe, "The Poetry of Henry Head (1861–1940)", this volume (2001), pp. 401–20.
8. S.W. Simon, The influence of the three Monros on the practice of medicine and surgery, *Annals of Medical History* **9**, 244 (1927).
9. J. Struthers, Historical sketch of the Edinburgh Anatomical School (1867) (Maclachlan Stewart), pp. 44–55.
10. R.E. Wright-St Clair, *Doctors Monro: A Medical Saga* (Wellcome Historical Medical Library, London, 1964).
11. Reproduced in 1994 by The Landmark Library, New York.
12. In 1851 J. Maclise published *Surgical Anatomy* (Churchill, London).
13. Published by Longman, Paternoster-Row, London.
14. Vol. I, p. 432.
15. Edinburgh, Cadell & Davies. Garrison Morton, 401.3.
16. Russell, No. 461, 1911–1987.
17. Edinburgh, London, T. Cadell & W. Davis. Garrison Morton, 5581.
18. Published by Blackwood, Edinburgh. One copy is inscribed "For James Jeffray, MD, Professor of Anatomy in the University of Glasgow, with the Author's most respectful compliments".
19. D.C. Godbee, Joseph Bell (1837–1911): a clinician's literary legacy, *Journal of Medical Biography* 7, 166–70 (1999).
20. A fine statue of Sherlock Holmes may be seen close to the John Lewis store in Edinburgh.
21. *Edinburgh Medical Journal* **22**, 135–7 (1876). Cited by Garrison Morton, 2127.1.

22. C. Bell (1798–9), *A System of Dissection, Explaining the Anatomy of the Human Body, the Manner of Displaying the Parts, and Their Varieties in Disease* (Edinburgh, Mundell & Son; Glasgow: J. Mundell [Part I]. Garrison Morton, 402).
23. Published by Longman of London.
24. For a history of William and his family, see: Samuel Foart Simmons and John Hunter, *William Hunter 1718–1783: A Memoir*, ed. by C.H. Brock (Glasgow University Press, 1983).
25. J.L. Thornton, *John Abernethy: A Biography*. Published by the author and distributed by Simpkin Marshall Ltd., London (1953).
26. On his gravestone her name is spelt "Maryon" and in the manuscript in the National Library of Scotland "Marion".
27. Alexander Cresswell wrote in *The Times* of 26 July 2000 ("Occupational Hazard", Letters, p. 17): "Sir, My household insurer has declined my policy renewal on the grounds of 'the nature of my occupation'; I am an artist, a painter in watercolours. Not being an Establishment figure I do not use unmade beds, dead sheep or formaldehyde—not even stolen body parts; just watercolours, brushes and a little water—high-risk stuff, clearly. Could this be a new tactic to winkle out traditionalist cells?"
28. Longman, London, 1806. Garrison Morton, 92, 6604. The original volume had 186 pages but later it was enlarged.
29. George Crabbe (1754–1832), *Tales of the Hall (1819): "Lady Barbara"*, **1**, p. 124.
30. See Garrison Morton, 5588.
31. Longman, London, 1807–9. Garrison Morton, 5583.
32. B. Perrett, *The Battle Book* (Cassell, London, 1992), p. 81. For a map of the battle see *British History Atlas*, by Martin Gilbert, published by Weidenfeld and Nicholson, p. 80.
33. *Archives of Universal Sciences*, **31**, pp. 172–9.
34. Strahan & Preston, London, 1811. Garrison Morton, 1254.
35. Five copies have been identified (British Museum, The Royal Society of London, Surgeons' General Library at Washington, The Royal Society of Medicine, and The Royal College of Surgeons of England, which has the copy presented by Lady Bell in 1863). This very rare privately printed pamphlet is reproduced in *Medical Classics*, **1**, 105–20 (1936) in facsimile reprint (London, 1966). Bell's own annotated copy, preserved in the library of The Royal Society of London, is reproduced in: Cranefield, *The Way in and the Way out: François Magendie, Charles Bell and the Roots of the Spinal Nerves* (Futura, New York, 1974). See No. 1588.9. Cranefield argues that Magendie (No. 1256) provided the Bell–Magendie Law.
36. Four of the original drawings are held at The Royal College of Surgeons in London. Other original drawings and paintings are held there too.
37. R. Porter, *The Greatest Benefit to Mankind: A Medical History of Humanity from Antiquity to the Present* (Fontana, London, 1999).

38. Specimen 111.1(14).B.24.
39. B. Perrett, *The Battle Book* (Cassell, London, 1992), pp. 310–2. Seen at Exeter Public Reference Library. For a map of the battle see *British History Atlas*, by Martin Gilbert, published by Weidenfeld and Nicholson, p. 81. Copy seen in Exeter Public Reference Library.
40. An editorial in the *British Medical Journal* of 12 June 1912, pp. 1327–8, is entitled "Sir Charles Bell and Waterloo" and comments on an article in the *Cornhill Magazine* entitled "One of the puzzles of Waterloo". The editorial notes: "Sketches in watercolours and oil were given to the Museum of The Royal College of Surgeons at Edinburgh. Lady Bell presented seventeen others, together with her husband's notebook, to The Royal Hospital, Netley, in 1867". Correspondence from Edwin Goodall follows on 15 June 1912.
41. "It is enough, gentlemen, that you have seen Charles Bell."
42. *A Description of the Anatomical Museum of the School of Great Windmill Street.* London; printed for Burgess & Hill, 55, Great Windmill Street, Haymarket, by J. Davy, 17, Queen Street, Seven Dials. 1819.
43. Longman, London, 1820–1. Garrison Morton, 5588. A second, undated issue appeared *c.* 1830. Copy seen at the Royal College of Surgeons in London.
44. *Philos. Trans.* **111**, 398–424 (1821). Garrison Morton, 4520.
45. *Ibid.*, p. 291.
46. The motor nerve of the face is the seventh cranial nerve. See also Bell's later paper, with more detailed description, in *Philosophical Transactions 1829*, **119**, 317–30 (1829). Reprinted in *Med. Classics* **1**, 152–69 (1936).
47. *Journal of Physiology and Experimental Pathology* **2**, 276–9 (1822). Garrison Morton, 1256.
48. Cranefield, No. 1588.9.
49. XVI Divn. Bell Cat.; 1823. Entered in an Obstetrical Catalogue in 1839. This is a catalogue of preparations, being those of the XVIth Division of Mr. Charles Bell's Museum; and calculated for the complete illustration of a course of lectures on Midwifery. London: printed by John McGowan, Great Windmill Street. A copy is held at the Royal College of Surgeons of Edinburgh.
50. The exhibits include Triceps brachii muscle—dissection of muscles attached to scapula; nerves from the brachial plexus, one partly dissected to show the funiculi and epinurium; carotid artery in the base of the skull, support from the right half of the base of the skull to show the internal carotid artery; skull-based cranial nerves, 1 January 1825; cranial nerves, 104; thoracic vertebrae, 11, 1825; hernia cerebri, 1825; spinal deformity, 11, 1825; cervical spine bone dislocation, spontaneous, 11, 1825; syphilitic skull osteotitis, 1825; brain corro plexus, 1825; and many others.
51. *The Anatomy of Expression* went to a third edition in 1844, the fourth was dated 1847 and published by John Murray of London, the sixth was published in 1872, and the seventh and last in 1893 by Bohn of London.

52. *The Anatomy and Philosophy of Expression as Connected with the Fine Arts*. Bohn, London, 1872. 6th ed.
53. *London Medical Gazette* **2**, 566–8 (1828).
54. The first and second editions were published in 1833, each in one volume, and the third edition in 1838 in one volume. The ninth edition appeared in 1874. A copy belonged to Robert Bentley Todd (1809–1860), an Irish physician who became Dean of King's College Hospital in London and who in 1854 described the paralysis which may follow an epileptic seizure and which is known as Todd's paralysis. Also reproduced in facsimile by The Classics of Medicine Library, Birmingham, Alabama, with Robert Knox's *A Manual of Artistic Anatomy for the Use of Sculptors, Painters, and Amateurs*.
55. C. Gardner-Thorpe (2002). William Paley (1743–1805): neuroanatomist? *Journal of Medical Biography* **10**, 215–23.
56. Copy of the 14th edition seen at the Devon and Exeter Institution. Shelf A19.10.
57. *The Library of Useful Knowledge*, 3rd ed. (1827). *Animal Mechanics: Treatise 1*, p. 1. Copy seen in the Harveian Library, Royal College of Physicians, where it is bound as Tract 321, part 15.
58. *Ibid.*, p. 119.
59. In 1845 *Knight's Weekly Volume for All Readers* was to publish (in four volumes) *Paley's Natural Theology with illustrative notes by Henry, Lord Brougham, FRS and Sir C. Bell KGH etc. and a discussion of Natural Theology by Lord Brougham: to which are added, supplementary dissertations and a treatise on mineral mechanisms, by Sir Charles Bell with numerous woodcuts, in Four Vols*. (Charles Knight and Co., Ludgate Street, London). Copy seen at the Devon and Exeter Institution, shelf Q1.38–41.
60. *Lancet* **i**, 89 (1835).
61. D.L. Gardner, *Charles Bell: Surgeon and Artist* (1997). Based on an invited address delivered to the Sections of Pathology and of the History of Medicine of the Royal Society of Medicine, 24 April 1997.
62. D.L. Gardner, *Charles Bell and the Faces of the Wounded* (1997). Based on an invited address delivered to the Sections of Pathology and of the History of Medicine of the Royal Society of Medicine, 24 April 1997.
63. In the RAMC/95 Collection at the Wellcome Institute, London.
64. Robert Knox, *A Manual of Artistic Anatomy, for the Use of Sculptors, Painters and Amateurs* (Renshaw, London, 1852). Published in facsimile by *The Classics of Medicine Library* in Birmingham in 1985, along with the 1833 publication of Bell's *Bridgewater Treatise*.
65. Noel Annan, *The Dons: Mentors, Eccentrics and Geniuses* (Harper Collins, London, 1999). *The Don as Scholar* (Frederic Maitland), pp. 79–97.
66. P. 525.
67. The old churchyard lies at the end of Church Lane, the first right hand turn to the north of the present Hallow church; there is a footpath into Church Lane

from the rear of the churchyard. The grave is on the far right when the yard is viewed from the gateway.

68. The grave is in Compound Y, 237'3"×136'3", in the second row when the Compound is viewed from the western path, approximately halfway along the west side. When entering the cemetery from the north, i.e. from the Old Brompton Road end, there is a map of the cemetery layout immediately on the left. Walk past this, ignoring the first turn to the left (where the memorial to John Snow may be found) but taking the second turn to the left. After taking this turn, ignore the path that crosses and then count on the left 11 graves, and when reaching the 11th look two further graves in, making the third grave in. Behind a large laurel bush there is a memorial flat to the ground but its inscription is almost illegible.
69. The 39-acre cemetery which was opened in 1840 lies between Old Brompton Road in the north and Fulham Road in the south. Details of burials in Brompton Cemetery are included in *Permanent Londoners: an Illustrated, Biographical Guide to the Cemeteries of London* by Judi Culbertson and Tom Randall, published in 1991 and republished in 2000 by Robson Books, London. Guides to burial sites are popular, and other publications include *Permanent Parisians: An Illustrated, Biographical Guide to the Cemeteries of Paris*, by the same authors; *Who's Buried Where in England*, by Douglas Greenwood, published in 1982 by Constable, London; *Stones Unturned: Memorials of Medical Significance in Exeter Cathedral*, by Christopher Gardner-Thorpe, published in Exeter in 2000; and doubtless many others.
70. A large white memorial, near the north end of the Cemetery, it bears the inscription (in capitals) "To John Snow, MD. Born at York on March 15th 1813, died in London June 16th 1858. In remembrance of his great labours in science and of the excellence of his private life and character this monument (with the assent of Mr William Snow) has been erected over his grave by his professional brethren and friends. Restored in 1895."
71. Compound Y, 59'O"×39'3". It is in the second row when the Compound is viewed from the western path, approximately halfway along the West side.
72. A.E.H. Emery and M.L.H. Emery, *The History of a Genetic Disease: Duchenne Muscular Dystrophy or Meryon's Disease* (Royal Society of Medicine Press, London, 1995). See also: V. Jay and J. Vajsar, The dystrophy of Duchenne, *Lancet* **357**, 550–2 (2001).
73. Henry Charlton Bastian (1837–1915) described peripheral facial palsy as Bell's paralysis. See: H.C. Bastian, *Paralyses Cerebral Bulbar and Spinal: A Manual of Diagnosis for Students and Practitioners* (H.K. Lewis, London, 1886), p. 445.
74. See *Medical Classics*, Oct. 1936, Vol. 1, No. 2; Sir Charles Bell. This was reprinted in *Classics of Neurology* by Robert Krieger, New York, in 1971. It includes "Idea of a new anatomy of the brain", "On the nerves", "On the nerves of the face" and "On the motions of the eye in illustration of the uses of the muscles and nerves of the orbit".

75. F. Clifford Rose, Charles Bell: the man—three early 19th century British neurological texts, *A Short History of Neurology: The British Contribution 1660–1910* (Butterworth Heinemann, Oxford, 1999), pp. 122–8. Frank Clifford Rose describes Bell and provides a list of 17 neurological texts.
76. J. Deng, N.M. Newton, M.A. Hall-Craggs, R.A. Shirley, A.D. Linney, W.R. Lees, C.H. Rodeck and D.A. McGrouther, Novel technique for three-dimensional visualisation and quantification of deformable, moving soft-tisssue body parts, *Lancet* **356**, 127–31 (2000).
77. O. Appenzeller, J.M. Stevens, R. Kruszynski and S. Walker, Neurology in ancient faces, *Journal of Neurology, Neurosurgery and Psychiatry* **70**, 524–9 (2001).
78. *The Penguin Book of English Verse*, ed. by John Hayward (Penguin, Middlesex, 1963), pp. 225–7.
79. Sir Gordon Gordon-Taylor, and E.W. Walls, *Sir Charles Bell: His Life and Times* (E. & S. Livingstone, Edinburgh, 1958).
80. E.W. Walls and D.L. Gardner, *Charles Bell 1774–1842: Surgeon, Physiologist, Artist and Author.* A booklet prepared to accompany an exhibition from 12th August to 31st August 1996 at the Royal College of Surgeons of Edinburgh, of Sir Charles Bell's books, drawings and 1809 Corunna oil paintings, together with photographic reproductions of his 1836 Waterloo watercolour drawings.

Chapter 7

Normal and Pathological Gait as Inspiration for the Artist

Geneviève Aubert

Introduction: Arthur Van Gehuchten

This reflection on the relationship between gait study and art has been prompted by a research on the leading figure of Belgian neurology around 1900, Arthur Van Gehuchten (1861–1914).[1] An anatomist of repute, he participated actively in the formulation of the neuron doctrine and worked in close collaboration with Cajal.[2–4] A shrewd neurologist, he proposed innovative surgical operations.[5,6]

An avant-garde teacher, he was a pioneer of cinematography in clinical neurology. This original aspect of Van Gehuchten has recently been highlighted.[7,8] He used cinematography extensively, from at least 1905 up to his death in 1914. He underlined the pedagogic and documentary interest of this technique in his publications.[9] Examination of the neurological patient, demonstration of clinical signs of neurologic disorders and evolution of symptoms after surgical treatment were among the many subjects which he documented in his films.[5,10,11] His original nitrate films, which are incunabula of cinematography, have recently been found. They have been the object of a meticulous restoration at the Royal Belgian Film Archive, in Brussels, where they are the oldest Belgian films surviving.[12] Not surprisingly, gait disorders form a considerable part of this cinematographic corpus.

De Putter and Van Gehuchten

The Film Archive is part of the Palais des Beaux-Arts, the most important fine arts centre in Brussels, which hosts theatres, concert halls and exhibitions. The

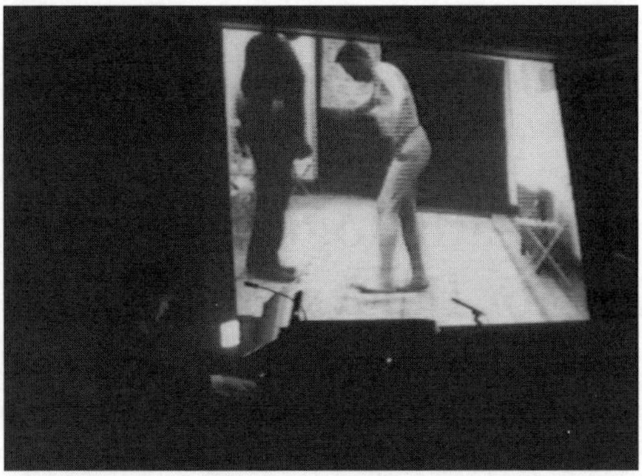

Fig. 1. *Chorée*, music composition by Renaud De Putter on films of Arthur Van Gehuchten, performed on the piano by Stéphane Ginsburg, Creation 12 Sep. 1998, Brussels.

Philharmonic Society, one partner of this centre, is the principal organiser of concerts in Brussels. In addition, it stages original musical events. In 1997, the Philharmonic Society asked nine young Belgian musicians to compose music on silent movies kept at the Film Archive. The creation of these works was scheduled at a special movie show for which each artist chose a short film which particularly inspired him. One of the composers, Renaud De Putter (born in Brussels, in 1967), was so struck by the power and the strangeness of Van Gehuchten's films that he thought about using them in his work. For different reasons, Van Gehuchten's films were finally discarded from the definitive programme of the event, and this project was given up.

Meanwhile, I had become acquainted with De Putter. I attended a piano concert of the pianist Stéphane Ginsburg, where another creation of De Putter, *Corymbe*, was played, alongside almost classical pieces of Charles Ives and Elliott Carter. I was captivated and proposed to De Putter that he should complete his project on Van Gehuchten's films. This composition was created at the symposium "Images du Cerveau, Images de la Neurologie", organised on the occasion of the retirement of Christian Laterre, head of the neurological department of the Cliniques Universitaires Saint-Luc in Brussels (Figure 1). As stated by the artist, he had been particularly interested by the questioning about movement and the spontaneity of gesture. The title chosen by the artist for his work, *Chorée*, has a double reference, to neurology and to art, through the Greek etymology of the word, meaning dance. To participate in the creation of this musical composition and in the reflection of the artist about neurological diseases, body reality, voyeurism and identification, has been for me a rewarding experience.

Artistic Legacy of Gait Studies

It was not the first time that I had met, in my research into the history of neuroscience, this resonance between two cultures, namely neurology and arts. My quest concerning the beginnings of photography and cinematography in neurology brought me to Marey and Muybridge, who played a pivotal role in the evolution from photography to cinematography.[13–15] The developments that occurred from photography to cinematography in the 19th century were a joint venture of photographers, technicians, scientists and physicians.[16] Gait recording and analysis were a recurrent theme in these researches and the object of great interest from physiologists as well as neurologists. Artists, and also the man in the street, were immediately fascinated by the images revealed by these new techniques. Examples of gait studies as a source of inspiration for the artist are to be found in almost any discipline, from painting to music and from sculpture to choreography.

Bacon, Muybridge and Dercum

A first example is a picture, *Paralytic Child Walking on All Fours (from Muybridge)*, by Francis Bacon (1909–1992), Irish-born British painter.[17] It is quite typical of the artist: a zoomorphic creature is crawling in the midst of the wide space of a dark canvas. This canvas, painted in 1961, belongs to the Gemeentemuseum of The Hague in The Netherlands.[18] The genesis of this painting is extremely interesting. Bacon's paintings were often based on images, paintings by other artists, or photographs. That is the case for this painting, which was directly inspired by Muybridge, one of the pioneers of the photographic analysis of movement. Three men played an important role in these developments: Muybridge (1830–1904), British-born American photographer; Marey (1830–1904), French physiologist and Professor at the Collège de France; and Londe (1858–1917), photographer at the Salpêtrière. These three men developed different methodological approaches and their work has had interesting neurological as well as artistic outcomes. During his whole life, Marey studied human and animal locomotion, first by graphic methods. In 1873, he published his book *La machine animale*, which was translated into English the following year.[19] At that time, Muybridge had succeeded in fixing for the first time the picture of a horse in motion. Marey's work definitely inspired Muybridge. The latter aligned a battery of 12, then 24 cameras, equipped with an ingenious electromagnetic tripping device. This yielded, in 1878, the first series of successive instantaneous photographs of a horse in motion. This picture aroused considerable excitement all over the world. In 1881, while touring and lecturing in Europe, Muybridge was received in Paris by Marey with such leading scientific and artistic experts as Helmholtz, Brown-Séquard, Meissonier and Nadar. This meeting had an extraordinary and fecund reciprocal effect on the two men.

Following the meeting with Marey, Muybridge designed the project of a systematic study of movement in man and animal.[15] Muybridge conceived of this work as being equally valuable to the painter, the sculptor, the photographer, the anatomist and the physiologist. Back in the US, he went looking for a sponsor for this venture. The University of Pennsylvania, in Philadelphia, agreed to support this huge programme. At that time, the provost of the university was a young physician, William Pepper. In order to supervise Muybridge and to guarantee the scientific quality of this vast undertaking, Pepper appointed a university commission. Among its members, two persons deserve a special mention: the painter Thomas Eakins and the neurologist Francis Xavier Dercum.[15,20] Eakins was a professor of drawing and painting at the academy, after having been an instructor in anatomy. He was also a photographer and would himself use the techniques developed by Muybridge and Marey, in order to document movement for artists.[21] Dercum, instructor in nervous diseases at the university, suggested that Muybridge should photograph a series of hospital patients with abnormal gait: locomotor ataxia, lateral sclerosis, chorea, etc. In 1897, Muybridge's monumental work, *Animal Locomotion*, was published by the University of Pennsylvania.[22] It contains about 800 series of sequential photographs of animals and men in motion. The patients with abnormal movements form the eighth volume. The plate "Infantile paralysis: child walking on hands and feet" shows a boy with poliomyelitis. The last picture of the series directly inspired the quadruped figure in Bacon's canvas (Figure 2). This painting dramatically conveys a poignant feeling of distress and pain, as experienced in neurological practice.

Chronophotography and Painting

When Marey met Muybridge in Paris in 1881, he immediately realised the potential of photography as an improvement for his recordings and, from

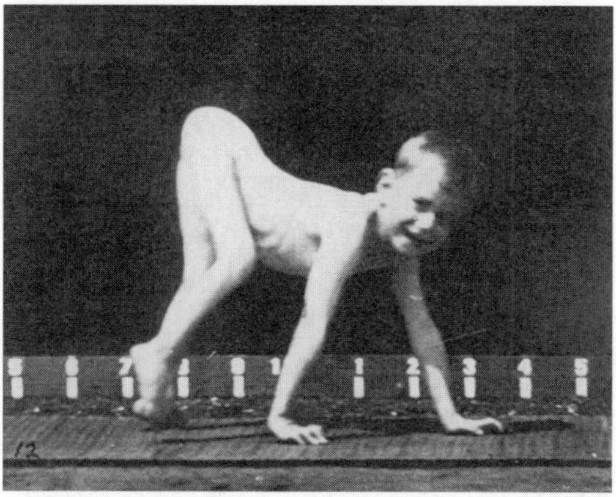

Fig. 2. Eadweard Muybridge, "Infantile paralysis: child walking on hands and feet", detail of plate 539 from *Animal Locomotion* (University of Pennsylvania, Philadelphia, 1887). From the Ecole Nationale Supérieure des Beaux-Arts, Paris.

then on, he adopted photography in his studies. At the same time, Marey was disappointed by the crudeness of Muybridge's method, which yielded a juxtaposition of frozen instantaneous moments extracted from an indivisible flux. Marey aimed at giving, through photography, a reflection of the continuity of movement as was translated in his graphic methods by a stylus on a revolving cylinder. He would therefore develop new tools, both more elegant and more detailed than those of Muybridge.

Marey's photographic investigations were inspired by one unifying principle: one single camera with one single lens.[13,14] First, as early as 1882, he developed a photographic gun, inspired by the method used by the French astronomer Janssen. This apparatus soon evolved into a new camera that could register the successive phases of movement on a fixed plate. Marey named this new method "chronophotography". For the first time, the successive parts of movement appeared on a single photograph. Not yet satisfied, Marey would still simplify the tracings by putting white bands and dots on the subject's black suit. With these photographic diagrams, he could very accurately record the continuous pattern of movement and measure its different mechanical components (Figure 3). The potential of this approach to studying pathological gait was soon investigated by clinicians.[23–25] The most comprehensive study was published by the Hungarian neurologist Jendrassik, who systematically evaluated gait by this technique, in 44 patients with various neurological diseases (Figure 4).[26]

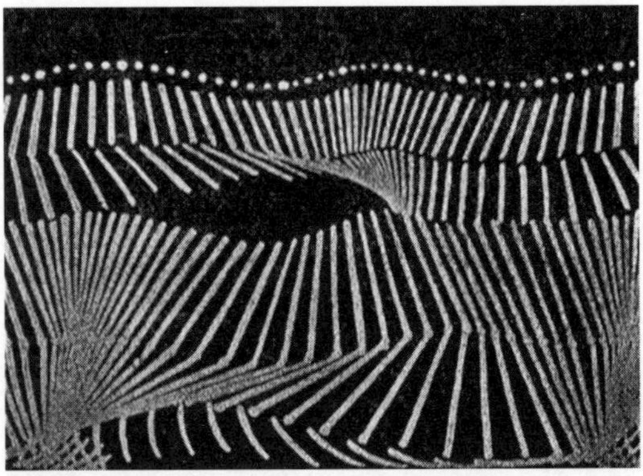

Fig. 3. Etienne-Jules Marey, "Chronophotography of man", in *La Nature*, 29 Sep. 1883 (private collection).

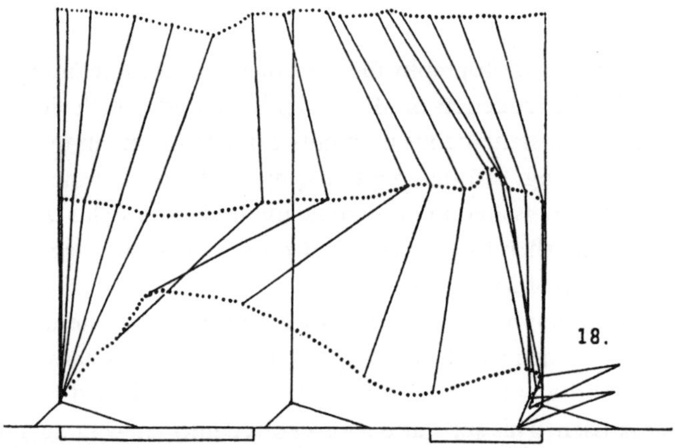

Fig. 4. E. Jendrassik, "Chronophotography of tabetic gait", in *Klinische Beiträge zum Studium der normalen und pathologischen Gangarten. Aus der II. medicinischen Klinik, Deutsches Archiv. f. klin. Medicin*. **LXX**, 81–132 (1901).

Not only were scientists and physicians fascinated by those images which showed more than what was immediately accessible to human vision, but the artists and the general public were taken aback by the images of decomposition of movement.[27] By giving a new dimension to time constraints and a simultaneous presentation of the stages of movement, chronophotography created a new artistic sensibility.[21,28] On the other hand, the excessive reality yielded by chronophotography was held by some to be a distortion of optical truth, and therefore pernicious to art. Indeed, in the frame of naturalism at the end of the 19th century, such abstract images of motion contained in them the germs of a fundamentally anti-naturalist art, which could substitute, by signs, more vital direct observation and recording of nature. They became the schemata of a new visual language for the representation of animated forms.[14]

At the beginning of the 20th century, different art circles studied and discussed Marey's work. The influence of Marey is particularly well documented in the work and statement of the Italian Futurists. This group of artists, led by the poet Marinetti, exalted everything dynamic.[28] In April 1910, they published in Milan a *Manifesto* outlining their programme for the renovation of painting. The parallel between Marey's or Jendrassik's diagrams and the study for *Girl Running on a Balcony* or *Dynamism of a Dog on a Leash*, by Balla, is evident.[14] Both pictures date from 1912.

In the same year, Marcel Duchamp's painting *Nude Descending a Staircase* thoroughly disturbed the Parisian art community. After being withdrawn from the Salon des Indépendants, the painting was sent to New York for the 1913 Armory show, where it was bought.[29] The stroboscopic passage down the stairs is literally dependent on Marey's photographs and diagrams. This direct legacy of Marey has been expressed by Duchamp himself.[30] Duchamp seems to have been introduced to Marey's work by his brother Raymond Duchamp-Villon, who had been a medical student at the Salpêtrière.[14]

One century later, Marey's gait analysis still haunts the imagination in amazing places. The façade of the French pavilion at the Hanover universal exhibition of 2000 was decorated with chronophotography of Marey. In a symbolic line, this choice was emblematic of the leading cultural, economical and strategic issues chosen by France for its promotion in the transition towards a new millennium.

Londe and Richer

The third actor in the developments of chronophotography was Albert Londe, head of the photographic department at the Salpêtrière in Paris.[31] This department, equipped with indoor and outdoor facilities, was one of the most famous annexes of Charcot's service.[32] Many close medical associates of Charcot were involved in this photographic activity. Not surprisingly, it was Paul Richer, probably Charcot's favourite disciple, who showed the greatest interest in this technique. During his whole career, he would stand on the cusp between art and medical science. At the Salpêtrière, he was in charge of the anatomopathological laboratory and the casting workshop. Later, in 1903, he would become professor of artistic anatomy at the Ecole Nationale Supérieure des Beaux-Arts and develop an ambitious programme of scientific aesthetics.[33]

Richer's conception of anatomy was quite revolutionary in the academic artistic circle of Paris. In this approach, he was very close to what Eakins had aimed at in Philadelphia. Richer based his teaching not solely on the classical data obtained from dissection, but also on the study of the exterior shapes of the living human body; not only from a static point of view, but also in a dynamic approach to the body in movement. This was achieved thanks to careful photographic studies made with Londe and Marey. This friendly collaboration is acknowledged by the famous medal of Marey, engraved by Paul Richer. It is a superb summary of the achievements of Marey in recording movement, from graphic methods to chronophotography.[34] Londe built several original models of photoelectric cameras equipped with 9 and later 12 lenses.[35] With these devices, he could obtain series of independent consecutive photographs. Richer used chronophotography not as a means of aesthetic expression, but as a crude document in order to reveal the truth of the human body. Through this method, he analysed the phases of walking and running, and the muscles at play. The first publication of these chronophotographic studies, *Physiologie artistique de l'homme en mouvement*, dealt with normal locomotion. In order to be able to study the muscular action in each body segment, athletes were the subjects of these plates.[36] Later, with Londe, he would also study neurological patients with pathological gait.[37]

Richer was a complete artist. He used every technical approach, in order to illustrate normal and pathological gait. Besides many well-known sketches and drawings, he made a series of extremely lively plaster figures, of athletes as well as of neurological patients.[38]

Gait Analysis and Choreography

An unexpected inspiration from these physiologic and neurologic studies is to be found in choreographic realisations. Two very original and ambitious experiences have recently been created. Actually, they encompass more than dance. Indeed, both examples are multidisciplinary projects, incorporating music, dance, theatre, plastic arts, with the new vocabulary proposed by modern multimedia technologies.

The first example is directly inspired by Muybridge and Marey, who played such a crucial role in the history of art, science and images. These two pioneers, in addition to having the same initials, were exactly contemporary: they were born and died in the same years. This explains the title of the production: *EJM1* and *EJM2*. It is a twin choreographic show created at the Opéra National de Lyon in France, in 1998. The two parts were presented in the course of a single evening. Later they toured separately in a longer version, in such places as Paris, Amsterdam and Tokyo. *EJM1*, "Man walking at ordinary speed", draws on the work of Muybridge and was created for the Belgian choreographic company Charleroi/Danses—Plan K (Figure 5). *EJM2* is a fiction centred on the work of Marey and was created for the French Ballet de l'Opéra National de Lyon. The Belgian choreographer Frédéric Flamand asked the two American architects Elisabeth Diller and Ricardo Scofidio to work with him on this project. As stated by Flamand:

> "Our aim, even though we were inspired by the works of these two 'techno-visionaries', was not simply to deliver a three-dimensional staged representation of the iconography of their universe that is already so familiar the world over. In the course of all the many discussions with Diller and Scofidio ahead of these rehearsals, it became apparent that the works of Muybridge and Marey which encompassed several spheres of learning (science, technology, economics and the history of art) have had a decisive influence on the emergence of the conception of the post-modern body and its ambiguous relationship with machinery."

The Belgian composer Renaud De Putter has expanded his first work on Van Gehuchten's neurological films, and asked a choreographer, Johanne Saunier, to add a dance part with songs. This creates a counterpoint between the filmed pictures, in a complex play of anticipation, duplication and commentaries. De Putter named this production "*Chorée, études de mouvement*", a "musichoreography". As stated by the artist, each of the 13 pieces is a reflection on a particular type of movement. The spoken and sung parts include extracts from Michaux and Fennetaux. Citations from the poet Henri Michaux are used as a comment on the dissociation between the abstract idea of movement and its reality. The same idea is evoked, in the pathological domain, by extracts of Fennetaux, a psychoanalyst affected by Parkinson's disease, who has transmitted in a highly literary text his patient experience.[39] The dance part has been directly inspired by the uncanniness of the pictures of Van Gehuchten. Both the abnormal gait of the patients, and the discretion, emotion and empathy with which those images were filmed, have had a direct creative impact.

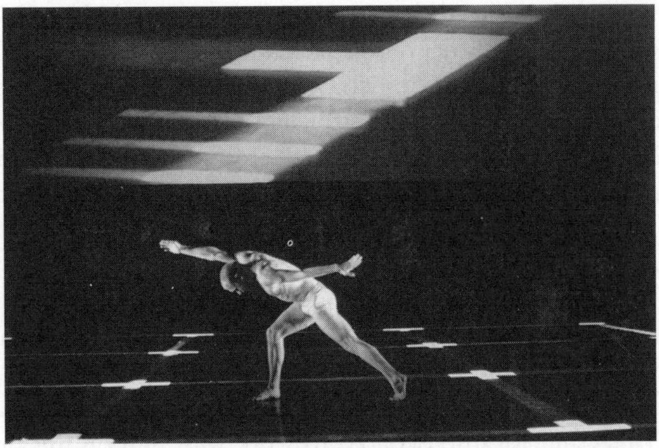

Fig. 5. *EJM1*, "Man walking at ordinary speed", choreography by Frédéric Flamand, scenography by Diller + Scofidio, Compagnie Charleroi/Danses—Plan K, Creation 16 Sep. 1998, Opéra de Lyon.

Whereas *EJM1* and *EJM2* convey the dynamism of normal human movement, in its physiological perfection and as a tool in a modern industrialised world *Chorée, études de mouvement* brings out both the awkwardness associated with gait disorders and the kindness of the caring physician.

Acknowledgements

I thank Laurent Mannoni (Paris), the Ecole Nationale Supérieure des Beaux-Arts (Paris), Renaud De Putter (Brussels), Charleroi/Danses (Brussels), the Centre d'Art Contemporain (Brussels) and the Maison du Spectacle La Bellone (Brussels) for the illustrations and many documents concerning the artistic part of this study, and UCB-Pharma (Belgium) for its support.

References

1. G. Aubert, Arthur Van Gehuchten (1861–1914), *J. Neurol.* **248**, 439–40 (2001).
2. A. Van Gehuchten, *Le système nerveux de l'homme* (Van In, Lierre, 1893).
3. S. Ramon y Cajal, *Recollections of My Life* (The MIT Press, Cambridge, Massachusetts, 1937).
4. G.M. Shepherd, *Foundations of the Neuron Doctrine* (Oxford University Press, New York, 1991).

5. A. Van Gehuchten, *Les maladies nerveuses* (Librairie Universitaire, Louvain, Uystpruyst, A, 1920).
6. P. Van Gehuchten, *Neuro-chirurgie d'hier et d'aujourd'hui. Arthur Van Gehuchten—Souvenirs et documents*, *Revue médicale de Louvain* **11–12**, 1–20 (1950).
7. P. Van Gehuchten, *The Scientific Work of Arthur Van Gehuchten* (Imprimerie des sciences, Bruxelles, 1974).
8. G. Aubert, *Photographie et cinématographie médicales avant 1914: rapports privilégiés avec les neurosciences*, *Bulletin et Mémoires de l'Académie royale de Médecine de Belgique* **155**, 130–140 (2000).
9. A. Van Gehuchten, *Coup de couteau dans la moelle lombaire. Essai de physiologie pathologique*, *Le Névraxe* **XI** 208–232 (1907).
10. A. Van Gehuchten, *La radicotomie postérieure dans les affections nerveuses spasmodiques (modification de l'opération de Foerster)*, *Bulletin de l'Académie royale de Médecine de Belgique* 1–43 (1910a).
11. A. Van Gehuchten, *Over myopatische ziekten. Voordracht met kinematographische lichtbeelden*. Lecture given in Antwerp, Sep. 1910, 1–8 (1910b).
12. *Belgian Cinema. Le Cinéma Belge. De Belgische Film* (The Royal Belgian Film Archive, 1999).
13. L. Mannoni, *Etienne-Jules Marey, la mémoire de l'oeil* (Mazzotta, Cinémathèque français, Paris, 1999).
14. M. Braun, *Picturing Time: The Work of Etienne-Jules Marey (1830–1904)*, The University of Chicago Press, Chicago, London, 1992).
15. A.V. Mozley, Introduction to the Dover edition. In *Muybridge's Complete Human and Animal Locomotion*, ed. A.V. Mozley (Dover, New York, 1979), pp. i–xxxviii.
16. V. Tosi, *Il cinema prima di Lumiere* (Edizioni Radiotelevisione Italiana (ERI), Torino, 1984).
17. J. Russell, *Francis Bacon* (Thames and Hudson, London, 1993).
18. E. Darley and H. Janssen, *Bacon* (Waanders Uitgevers, Zwolle, 2001).
19. E.J. Marey, *Animal Mechanism: A Treatise on Terrestrial and Aerial Locomotion* (Henry S. King and Co., London, 1874).
20. M.R. McVaugh, Francis X. Dercum and animal locomotion, *Caduceus* **3**, 1–35 (1987).
21. J.-L. Daval, *La photographie. Histoire d'un art* (Skira, Paris, 1982).
22. *Muybridge's Complete Human and Animal Locomotion* (Dover, New York, 1979).
23. G. Demenÿ and E. Quénu, *De la locomotion dans l'ataxie locomotrice*, *Comptes Rendus des Séances de l'Académie des Sciences* **108**, 963–4 (1888a).
24. G. Demenÿ and E. Quénu, *Etude de la locomotion humaine dans les cas pathologiques*, *Comptes Rendus des Séances de l'Académie des Sciences* **107**, 1550–64 (1888b).

25. G. Marinesco, *Un cas d'hémiplégie hystérique guéri par la suggestion hypnotique et étudié à l'aide de la chronophotographie*, *La Semaine Médicale* 421 (1899).
26. E. Jendrassik, *Klinische Beiträge zum Studium der normalen und pathologischen Gangarten. Aus der II. medicinischen Klinik*, *Deutsches Archiv. f. klin. Medicin.* **LXX**, 81–132 (1901).
27. A. Scharf, Painting, photography, and the image of movement, *The Burlington Magazine* **104**, 186–195 (1962).
28. J.-L. Prat, Préface. In *L'art en mouvement* (Fondation Maeght, Saint-Paul, 1992), pp. 11–7.
29. Y. Arman, *Marcel Duchamp Plays and Wins* (Marval, Paris, 1984).
30. P. Cabanne, *Entretiens avec Marcel Duchamp* (Pierre Belfond, Paris, 1967).
31. D. Bernard and A. Gunthert, *L'instant rêvé. Albert Londe* (Jacqueline Chambon, Nimes, 1993).
32. C.G. Goetz, M. Bonduelle and T. Gelfand, *Charcot: Constructing Neurology* (Oxford University Press, New York, Oxford, 1995).
33. M. Poivert, *Variété et vérité du corps humain, l'esthétique de Paul Richer*. In *L'art du nu au XIXe siècle, le photographe et son modèle* (Hazan/Bibliothèque Nationale de France, Paris, 1997), pp. 164–75.
34. A.R. Michaelis, E.J. Marey: physiologist and first cinematographer, *Medical History* **10**, 201–3 (1966).
35. A. Londe, *La photographie médicale. Application aux sciences médicales et physiologiques* (Gauthier-Villars et fils, Paris, 1893).
36. P. Richer, *Physiologie artistique de l'homme en mouvement* (Octave Doin, Paris, 1895).
37. A. Londe, *Notice sur les titres et les travaux scientifiques de M. Albert Londe* (A. Gauthier-Villars, Masson et Cie, Paris, 1911).
38. N. Simon-Dhouailly, *La leçon de Charcot. Voyage dans une toile* (Musée de l'Assistance publique, Paris, 1986).
39. M. Fennetaux, *et dès lors ma guerre commença* (Verticales, 1997).

Chapter 8

Epilepsy in Pictorial Art

Bernt A. Engelsen

Introduction

Epileptic seizures represent sudden losses of control. As they are perceived, something or someone takes over and controls behaviour which the individual wants to control himself. Epilepsy is derived from the Greek "*epilambanein*", i.e. "to be seized or attacked",[1] and was re-introduced in medical terminology by Avicenna of Baghdad (980–1037 A.D.).[1,2]

Seizures may appear as loss of consciousness, convulsions, anxiety, confusion, delusion, forced thoughts, hallucinations, religious experiences, autonomic symptoms with sweating, incontinence, etc. Since seizures may appear dramatic and as intrusions, they often need to be interpreted. They occur in people with different personalities, and different religious, ideological or political convictions. Personal interpretation(s) of seizures, therefore, may be loaded with personal values in a situational context and in a broader personal delineation.

Historically, epileptic seizures have mainly been synonymous with convulsions, although early historical sources mention different seizure types such as focal seizures, status epilepticus, etc.[1,3] Non-convulsive seizures of cerebral origin were known to Avicenna[1] but were first described in the late 19th century, and the full semiology of seizures was established in the late 20th century.[4]

The Epileptic as Being Seized or Possessed

For the Babylonians, *antasubba*, a Sumerian term meaning "the falling disease", was a manifestation of demons and ghosts that seized or possessed (*sabatu*) the person.[3] The *sakikku* ("all diseases") stone tablets describe different seizure types and symptom development suggesting that the demons depart the body during the clonic stage of a tonic–clonic seizure.[3] The Hippocratic school and Galen (200 A.D.) tried to explain epilepsy as symptoms of bodily disease, involving the brain.[1] In the Christian religion, the act of Jesus driving out the unclean spirit of the epileptic boy emphasizes that epileptic persons are seized or possessed. Therefore, they need healing through exorcism by Jesus or a priest.

In the prayer book of Duke de Barry, by the Limbourg brothers, from approximately 1410, folio 166 shows a possessed boy held by his mother, as Jesus drives out the unclean spirit, which leaves from the head as a dark dragon.[5,6] The unclean spirit can also leave from the mouth, as shown in an altar piece by Pesellino (in the National Gallery, London[7]), where St. Zenobius of Florence drives out an unclean spirit from the mouth of a woman. The treatment was the same for some mental as well as epileptic symptoms but, in this case, the distorted facial expression suggests an epileptic seizure. As late as 1720, the Bible portrays Jesus driving out an unclean spirit in this way (Figure 1).[8]

The most beautiful picture describing such an exorcism by Jesus is Raphael's well-known painting *The Transfiguration* (Figure 2). It was his last painting and was almost completed before his death on Good Friday in 1520. It is in the Vatican, with a copy in St. Peter's Dome. A painting of the same scene but by another painter is in the Prado Museum, Madrid.

A part of this picture was used by Lennox as a frontispiece in volume 2 of his book *Epilepsy and Related Disorders* (1960).[2] The full painting has been discussed by epileptologists and other doctors.[9–11] There is a peculiar axis between the epileptic boy and Jesus. At the top, Jesus is on Mount Tabor in the company of Moses and Elijah (representing law and promise), and the three disciples Peter, James and John. Jesus is transformed; his face shines like the sun and his clothing becomes as white as the light. At the bottom right a boy in the tonic phase of a seizure is presented by his father to the disciples and Jesus. Whether the boy has or has had a seizure, relieving the spirits through his open mouth, or is crying, is not important for us today.[9] However, I believe that the painting portrays a focal seizure, and that the scene may indeed reflect types of transformations, so that the epileptic seizure is a simile for Christ's transfiguration through suffering, death and resurrection. Many consider the picture Raphael's best.

Historically, Raphael seems to have contributed more to this picture/scene than usual for artists of that time, possibly since he competed with such

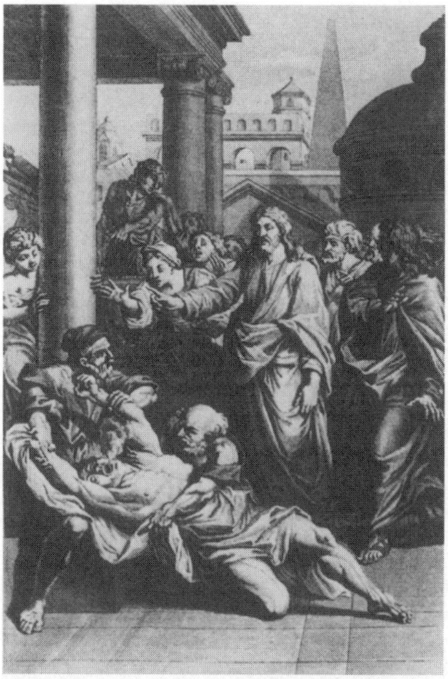

Fig. 1. Possession. Bible from 1720; Jesus driving out an unclean spirit. (Reference 8, quoted from Ref. 1, p. 88.)

established artists as Michelangelo.[10] Since "Rapha-el" means "he/God has healed",[10] some have asked whether his last picture might contain a hidden reference to himself. There is, however, some controversy as to whether the picture with the epileptic boy represents an icon of healing[10] or a simile for Christ's transfiguration.[9]

St. Valentine

People with epilepsy also received empathy in the Church, reflected in the well-known woodcut from 1480 of St. Valentine, the patron saint of epileptics, at a priory in Rufah, Elsass, where people with epilepsy pilgrimaged for a cure.[1,2,12] Bishop Valentine with his typical robe, mitre and crozier (stick) is approached by two pilgrims, while two persons lie outstretched as in a seizure at the bottom right. A pig at the lower left indicates the presence of evil, the Devil, or uncleanliness.

According to Duchet-Suchaux and Pastoreau,[13] the Roman priest Valentine, who was beheaded in 273 A.D., has been confused with another bishop

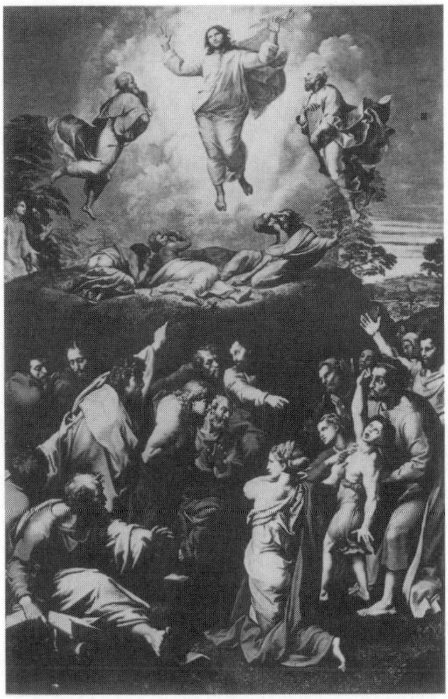

Fig. 2. Raphael, *Transfiguration*. From the Vatican Museum. (Can be viewed at http://www.christusrex.org/www1/vaticano/P5-Pinacoteca.html)

Valentine (of Terni), both celebrated on the 14th of February. A third Valentine, bishop of Rheatia, who lived in the fifth century A.D., was buried close to Merano in the Italian Tyrol, but his body was transported to Passau in Bavaria in the eighth century. This Rheatian Valentine was evoked in Germany against epilepsy.[13]

Lucas Cranach the elder (1472–1540) made a woodcut of St. Valentine with a dramatic depiction of an epileptic in 1509 (Bavarian State Library, Munich).[5] Less well known is his painting of St. Valentine with a "stifter" (i.e. the commissioner of the painting) and most likely an epileptic, from 1502 (Figure 3). It was painted during his brief stay in Vienna, were he met Johannes Cuspinian, the liberal dean of the medical faculty.[14] Most likely, the painting portrays a young person healed of epilepsy, ordering the painting as an act of gratitude. Cranach knew and painted Martin Luther,[14] who supposedly suggested that St. Valentine's name showed his connection with epilepsy. St. Valentine is pronounced "St. *Fallen*tin" in German dialects, giving an immediate association with the falling sickness.[5]

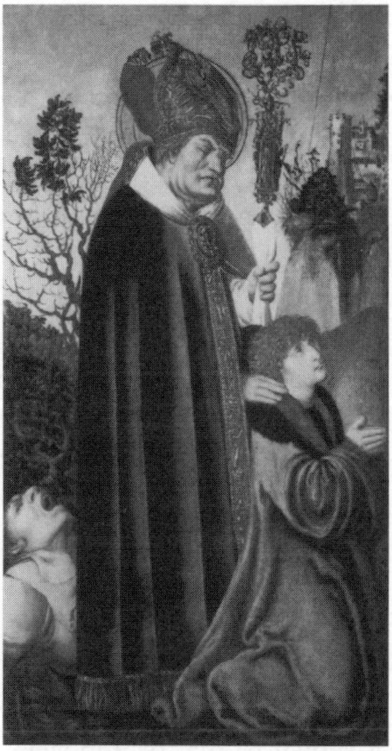

Fig. 3. Black-and-white copy of a painting of St. Valentine with a "stifter". Table 9 in Ref. 14, Vienna. Akademie der Bildende Künste. Gemäldegalerie (Inv.-Nr.549).

Treatment of Epilepsy

Mediaeval treatments were portrayed in medical sources. A picture of cauterization from the book "*Metodus curandi morbus*", by Rondelius of Frankfurt (1592), is shown in both Temkin's and Blakemore's books.[1,7] Usually a hot iron was applied to the occiput, and to the bregma.

The establishment of universities led to more neutral descriptions of medical conditions, including epilepsy, as demonstrated by a person lying outstretched on the ground in a 12th century miniature from "*De Proprietatibus Rerum*", which describes differing states of health.[15]

The belief in ritualistic cures for epilepsy is portrayed in a drawing based upon a lost original drawing by Breughel the elder (1520?–1569). People with epilepsy pilgrimaged to the church of St. John at Moolenbeck, outside Bruxelles, where Breughel had recently moved due to his marriage in 1564. The epileptic persons danced or "were danced" over a bridge, to the sound of bagpipes, on St. John's Day in order to relieve the epilepsy for the following 12 months.

Based on Peter Breughel's drawings from 1564, Hendrik Hondius made two engravings in 1642,[16] representing St. Vitus' dance, ergotism, folly and epileptics.[17,18] In my opinion the women pertain to epilepsy. If the engravings portray choreomanic dancing, they may still refer to epilepsy, since many dancers ended up literally convulsing.[16]

The social aspect of epilepsy was occasionally addressed in pictures or drawings, as when Thomas Harman met the *Counterfet Cranke*, or a beggar simulating an epileptic, in 1566.[1,12] "The pretended epileptic was clad in rags, his face smeared with blood, and he gave the following fraudulent account of himself; 'Sir, say the he, I was born at Leycestar, my name is Nycholas Genings, and I haue had this falling sickness viii. years, and I can get no remedy for the same.' "[1,12] The man was exposed as fraudulent and put in necklock.[1,12]

Post-Renaissance Painters

In 1604–5, Peter Paul Rubens painted a version of the Transfiguration, during his stay in Mantua after a visit to Rome.[19] It shows an epileptic boy in the arms of his father, with an axis similar to that of Raphael's painting, but the boy's and Jesus' eyes do not meet. The outline of the painting has many similarities to Raphael's painting.

Rubens, the great master of drama, movement and epic pictorial storytelling, may have found this human drama of convulsing and being obsessed particularly interesting, as three further pictures of his contain scenes of people with epilepsy (Figure 4(a)).

St. Ignatius of Loyola (healing the possessed)[19,20] reveals his dramatic force, but also probably a personal knowledge of seizures. It is the first painting for an altar in the Jesuit church of Antwerp, finished in 1619. This and the following detail of a second version (Figure 4(b)), which alternated as the altar painting, both reveal an unusually moving and telling presentation.

Both pictures were transferred to Austria in 1776, three years after the brotherhood of Jesus was abolished in the Netherlands. A third version of this event/picture is at St. Ambrosio, Genoa.[19]

These pictures are also interesting since St. Ignatius, in his autobiography, described episodes with visual hallucinations and impaired consciousness, which might suggest epilepsy.[21]

In 1985, I toured some galleries in London and stumbled upon Edward Lear (1812–1888) at the Royal Academy of Art. His many beautiful pictures, including one of Jerusalem at sunrise seen from the Mount of Olives (1859),

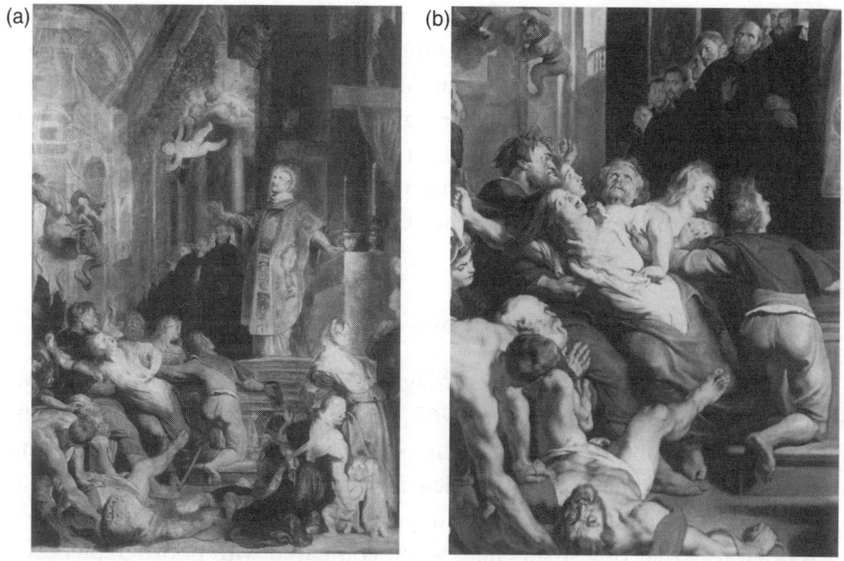

Fig. 4. Peter Paul Rubens. A detail of *The Miracles of St. Ignatius of Loyola*. Originally for the high altar of the Church of the Jesuits in Antwerp. Most likely completed by 1618 (Ref. 20). It is located in the Gemäldegalerie, Kunsthistorisches Museum, Vienna.

made me buy the catalogue, which revealed his epilepsy.[22] Lear was deeply humiliated by his possible temporal lobe epilepsy, which started in early boyhood, and which he was able to conceal from most of his friends. He referred to it in his diaries. It attacked him 10–15 times a month, sometimes several times a day.[23,24] It may have been directly responsible for his sensitivity to the needs of children, whom he addressed in his lovely work with pictures, rhymes and songs.

In 1873, Lear was bedridden with bronchitis at San Remo as he made his first draft for a most personal and sad poem called "Some Incidents in the Life of My Uncle Arly"—in Steven Runciman's words, a brief, transmuted autobiography, with symbols too well disguised for interpretation.[22]

Another historic person supposedly afflicted with epilepsy was Joan of Arc (1410–1431).[17,25,26] In a well-known picture from the Mansell collection.[7] She is portrayed at Domremy reciving angelic instructions. She experienced from 13 years of age episodes with flashes of light, and heard voices, initially from unknown people, later identified as the saints Gabriel, Margaret and Catherine. She also had visions of angels. Based on her own information, symptoms seemed to be triggered by church bells, and history tells us that she often let them ring for a prolonged time.[25,26] Francois Rude's (1784–1855) sculpture of Joan of Arc from 1845, in Musée de Dijon, is more correct, since she is listening to the voices from the right.[27] According to official texts from her trial at Rouen (1431), she stated: "I heard this voice to my right towards the church; rarely do I hear it without it being accompanied by a light. The light comes from the same side as the voice."[25]

Artists with Declared Epilepsy

According to Oliver Sacks, Franco Magnano (1934–?)[28] left his hometown, Pontito, in 1946 and has since 1965 lived in San Francisco. He saw his hometown in ecmnestic hallucinations, or "dreamsights", and started painting scenes from his hometown with a view from his room. The interpretation of the scenes as epileptic seizures was supported by the fact that the perspective was obviously that of a small child, when compared with photographs taken from Pontito's original room.[28]

During the last decade new artists have declared their epilepsy and tried to explain the different impacts on their lives and art, such as the group "From the Storm: Artists with Temporal Lobe Epilepsy",[29] who exhibited during the International Epilepsy Congress in Sydney in 1995.

Jennifer Hall, in her own words, used "the imagery of performances called; out of the body theater, drawn from the world in which I exist during seizures". During these, her visions flourished and she had indescribable smells. Her picture *Transcending* expresses a feeling of leaving the body (Figure 5). The artist Juliane Ahrens called one of her pictures "seizures like a dream".

The Australian photographer Kellyann Geurts portrayed her impressions due to her possible primary generalized epilepsy in the booklet *Of Mind*, presented at the International Epilepsy Congress in Dublin in 1997.[30]

Reflections

No medical disease or symptom can explain artistic temperament, and in artists of historical interest medical diagnoses will often remain uncertain or controversial.

Nevertheless, single works of art may be relevant for understanding thematic or technical aspects and developments in individual artists. For instance,

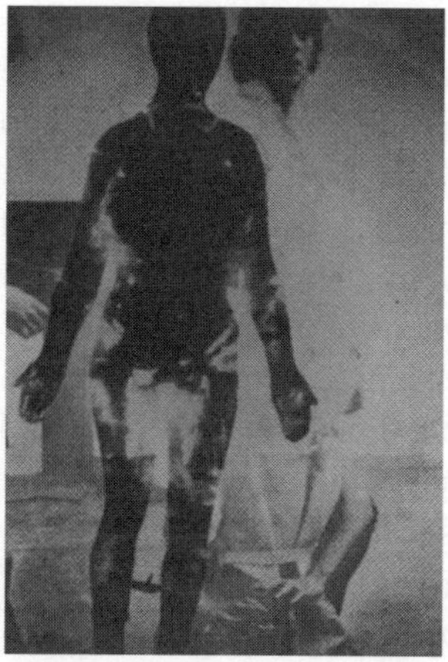

Fig. 5. Jennifer Hall, *Transcending*. Black and white copy of original black, yellow, green and orange picture. Reprinted with permission of the artist, who stated: "The imagery is drawn from the world in which I exist during seizures, with flourishing visions and hallucinations of indescribable smells." (Can be viewed at http://www.dowhile.org/physical/projects/storm/jenhall.html)

the obvious hallucinations of Charles Meryon (1821–1868) which were incorporated into his etchings during psychotic illness in the 1860s[30] show that art may reflect disease.

In a self-portrait of Ernst Kirshner (1880–1938) in military uniform and with a severed right hand, he refers to his rather prolonged nervous problems with functional/nonorganic hand paralysis hindering his artistic work during a few years between 1915 and 1917.[32] His contribution was a conscious artistic declaration.

Migraine aura was an artistic inspiration for Hildegard of Bingen,[33] and possibly also in a few cases for the modern surrealist de Chirico.[34]

Whether van Gogh had temporal lobe epilepsy, manic-depressive disease, both, Meniere's disease, acute intermittent porhyria, or was subject to absinthe intoxication may remain essentially unresolved.[35,36] Most likely he had a temporal lobe epilepsy, as stated officially by a plate at the van Gogh museum in Amsterdam. Seizures may often not evolve out of a vacuum, but in a context. Thus, the cutting of his ear most likely had a deep personal meaning, and was no mere accident or mishap, although related to his epilepsy. In 1882 van Gogh read Emile Zola's book *The Sin of Father Mouret*,[35] about the village vicar who had an ecstatic religious experience, a nervous breakdown, and a subsequent rescue by Brother Archangais. The latter pinched the choirboys, specifically one named Vincent, on their ears. Since Father Mouret made the 15-year-old Albine pregnant, and she took her life, her father cut off Mouret's right ear in rage. Moreover, van Gogh knew Fernando Gallego's painting from 1440—*The Betrayal of Christ*, portraying Simon Peter cutting off the ear of Malcus, the servant of the high priest, by means of a sword. Subsequently Jesus healed the ear by his touching hand.[35]

The surrealist René Magritte altered his style of painting markedly during a brief period of hypomanic excitement,[37] and Ernst Josephson's mental instability was reflected in a well-known portrait of his uncle, from 1893.[38,39]

Thus, disease may influence pictorial art, and pictorial art may reflect disease or health problems as artistic inspiration, such as for Goya[36] and Frida Kahlo.[40]

Considering that approximately 1% of the world's population has or has had epilepsy, it is a comparatively rare topic in pictorial art. Indeed, it is my opinion that artists often do not reveal information about their health. Most biographies of painters and artists lack references to health problems, which are most likely as important to artists as to any other person. However, for some artists an aquired health problem like traumatic epilepsy may simply not influence their art.[41]

The initiatives of Jennifer Hall and other artists at the Do While studio and of artists like Kellyann Geurts should be gratefully acknowledged. They increase interest in and communication about art. Moreover, they are important for a better understanding of epilepsy as a medical problem, but even more so as an integral part of individuals who happen to be artists. In this context it is praiseworthy that Dr. Schachter of Harvard has initiated a calendar exibition by artists with epilepsy, sponsored by a pharmaceutical company.

In conclusion, no artistic disposition can be explained or should be analysed in terms of medical problems. Health problems do, however, most likely affect technical or thematic aspects of at least individual art products in many artists. There are, however, no means by which we can analyse pictorial contents or pictures relevant to epilepsy without knowing the medical facts.

For the sake of epileptology and art, it is important to obtain further contributions concerning artists with epilepsy and epilepsy in art, from various cultures and traditions around the world.

Acknowledgments

The author is grateful to Jennifer Hall, who allowed the inclusion of her work *Transcending* in this chapter. Patricia Pedracini, at the Musée des Beaux-art de Nancy, is thanked for supplying a colour slide copy of Ruben's *Tranfiguration*.

References

1. O. Temkin, *The Falling Sickness*, 2nd ed. (Johns Hopkins University Press, Baltimore, 1971, 1994).
2. W.G. Lennox and M.A. Lennox, *Epilepsy and Related Disorders*, Vol. 1 (Little, Brown & Co., Boston, 1960), p. 40.
3. J.V.K. Wilson and E.H. Reynolds, Text and documents: translation and analysis of a cuneiform text forming part of a Babylonian treatise on epilepsy, *Medical History* **34**, 185–98 (1990).
4. Commission on Classification and Terminology of the International League Against Epilepsy: proposal for revised clinical and electro-encephalographic classification of epileptic seizures, *Epilepsia* **22**, 489–501 (1981).
5. W. Kosenow, *Über Epilepsie und deren Geschichte, Kinderkrankenschwester* **13**, 377–381 (1994).
6. http://www.christusrex.org/www2/berry/f166r.html
7. C. Blakemore, *Mechanics of the Mind* (Cambridge University Press, Cambridge, 1977).
8. O. Rosenthal, *Wunderheilungen und ärztliche Schutzpatrone in der bildenden Kunst* (F.C.W. Leipzig, Vogel, 1925).
9. D. Janz, Epilepsy, viewed metaphysically: an interpretation of the biblical story of the epileptic boy and of Raphael's *Transfiguration*, *Epilepsia* **27**, 316–322 (1986).
10. G. Bendersky, Decoding Raphael's *Transfiguration*, *Pharos* **60**(4), 26–30 (1997).
11. J. De Toledo, R.E. Ramsay and C.A. Marsan, The lunatic and his seizure, *Neurology* **47**, 292–293 (1996).
12. G. Ritter, *Epilepsie und soziales Vorurteil in historischer sicht*, *Psychiat. Neurol. Med. Psychol. (Leipzig)* **25**, 754–61 (1973).
13. G. Duchet-Suchaux and M. Pastoureau, *The Bible and the Saints* (Flammarion, Paris, 1994).
14. W. Schade, *Die Malerfamilie Cranach* (Prisma Verlag, Gütersloh, 1983).
15. R.J. Petrucelli, The rise of the universities. In: A.S. Lyons, and R.J. Petrucelli, *Medicine: An Illustrated History* (Abraham, New York, 1987).
16. N.H. McAlister, The dancing pilgrims at Muelenbeek, *Journal of the History of Medicine* cc: 315–9 (1977).
17. M.R. Trimble, Women and epilepsy: famous and not so famous. In: M.R. Trimble, ed., *Women and Epilepsy* (John Wiley, Chichester, 1991), 263–73.
18. L.C. McHenry Jr. Neurology and art. In: F. Clifford Rose and W.F. Bynum, eds., *Historical Aspects of the Neurosciences* (Raven, New York, 1982), pp. 481–510.
19. J. Burckhardt, *Rubens* (*Erinnerungen aus Rubens*) (Grosse Illustrierte Phaidon-Ausgabe, Vienna, Dr. Horovitz, 1938).
20. F. Baudouin, *Pietro Paolo Rubens* (Bracken, London, 1987).

21. W.G. Lennox and M.A. Lennox, Epileptics of worth and fame. In: W.G. Lennox and M.A. Lennox, *Epilepsy and Related Disorders*, Vol. 2 (Little, Brown & Co., Boston, 1960), pp. 700–11.
22. V. Noakes, *Edward Lear 1812–1888* (Royal Academy of Arts, London, 1985).
23. P. Levi, *Edward Lear: A Biography* (Scribner, New York, 1995).
24. H.M. de Boer, Edward Lear, poet and painter. Abstract. *Epilepsia* **38**(Supp. 13), 281 (1997).
25. E. Foote-Smith and L. Bayne, Joan of Arc, *Epilepsia* **32**, 810–5 (1991).
26. E. LaPlante, *Seized* (Harper Collins, 1993).
27. W. Fleming, *Arts and Ideas*, 8th ed. (Fort Worth, Holt, Rinehart and Winston, 1991).
28. O. Sacks, *An Anthropologist on Mars*, Swedish transl. (Bromberg, Köping, 1995).
29. J. Hall (curator), *From the Storm: Artists with Temporal Lobe Epilepsy* (The Do While Studio, Boston, 1993).
30. K. Geurts, *Of Mind—An Emotional Matter* (Imerge, Victoria, Sandy Point, Australia, 1996).
31. J.L. Yarnall, Meryon's mystical transformations, *Art Bulletin* **61**, 289–300 (1979).
32. D. Elger, *Expressionism: A Revolution in German Art* (Benedikt Taschen, Cologne, 1989).
33. C. Singer, The visions of Hildegard of Bingen. In *From Magic to Science* (Ernst Benn., London, 1928), pp. 199–239.
34. G.N. Fuller and M.V. Gale, Migraine as artistic inspiration, *Br. Med. J.* **297**, 1670–2 (1988).
35. W.N. Arnold, *Vincent van Gogh: Chemicals, Crises, and Creativity* (Birkhäuser, Boston, 1992).
36. A. Neumayr, *Kunst und Medizin* (Pichler Verlag, Wien, 1996).
37. J.E. Gedo, *The Artist and the Emotional World* (Columbia University Press, New York, 1996).
38. E. Blomberg, *Ernst Josephson. Hans Liv* (Wahlström og Widstrand, Stockholm, 1951), Swedish.
39. P. Sandblom, *Creativity and Disease*, 7th ed. (Marion Boyars, New York, 1992).
40. A. Kettenmann, *Frida Kahlo 1907–1954: Pain and Passion* (Benedikt Taschen, Cologne, 1992).
41. E.O. Hjelle, *Rolf Nesch* (Gyldendal Norsk Forlag, Oslo, 1998), Norwegian.

Chapter 9

Brain Mapping in Musicians

Michael E. Charness and Gottfried Schlaug

Introduction

Several studies have shown that musicians differ from nonmusicians in brain structure and function. These differences could be due to the intense motor and musical training that musicians typically undergo; alternatively, some individuals may be self-selected to become musicians, because they possess the necessary brain structure for acquiring and executing skillful, bimanual motor tasks. Musicians develop their remarkable skills through long, regular practice, often beginning in early childhood. Brain mapping in musicians therefore provides a glimpse of the central nervous system processes that underlie the development of skill. In this chapter, we explore the effects of musical training on the unique structural and functional organization of musicians' brains. We also review a nascent literature on the existence of critical periods for the development of musical skills. Finally, we examine changes in the functional organization of the brain associated with the acquisition and loss of advanced musical skills, focusing on a disorder of skill—task-specific dystonia.

Nature and Nurture: The Development of Absolute Pitch

Absolute pitch (AP) is the ability to identify the pitch of any tone in the absence of a musical context or a reference tone. AP musicians can accurately name an electronically generated pure tone, a note played on a musical instrument, or a car horn. AP develops almost exclusively in musicians who begin training at age 7 or younger and almost never develops in musicians who begin training after age 11. However, only a small proportion of musicians with early training develop AP, which argues for the involvement of additional factors besides early musical training in the expression of this ability. One of those factors could be genetic predisposition, because there is evidence for a higher-than-expected prevalence of AP in family members of AP musicians, even if one controls for early exposure to music.[1–3] One other factor could be a unique configuration of brain structure and function that enables only the possessor to acquire AP. Profita *et al.*[1] identified pedigrees of AP musicians in which the pattern of inheritance appeared to be autosomal dominant with incomplete penetrance, the degree of penetrance influenced by early training. This study highlights the importance of controlling for early music training in examining the genetic aspects of AP. Taken together, these observations suggest that the development of AP is dependent on both a heritable factor and the commencement of musical training during a critical period of development.

The identification and naming of musical pitch requires both auditory and language processing. One region that might be involved in these tasks is the planum temporale (PT). The left PT lies within the superior temporal gyrus, adjacent to Heschl's gyrus and Wernicke's area. Located at the juxtaposition of language and auditory processing regions, the PT is ideally positioned to play a role in pitch identification. Right-handers typically show a leftward dominance of the PT, and this leftward PT asymmetry has been taken to be a structural marker of hemispheric dominance for language.[4] The PT asymmetry is established very early during development.[5] Schlaug *et al.*[6] used structural MRI to measure the surface area of the PT in a group of musicians and nonmusician controls. The musicians as a group had a stronger leftward PT asymmetry than the nonmusicians; however, the group difference was explained by a subgroup of musicians with AP. In a subsequent study, Keenan *et al.*[7] compared subgroups of AP and non-AP musicians with similar early music training; only the AP musicians showed extreme leftward PT asymmetry. Furthermore, Keenan *et al.*[7] found that a decrease in the surface area of the right PT, rather than an increase in the surface area of the left PT, determined the leftward asymmetry of the PT. Zatorre *et al.*[8] confirmed the finding of leftward asymmetry of the PT in a small group of AP musicians compared to a large group of unselected controls. These findings indicate a role for PT asymmetry in the development of AP. It seems likely that the increased leftward PT asymmetry is a requirement for the development of AP, rather than a consequence of early musical training.[7]

Critical periods also exist for the acquisition of accent-free language[9] or for the learning of the characteristic songs of a variety of avian species.[10] In songbirds, singing causes the release of the brain-derived neurotrophic factor in brain regions that subserve birdsong, which in turn leads to the increased survival of new neurons in these brain regions.[11] This is an example of musical experience altering the function as well as the structure of the developing nervous system. There is as yet no information on what structural change might occur in the human brain after ages 7–11 that hinders the acquisition of AP.

Whereas a leftwardly asymmetric PT appears to be required for the development of AP, the task of listening to pitches activates other brain regions as well. Zatorre *et al.*[8] compared brain activation while listening to tones versus noise to investigate differences in auditory processing between AP and non-AP musicians. Both groups of musicians activated the bilateral superior temporal gyrus while listening to tones versus noise or while discriminating tone pairs at an interval of a major or minor third. In listening to tones versus noise, the AP musicians showed a strong and unique activation of the left posterior dorsolateral frontal cortex, a brain region implicated in associative learning, perhaps because they were associating the tones with their note names. In contrast, during interval analysis, a task done equally well by the two groups, both AP and non-AP musicians activated the left posterior dorsolateral frontal cortex, consistent with the naming aspect of the task, but only the non-AP musicians activated the right inferior frontal cortex. Activation of the right inferior frontal cortex might therefore reflect the retention of pitches in working memory to allow their comparison, a process that the AP musicians could omit by simply remembering the names of the test notes. More recently, Ohnishi *et al.*[12] were able to demonstrate the involvement of the PT in music perception in trained musicians, with particularly strong PT activation observed in AP musicians.

Effect of Musical Training on the Functional Organization of the Auditory Cortex

Musical experience may influence the functional organization of the auditory cortex. Pantev *et al.*[13] used magnetic source imaging (MEG) to study the auditory evoked responses to piano and pure tones in a group of AP musicians, relative pitch (RP) musicians, and controls. MEG uses sensitive magnetic detection devices to record magnetic impulses from the cortical surface, and the strength of the dipole moment is proportional to the degree of synchrony of neuronal activation and to the number of neurons activated. Most of the musicians played the piano, either as a primary or as a secondary instrument. The current dipole in the auditory cortex was significantly larger in response to piano tones than to pure tones in the RP and AP musicians, but not in the controls. The strength of the dipole moment was inversely correlated with the age at inception of musical training. To test whether these changes are instrument-specific, Pantev *et al.*[14] used MEG to evaluate auditory responses in violinists and trumpet players. Violin timbres activated larger areas of the auditory cortex than pure tones in violinists, but not in trumpet players. Conversely, trumpet timbres produced larger activations than pure tones in trumpet players, but not in violinists. These findings are consistent with the hypothesis that early musical training causes instrument-specific changes in the functional organization or structure of the auditory cortex.

The auditory cortex also exhibits rapid adaptation in response to changes in the acoustic environment.[15] When musicians listened for 3 h to music that was engineered to remove frequencies of 1 kHz, auditory cortical responses to 1 kHz tones were subsequently diminished. The response reverted to normal the following day. These data suggest that the auditory system is capable of both long-term and short-term plastic responses. This dynamic neural plasticity may enable rapid adaptation to changes in the acoustic environment. The repetition of certain acoustic experiences, particularly in the setting of early musical training, may lead not only to short-term but also to long-term functional or structural changes associated with the development of musical skills.

Acquisition of Motor Skill in Musicians

Functional Reorganization of the Brain

Like auditory experience, motor learning in humans is associated with both short-term and long-term plasticity in the brain, each in turn associated with different patterns of brain activation.[16–18] Initial learning of a motor task engages the sensorimotor cortex and the prefrontal cortex. Within hours, strengthening and stabilization of the motor program is associated with a shift in regional brain activation to the premotor area (PMA), cerebellum, and posterior parietal cortex. Using transcranial magnetic stimulation (TMS), Pascual-Leone *et al.*[19] showed that corticomotor output is potentiated during the learning of a five-finger scale. Interestingly, even imagining the movement of the five fingers led to a measurable increase in skill and an enlargement of the cortical regions subserving finger movements. Expansion of areas of cortical activation subserving movement was also observed using fMRI.[20] Reversible changes in the motor representation of thumb movements can be demonstrated by TMS after 15–30 min of training and, in a few cases, in as little as 5–10 min.[21] This rapid and reversible plasticity may be an antecedent of the more permanent changes in cortical representation that characterize motor learning.[17,18,20] The cortical representation of skilled movement is highly dynamic, and the timing of testing is therefore important. For example, the cortical representation of the first dorsal interossous muscle in Braille readers was significantly larger after reading for 6 h than before reading after a two-day break.[22]

The observation that motor training provokes long-term changes in brain regions that subserve movement predicts that patterns of brain activation induced by finger movements will differ between instrumental musicians and nonmusicians. It is still an open question whether the execution of overlearned motor skills requires more activation of the motor cortex and less activation of motor control regions or vice versa in musicians compared with controls. Results from motor learning experiments do suggest a specialized role for the primary motor cortex in motor learning. Jancke *et al.*[23] observed a marked decrease in activation of the presupplementary motor area (SMA), the cingulate motor area (CMA), and a mild decrease in the primary motor cortex (M1) during a tapping task in a group of two pianists compared with a larger group of controls. They concluded that extensive motor training in musicians leads to greater efficiency of cortical neurons that control movement. Krings *et al.*[24] used fMRI to study the network of motor activation in four pianists and four control subjects. Brain imaging was obtained during six 32 s epochs of movement alternating with rest (total of 3 min). The task, a self-paced, complex pattern of alternate tapping of the thumb to various fingers of the dominant right hand (5-4-3-5-4-2-5-3-2-4-3-2), was practiced prior to scanning to avoid learning effects during the course of the scan. The pianists had a higher rate of tapping than the nonmusicians and rated the tapping task as easier, although performance accuracy did not differ between the two groups. Compared to the nonmusicians, the pianists showed a significantly smaller number of activated voxels for the primary sensorimotor cortex (SM1), SMA, and PMA. The correlation of activated voxels among different brain regions did not differ between the two groups, suggesting that the two groups activated similar neural networks. The authors concluded that the advanced training of the pianists allowed them to control complex finger movements through activation of a smaller number of neurons than in nonmusicians. These findings differ somewhat from those of Karni *et al.*[20] who found that learning of a complex motor task increased activation of M1. The difference may reflect subtle differences in test protocols and image acquisition.

The previous experiments indicate that brain activation differs between musicians and nonmusicians during finger movements. A second important question is whether brain activation differs between instrumental musicians and nonmusicians during the learning of a new motor task. During the first 7 min of task-training, tapping in pianists caused a smaller activation of ipsilateral M1 and secondary motor areas (PMA, bilateral SMA, and cerebellum) than in nonmusicians.[25] Activation of contralateral M1, SMA, and bilateral PMA declined during 35 min of training in nonmusicians. Pianists tapped faster than nonmusicians, and this might have contributed to an increase in contralateral M1 activation during training.[26] These data indicate that previous motor training influences the pattern of brain activation during the learning of a new motor task.

The manual skills of musicians are dependent on the integration of somatosensory and motor systems. Elbert *et al.*[27] used MEG to study the somatosensory representation of the digits in string players. The demands placed on the left and right hands of string players are highly asymmetric. Very little fine movement of the fingers is required for the right hand, which holds the bow. In contrast, the four fingers of the left hand are in constant motion on the fingerboard, whereas the thumb is relatively quiescent. The somatosensory representation of the second and fifth digits (D2 and D5) were significantly larger in the left hand of string players than in nonmusicians. The magnitude of the dipole moment for the left fingers was inversely correlated with the age at which musical lessons began. There were no such differences between musicians and nonmusicians for the left thumb or the right hand. Taken together, these data indicate that unique patterns of hand and finger activity in musicians shape the functional organization of the nervous system, particularly when musical training begins early.

Structural Alterations in the Nervous System Associated with Musical Training

The previous studies indicate that the highly developed skills of musicians are associated with task-specific differences in patterns of brain activation, particularly when training begins at an early age. Because brain development is influenced by neuronal activity, it is reasonable to ask whether musical training also leads to differences in brain morphology. Studies so far have focused on brain regions that are involved in motor learning and the integration of bimanual motor activities. The corpus callosum interconnects the two cerebral hemispheres and plays an important role in the coordination of bimanual tasks. Because development of the corpus callosum continues throughout childhood and adolescence,[28] it is reasonable to ask whether the morphology of the corpus callosum is influenced by early bimanual activity. Schlaug *et al.*[29] used structural MRI to measure the cross-sectional area of a mid-sagittal section of the corpus callosum in a group of 21 musicians who began training before the age of 7, 9 musicians who began after the age of 7, and 30 nonmusicians. The anterior half of the corpus callosum was significantly larger in musicians with early training than in musicians with late training or in nonmusicians. These data provide evidence that early musical training might be responsible for the structural differences in the mid-sagittal size of the corpus callosum. The cerebellum is involved in the learning and control of complex sequences of movement. The absolute and percent volume of the cerebellum in male musicians was 5% larger than that of male nonmusicians, but there was no difference in overall brain volume.[30] A small sample size may have precluded the observation of significant differences between female musicians and controls. The sample groups were not analyzed according to the age at which musical training began, so it is not clear whether the differences in cerebellar volume were a consequence of early musical training. Nonetheless, animal studies provide abundant evidence that rearing in an enriched environment is associated with an increase in neuronal numbers.[31] Similarly, many animal studies have shown an increase in synapses, glial cells, and capillaries in animals undergoing long-term programs of motor learning.[32]

Musicians show less motor asymmetry than nonmusicians in learning a tapping task.[33] Musicians can tap the nondominant hand more rapidly than nonmusicians, and this difference is greatest in those musicians with early musical training. Amunts *et al.*[34] measured the intrasulcal length of the posterior precentral gyrus (ILPG) as a gross anatomical marker of primary motor cortex size in musicians and in nonmusicians. The ILPG was less asymmetrical in musicians than in nonmusicians. This increased symmetry in musicians was found primarily in motor regions controlling hand movements and it was due to a larger ILPG of the nondominant hand. The overall size of this motor cortex marker correlated with the age of commencement of music training. Overall these data indicate that early musical training alters both the functional organization and the structure of the brain.

Focal Hand Dystonia, a Disorder of Skill

Dystonia is a movement disorder characterized by involuntary, sustained contraction of muscles, resulting in tremor, repetitive movements, or abnormal postures. Focal dystonias affect a single body region, such as the face (Meige syndrome), neck (torticollis), or upper extremity (writer's cramp or musician's cramp). Task-specific dystonias or occupational cramps are involuntary movements elicited by the performance of skilled, stereotyped, repetitive movement. In some musicians, focal hand dystonia may be elicited only by the performances of a particular sequence of musical notes. Though unable to play music at the most elementary level, these musicians may function normally in all other respects. In others, focal dystonia may invade all aspects of musical performance as well as writing and daily activities. Task-specific dystonia is a disorder of skill. As such, this focal dystonia may be associated with or result from the cerebral plasticity that accompanies the acquisition of skilled movement. The rapid repetitive hand movements involved in the acquisition of skill may independently contribute to the development of focal dystonia by producing peripheral nerve or soft tissue injury,[35] by activating sensory pathways that influence motor programs,[36,37] or by changing the local balance of inhibition and excitation.

Focal dystonia often arises when a long-established motor program is changed to compensate for weakness or pain. The new, dystonic motor program is extremely persistent and difficult to eradicate. Focal dystonia tends to worsen and stabilize without involving other body segments. Only rarely is there spontaneous remission. In many instances, focal dystonia significantly limits or ends the careers of professional musicians.

We observed a high prevalence of nerve entrapment and soft tissue injury among 73 cases of focal dystonia in 69 musicians.[35] The study cohort included international artists, symphony musicians, freelance musicians, students, and amateurs. All of the patients were highly skilled performers and many of the professionals were at the apex of their careers. There was evidence of nerve entrapment ipsilateral to the dystonia in 40 of 73 cases (55%). We identified 28 patients with focal dystonia and clinical or physiological evidence of ulnar neuropathy. Symptoms of ulnar nerve entrapment included medial elbow pain in 10 patients (36%), numbness or tingling in the ulnar territory in 14 (50%), and weakness of the little and ring fingers in 13 (46%). All 28 patients had mild weakness in ulnar-innervated muscles and 21 of 28 (75%) had findings that localized the ulnar nerve entrapment to the elbow region. In contrast, sensory abnormalities on clinical examination were observed in only 4 of 28 patients (14%). Using the near nerve recording technique, 27 (63%) patients with dystonia and ulnar neuropathy had electrophysiologic findings that localized the ulnar neuropathy to the elbow, while 20 of 27 (74%) had denervation or prolonged minimal conduction velocity.

The presence of ulnar neuropathy strongly predicted the pattern of the dystonic movements. Playing-induced flexion of D4,5 was evident in 24 of

28 (86%) cases of dystonia with ulnar neuropathy and only 8 of 45 (18%) cases without ulnar neuropathy. Conversely, ipsilateral ulnar neuropathy was diagnosed in 24 of 31 (77%) patients with dystonic flexion of D4,5. These findings suggest that ulnar neuropathy predisposes to the development of a specific focal dystonia involving flexion of the fourth and fifth proximal interphalangeal joints.

How might weakness in ulnar-innervated muscles initiate a dystonia mediated by the median-innervated superficial flexors? Focal dystonia develops predominantly in highly skilled musicians and arises rarely during the acquisition of the skill. Therefore, the plastic neural changes that underlie the acquisition of skilled movement may also contribute to the development of focal dystonia. An additional mechanism may be related to the muscle substitutions that sustain musical performance in the presence of neuropathic weakness. In musicians with isolated ulnar neuropathy, mild weakness of the lumbricals and interossei impairs flexion–extension movements at the fourth and fifth metacarpophalangeal joints. To compensate for this weakness, many musicians recruit the median-innervated superficial flexors to activate flexion–extension movements from the fourth and fifth proximal interphalangeal joints. The focal dystonia that sometimes develops in patients with ulnar neuropathy appears to be an involuntary, maladaptive, and exaggerated version of this compensatory maneuver. The development of dystonic flexion of D4,5 in musicians with ulnar neuropathy may therefore be a specific occurrence of a focal dystonia resulting from the modification of a stable motor program.[38] Consistent with these findings, Straube *et al.*[39] described the development of writer's cramp during recovery from a brachial plexus lesion in a patient with hereditary susceptibility to pressure palsy.

Ulnar neuropathy may also predispose to focal dystonia by inducing cortical reorganization. Section of the median nerve in adult monkeys causes an expansion of somatosensory cortical representation of the radial and ulnar cutaneous territory into the territory of previous median representation.[40] Injury to the facial nerve, a purely motor nerve, results in enlargement of the cortical representation of the hand into regions that normally subserve movement of the face.[41] Perhaps analogously, ulnar nerve injury increases the cortical representation of the median superficial flexors, predisposing to flexion dystonia of D4,5.

Electrophysiological studies in patients with isolated ulnar neuropathy support the hypothesis that ulnar nerve injury predisposes to the development of focal hand dystonia. In a simple task of repetitive tapping of D4, 9 of 10 patients with uncomplicated ulnar neuropathy exhibited a pattern of prolonged bursting activity in antagonist muscles similar to that of 7 patients with focal dystonia.[42] Girlanda *et al.*[43] also observed loss of alternating bursting in FDS4 and EDC4 in 11 of 12 patients with uncomplicated ulnar neuropathy. These patients also demonstrated reduced inhibition of the H reflex, consistent with an increase in spinal cord excitability, but there was no concomitant increase in the excitability of the motor cortex, as determined by TMS. Thus, simple nerve entrapment causes two physiological abnormalities that are also observed in patients with focal dystonia: cocontraction of agonists and antagonists (44) and reduced reciprocal inhibition of the H-reflex.[45–47]

The absence of increased cortical excitability in patients with ulnar neuropathy suggests that additional physiological events are required to trigger the progression from ulnar nerve entrapment to focal dystonia. Genetic factors may play a role, but have yet to be identified. Some first degree relatives of patients with generalized dystonia develop only focal dystonia; however, the great majority of musicians with focal dystonia do not have a positive family history, and those whom we have examined are negative for the GAG deletion on the DYT1 gene.[48] We did identify two sisters, a violinist and a flutist, with focal dystonia, so it is conceivable that a different gene mutation contributes to this predisposition.

Pathophysiology of Focal Limb Dystonia

Until recently, focal dystonia was regarded by some to be a psychological disorder. There is no evidence that psychiatric disorders are more common in patients with focal dystonia than in normal controls, and, as mentioned, focal dystonia may be the sole manifestation of genetic disorders that more commonly cause generalized dystonia. Physiological studies of patients with focal dystonia provide evidence for alterations in the planning of movement, the anatomical organization of sensorimotor function, and the integration of sensory information that guides motor processes.[45,46,49–51] In many instances, these physiological abnormalities are bilateral, despite the fact most focal limb dystonias are unilateral. The pathophysiology of focal dystonia, as determined by physiological and imaging studies, is presented below.

Sensory Contributions to Focal Dystonia

Sensory input to the resting limb of patients with focal dystonia can provoke dystonic limb contraction.[52–54] Vibration-induced muscle contraction in patients with focal dystonia was diminished by small doses of locally injected lidocaine, which reduce muscle spindle afferent activity without causing paralysis. Musicians with focal dystonia also show evidence of abnormal central nervous system integration of muscle spindle 1a afferent activity. Muscle vibration in the resting, silent flexor carpi radialis caused facilitation of flexor carpi radialis motor evoked potentials (MEPs) and inhibition of extensor carpi radialis MEPs in normal musicians and normal nonmusicians following cortical activation by TMS.[55] These changes were reduced in musicians with focal dystonia. Murase *et al.*[56] measured median-evoked SEPs at rest, just prior to hand movement and during hand movement in normal controls and patients with writer's cramp. In normal controls, the median-evoked SEP was attenuated over the frontal regions prior to the initiation of hand movement, consistent with gating of sensory input during the intent to move. Gating of the SEP was absent in patients with writer's cramp. These data suggest that writer's cramp is associated with abnormal gating of sensory input during the planning of movement, but not during movement itself. The authors speculated that sensory tricks may alleviate dystonia in some patients by normalizing sensory gating.

Transcutaneous stimulation (50 Hz) over the biceps selectively activates Ia muscle fiber spindle afferents, resulting in elbow flexion. Tracking of the stimulated arm, but not identification of limb position, was reduced in patients with focal limb and cervical dystonia compared with normal controls, suggesting that there was an abnormality in the perception of limb movement rather than in the perception of limb position.[57] Yoneda *et al.*[58] found that perception of the tonic vibration reflex was reduced at multiple levels of the nervous system in patients with focal dystonia. These studies provide evidence for widespread abnormalities in the processing of muscle spindle afferents in focal dystonia.

Processing of simultaneous sensory input is also altered in focal dystonia. Tanizzi *et al.*[59] studied the somatosensory evoked potentials (SEPs) at multiple levels of the nervous system in response to separate and simultaneous stimulation of the median and ulnar nerves. In normal subjects, the evoked responses to simultaneous stimulation of these two nerves is less than the arithmetic sum of the stimulation of each nerve, reflecting lateral surround inhibition during sensory processing. The magnitude of the suppression in SEPs during dual nerve stimulation was less in patients with generalized dystonia than in normal controls, particularly for cortical SEPs. These findings suggested that there is a deficit in lateral surround inhibition within the somatosensory system of dystonic patients. The authors speculated that the motor system in dystonic patients transforms poorly filtered sensory input into exaggerated motor responses.

Mapping Sensory Processes in Focal Dystonia

Tempel and colleagues[60,61] studied activation of the primary sensorimotor cortex during vibration of the hand using PET in 11 patients with focal dystonia and 18 normal controls. Vibration of the affected or the unaffected hand produced significantly less activation of the contralateral sensorimotor cortex and SMA in the dystonic patients than in the normal controls. Vibration produced dystonic muscle contraction in 6 of the 11 dystonic patients; however, vibration with voluntary cocontraction of the same muscle groups in normal controls produced an increase, rather than a decrease, in sensorimotor cortical activation,[60] suggesting that muscle contraction alone is not responsible for the reduced activation of sensorimotor cortex. In a related study, Feiwell *et al.*[62] found that activation of the primary somatosensory cortex by unilateral facial stimulation was reduced in patients with blepharospasm. Somatosensory cortex activation was also diminished in response to vibration of the normal hands in these patients, providing further evidence for a generalized abnormality of sensorimotor integration in focal dystonia. Because inhibitory synaptic activity is associated with an increase in regional cerebral metabolism, these data are consistent with physiological studies showing reduced cortical inhibition in patients with focal dystonia.

Frank distortions in the cortical representations of the digits have also been identified by brain imaging in patients with focal dystonia. Bara-Jiminez and colleagues[63] used somatosensory evoked responses to map the cortical S1 representation of the digits in 6 patients with focal dystonia of the hand, including 1 musician. The electrophysiological data were mapped onto MR images and analyzed. In 6 control subjects, sensory stimulation of right D1 mapped to the left postcentral gyrus at a location that was an average of 12.7 mM inferior and lateral to that of right D5. In the dystonic patients, the average distance between D1 and D5 representations was greatly reduced at 6.5 mm, and in half the patients, the position of D1 and D5 were inverted. The magnitude of this abnormality was positively correlated with the severity of the dystonia. It is not clear whether this distortion of the sensory homunculus is congenital or acquired, but the data are consistent with observations in monkeys that alterations of sensory input can lead to a reorganization of the sensory cortex.[37,64] Indeed, patients with focal hand dystonia showed a defect in the discrimination of temporally and spatially related sensory input to the hand.[50,51]

Elbert *et al.*[65] used MEG to map the cortical sensory representation of the digits in 7 musicians with focal dystonia, in 8 nondystonic musicians, and in 9 normal controls. The distance between the cortical representation of digit pairs was smaller in the dystonic patients than in the nondystonic musicians or in the normal controls, consistent with the findings of Bar-Jiminez *et al.* (above). In contrast, the topographic localization of each digit was not reordered. Interestingly, 4 of 7 dystonic musicians showed fusion of the cortical digital representation contralateral to the nondystonic hand. The investigators speculated that fusion of the sensory fields of the digits results from repetitive movements and contributes to the genesis of task-specific dystonia in musicians. In some musicians with unilateral dystonia, fusion of the sensory fields of the digits is present bilaterally, implying that this change predisposes to and antedates focal dystonia.

Lenz and Byl[66] mapped sensory fields of the ventral caudal *thalamic nucleus* in 11 patients undergoing stereotactic thalamotomy for dystonia. Fifteen patients undergoing similar surgery for essential tremor served as controls. The proportion of receptive and projective fields subserving multiple body parts was greater in the dystonic patients than in patients with essential tremor. This study confirmed the presence of an abnormal sensory map in patients with focal dystonia, and extended the area of abnormal sensory representation to include the sensory thalamus.

Motor System Abnormalities

Cocontraction of agonist and antagonist muscles is a hallmark of focal limb dystonia, consistent with a loss of Sherringtonian reciprocal inhibition.[45,46] Chen *et al.*[47] showed that reciprocal inhibition of the H reflex is reduced, in both the dystonic and the nondystonic hand. They postulated a generalized predisposition to task-specific dystonia in dystonic patients, which might account for the increased incidence of focal dystonia after switching to use of the nonaffected hand.

One apparent locus for the loss of reciprocal inhibition is the motor cortex. Siebner *et al.*[67] used repetitive TMS (rTMS) to study the excitability of the motor cortex in patients with focal hand dystonia and in controls. They found that rTMS caused a significant increase in motor unit potentials in dystonic patients, but a significant decrease in controls. They concluded that corticomotor excitation is significantly greater in patients with focal hand dystonia than in controls. Using TMS, Ikoma *et al.*[68] also found evidence of increased cortical excitability in patients with task-specific dystonia. Increased cortical excitability may result from reduced intracortical inhibition, as suggested by physiological studies using a paired pulse TMS paradigm.[69] Subthreshold, low frequency rTMS of the motor cortex diminished the increased excitability of the motor cortex in patients with writer's cramp and produced a concomitant, transient improvement in writing.[70] The observation of increased cortical excitability in patients with focal dystonia is interesting in light of similar findings in some studies of nondystonic subjects after the learning of new motor skills (above).

Patients with focal hand dystonia also show alterations in the organization of the motor cortex. Using TMS, Byrnes *et al.*[71] mapped the corticomotor projections to APB and FDI in patients with writer's cramp and in normal controls. Patients with writer's cramp showed displacement of the maps for the APB and FDI, which normalized transiently following treatment with botulinum toxin. Abnormal maps were sometimes evident in clinically unaffected muscles, consistent with a generalized abnormality of motor control in patients with focal dystonia. The magnitude of displacement of the corticomotor maps was a function of the duration and severity of the focal dystonia. The plasticity of cortical maps following botulinum toxin injection suggests that the abnormal cortical maps arise from altered sensory feedback from dystonic muscles.

There is also evidence that focal dystonia is associated with abnormalities in the planning of movement. Deuschl *et al.*[72] studied movement-related cortical potentials in a self-paced finger abduction task. The amplitude of the early portion of the negative slope peak, the Bareitschaft potential, was reduced in patients with simple or dystonic writer's cramp. Because this activity precedes electromyographic activity, the authors concluded that patients with focal dystonia have a deficiency in motor cortex activation just prior to movement.

Mapping Motor System Abnormalities in Focal Dystonia

Only one study has employed brain imaging during playing-induced dystonia in musicians. Pujol *et al.*[73] used a specially constructed guitar that could be played in the MRI scanner. Importantly, their patients practiced with this modified instrument so that playing would reliably induce dystonia. They studied 5 guitarists with playing-induced hand dystonia and 5 normal guitarists. Playing the guitar in the normal subjects contralaterally activated the somatosensory cortex and bilaterally activated the PMA, SMA, and posterior parietal lobe. In contrast, dystonia inducing guitar playing resulted in a greatly reduced activation of the PMA and a significantly increased activation of the primary sensorimotor cortex. There was also a trend toward a reduced activation of the SMA and posterior parietal lobe during dystonic playing. These findings are in contrast to those of Caballo-Bauman *et al.*,[74] who used fMRI to study patients with writer's cramp. Compared to writing in normal subjects, writing-induced dystonia decreased activation of the primary somatosensory cortex and enhanced activation of the PMA and SMA. These discrepant findings may reflect differences in the motor organization of guitar playing and writing. Alternatively, there may be differences in the pathophysiology of different task-specific dystonias.

Odergren *et al.*,[75] using PET, studied the progression of brain activation during 30 or 120 s of writing in patients with writer's cramp. The initiation of writing was associated with diminished activation of the primary motor cortex in patients with writer's cramp compared with age-matched controls. However, as the duration of writing increased, there was a progressive increase in the activation of the contralateral sensorimotor cortex, PMA, thalamus, and cerebellum. Based on these studies, Pujol *et al.*[73] speculated that in dystonic patients, nondystonic hand movements result in decreased activation of the sensorimotor cortex, whereas dystonic-producing tasks trigger brain networks that increase activation of the sensorimotor cortex.

PET was used to evaluate regional cerebral blood flow (rCBF) in 7 patients with simple writer's cramp and 7 age- and gender-matched controls during writing, sustained contraction, or tapping with the right hand.[76] During the writing task, patients with focal dystonia showed decreased activation of PMA and a reduced correlation between activation of the putamen and the PMA network. There was a reduction in sensorimotor cortex activation in the dystonic patients compared to the controls during the sustained contraction task. In contrast, there was no significant difference between patients with writer's cramp and controls in the pattern of activation during rapid, alternate tapping of the fingers to the thumb.[76] These findings are consistent with those of others showing reduced activation during writing in patients with focal dystonia of a frontal network including the sensorimotor cortex, PMA, and caudal SMA.[76] Reduced inhibition of the motor cortex by the somatosensory cortex and premotor regions could result in the development of cocontraction of agonists and antagonists during the performance of skilled movements.

The pattern of increased cortical activation and reduced intracortical inhibition suggests that inhibition of cortical activity by the basal ganglia is reduced in patients with focal dystonia. To understand the relation between abnormal basal ganglia function and cortical activation, Ceballos-Baumann *et al.*[77] studied rCBF in 5 patients with hemidystonia due to lesions of the contralateral basal ganglia or posterior thalamus. Paced movements of a joystick with the affected hand of dystonic patients was associated with increased activation of the contralateral prefrontal, lateral PMA, rostral SMA, anterior cingulate, bilateral sensorimotor cortex, insula, medial parietal cortex, and ipsilateral cerebellum compared with controls. Movements of the nonaffected hand produced similar hyperactivity of the frontal cortex, except that enhanced activity of the SMC and insula was observed only on the contralateral side. The authors postulated that movement-induced cortical hyperactivity results from loss of inhibitory control of the thalamofrontal system by the damaged basal ganglia. Interestingly, this study suggested that unilateral lesions of the basal ganglia produced bilateral disinhibition.

Acknowledgments

The authors have been supported in part by a grant from the Milton Foundation, the International Foundation for Music Research (IFMR), a Clinical Scientist Development Award from the Doris Duke Charitable Foundation, the Harvard Medical School and the Research Service, Department of Veterans Affairs.

References

1. J. Profita and T.G. Bidder, Perfect pitch, *Am. J. Med. Genet.* **29**, 763–71 (1988).
2. S. Baharloo, P.A. Johnston, S.K. Service, J. Gitschier and N.B. Freimer, Absolute pitch: an approach for identification of genetic and nongenetic components [see comments], *Am. J. Hum. Genet.* **62**, 224–31 (1998).
3. S. Baharloo, S.K. Service, N. Risch, J. Gitschier and N.B. Freimer, Familial aggregation of absolute pitch, *Am. J. Hum. Genet.* **67**, 755–8 (2000).
4. A.L. Foundas, C.M. Leonard, R. Gilmore, E. Fennell and K.M. Heilman, Planum temporale asymmetry and language dominance, *Neuropsychologia* **32**, 1225–31 (1994).
5. J.G. Chi, E.C. Dooling and F.H. Gilles, Left–right asymmetries of the temporal speech areas of the human fetus, *Arch. Neurol.* **34**, 346–8 (1977).
6. G. Schlaug, L. Jancke, Y. Huang and H. Steinmetz, In vivo evidence of structural brain asymmetry in musicians [see comments], *Science* **267**, 699–701 (1995).
7. J.P. Keenan, V. Thangaraj, A.R. Halpern and G. Schlaug, Absolute pitch and planum temporale, *Neuroimage* **14**, 1402–8 (2001).
8. R.J. Zatorre, D.W. Perry, C.A. Beckett, C.F. Westbury and A.C. Evans, Functional anatomy of musical processing in listeners with absolute pitch and relative pitch, *Proc. Natl. Acad. Sci. U.S.A.* **95**, 3172–7 (1998).
9. H.J. Neville and D. Bavelier, Neural organization and plasticity of language, *Curr. Opin. Neurobiol.* **8**, 254–8 (1998).

10. A.J. Doupe and P.K. Kuhl, Birdsong and human speech: common themes and mechanisms, *Annu. Rev. Neurosci.* **22**, 567–631 (1999).
11. X.C. Li, E.D. Jarvis, B. Alvarez-Borda, D.A. Lim and F. Nottebohm, A relationship between behavior, neurotrophin expression, and new neuron survival, *Proc. Natl. Acad. Sci. U.S.A.* **97**, 8584–9 (2000).
12. T. Ohnishi, H. Matsuda, T. Asada, M. Aruga, M. Hirakata, M. Nishikawa, A. Katoh and E. Imabayashi, Functional anatomy of musical perception in musicians, *Cereb. Cortex* **11**, 754–60 (2001).
13. C. Pantev, R. Oostenveld, A. Engelien, B. Ross, L.E. Roberts and M. Hoke, Increased auditory cortical representation in musicians, *Nature* **392**, 811–4 (1998).
14. C. Pantev, L.E. Roberts, M. Schulz, A. Engelien and B. Ross, Timbre-specific enhancement of auditory cortical representations in musicians, *Neuroreport* **12**, 169–74 (2001).
15. C. Pantev, A. Wollbrink, L.E. Roberts, A. Engelien and B. Lutkenhoner, Short-term plasticity of the human auditory cortex, *Brain Res.* **842**, 192–9 (1999).
16. A. Pascual-Leone, J. Grafman and M. Hallett, Modulation of cortical motor output maps during development of implicit and explicit knowledge [see comments], *Science* **263**, 1287–9 (1994).
17. R. Shadmehr and H.H. Holcomb, Neural correlates of motor memory consolidation, *Science* **277**, 821–5 (1997).
18. A. Karni, G. Meyer, C. Rey-Hipolito, P. Jezzard, M.M. Adams, R. Turner and L.G. Ungerleider, The acquisition of skilled motor performance: fast and slow experience-driven changes in primary motor cortex, *Proc. Natl. Acad. Sci. U.S.A.* **95**, 861–8 (1998).
19. A. Pascual-Leone, D. Nguyet, L.G. Cohen, J.P. Brasil-Neto, A. Cammarota and M. Hallett, Modulation of muscle responses evoked by transcranial magnetic stimulation during the acquisition of new fine motor skills, *J. Neurophysiol.* **74**, 1037–45 (1995).
20. A. Karni, G. Meyer, P. Jezzard, M.M. Adams, R. Turner and L.G. Ungerleider, Functional MRI evidence for adult motor cortex plasticity during motor skill learning, *Nature* **377**, 155–8 (1995).
21. J. Classen, J. Liepert, S.P. Wise, M. Hallett and L.G. Cohen, Rapid plasticity of human cortical movement representation induced by practice, *J. Neurophysiol.* **79**, 1117–23 (1998).
22. A. Pascual-Leone, E.M. Wassermann, N. Sadato and M. Hallett, The role of reading activity on the modulation of motor cortical outputs to the reading hand in Braille readers, *Ann. Neurol.* **38**, 910–5 (1995).
23. L. Jancke, M.J. Shah and M. Peters, Cortical activations in primary and secondary motor areas for complex bimanual movements in professional pianists, *Brain Research. Cognitive Brain Research* **10**, 177–83 (2000).

24. T. Krings, R. Topper, H. Foltys, S. Erberich, R. Sparing, K. Willmes and A. Thron, Cortical activation patterns during complex motor tasks in piano players and control subjects: a functional magnetic resonance imaging study, *Neurosci. Lett.* **278**, 189–93 (2000).
25. M. Hund-Georgiadis and D.Y. von Cramon, Motor-learning-related changes in piano players and non-musicians revealed by functional magnetic-resonance signals, *Exp. Brain Res.* **125**, 417–25 (1999).
26. G. Schlaug, J.M. Sanes, V. Thangaraj, D.G. Darby, L. Jancke, R.R. Edelman and S. Warach, Cerebral activation covaries with movement rate, *Neuroreport* **7**, 879–83 (1996).
27. T. Elbert, C. Pantev, C. Wienbruch, B. Rockstroh and E. Taub, Increased cortical representation of the fingers of the left hand in string players, *Science* **270**, 305–7(1995).
28. J. Pujol, P. Vendrell, C. Junque, J.L. Marti-Vilalta and A. Capdevila, When does human brain development end? Evidence of corpus callosum growth up to adulthood, *Ann. Neurol.* **34**(1), 71–5 (1993).
29. G. Schlaug, L. Jancke, Y. Huang, J.F. Staiger and H. Steinmetz, Increased corpus callosum size in musicians, *Neuropsychologia* **33**, 1047–55 (1995).
30. G. Schlaug, The brain of musicians: a model for functional and structural adaptation, *Ann. N.Y. Acad. Sci.* **930**, 281–99 (2001).
31. H. van Praag, G. Kempermann and F.H. Gage, Neural consequences of environmental enrichment, *Nature Rev. Neurosci.* **1**(3), 191–8 (2000).
32. J.E. Black, K.R. Isaacs, B.J. Anderson, A.A. Alcantara and W.T. Greenough, Learning causes synaptogenesis, whereas motor activity causes angiogenesis, in cerebellar cortex of adult rats, *Proc. Natl. Acad. Sci. U.S.A.* **87**(14), 5568–72 (1990).
33. L. Jancke, G. Schlaug and H. Steinmetz, Hand skill asymmetry in professional musicians, *Brain & Cognition* **34**, 424–32 (1997).
34. K. Amunts, G. Schlaug, L. Jancke, H. Steinmetz, A. Schleicher, A. Dabringhaus and K. Zilles, Motor cortex and hand motor skills: structural compliance in the human brain, *Human Brain Mapping* **5**, 206–15 (1997).
35. M.E. Charness, M.H. Ross and J.M. Shefner, Ulnar neuropathy and dystonic flexion of the fourth and fifth digits: clinical correlation in musicians, *Muscle Nerve* **19**, 431–7 (1996).
36. M. Byl, F. Wilson, M. Merzenich, M. Melnick, P. Scott, A. Oakes and A. McKenzie, Sensory dysfunction associated with repetitive strain injuries of tendinitis and focal hand dystonia: a comparative study, *J. Orthop. Sports Phys. Ther.* **23**, 234–44 (1996).
37. N.N. Byl, M.M. Merzenich and W.M. Jenkins, A primate genesis model of focal dystonia and repetitive strain injury: I. Learning-induced dedifferentiation of the representation of the hand in the primary somatosensory cortex in adult monkeys, *Neurology* **47**, 508–20 (1996).

38. F.R. Wilson, C. Wagner and V. Homberg, Biomechanical abnormalities in musicians with occupational cramp/focal dystonia, *J. Hand Ther.* **6**, 298–307 (1993).
39. A. Straube, N. Mai, E. Walther and M. Mayer, Persisting "writer's cramp" as a result of compensation of a temporary palsy due to a hereditary neuropathy with liability to pressure palsies, *Movement Disorders* **11**, 576–9 (1996).
40. M.M. Merzenich, J.H. Kaas, J.T. Wall, M. Sur, R.J. Nelson and D.J. Felleman, Progression of change following median nerve section in the cortical representation of the hand in areas 3b and 1 in adult owl and squirrel monkeys, *Neuroscience* **10**, 639–65 (1983).
41. M. Rijntjes, M. Tegenthoff, J. Liepert, G. Leonhardt, S. Kotterba, S. Muller, S. Kiebel, J.P. Malin, H.C. Diener and C. Weiller, Cortical reorganization in patients with facial palsy, *Ann. Neurol.* **41**, 621–30 (1997).
42. M.H. Ross, M.E. Charness, D. Lee and E.L. Logigian, Does ulnar neuropathy predispose to focal dystonia? *Muscle Nerve* **18**, 606–11 (1995).
43. P. Girlanda, A. Quartarone, F. Battaglia, G. Picciolo, S. Sinicropi and C. Messina, Changes in spinal cord excitability in patients affected by ulnar neuropathy, *Neurology* **55**, 975–8 (2000).
44. L.G. Cohen and M. Hallett, Hand cramps: clinical features and electromyographic patterns in a focal dystonia, *Neurology* **38**, 1005–12 (1988).
45. M.E. Panizza, M. Hallett and J. Nilsson, Reciprocal inhibition in patients with hand cramps, *Neurology* **39**, 85–9 (1989).
46. M. Panizza, S. Lelli, J. Nilsson and M. Hallett, H-reflex recovery curve and reciprocal inhibition of H-reflex in different kinds of dystonia, *Neurology* **40**, 824–8 (1990).
47. R.S. Chen, C.H. Tsai and C.S. Lu, Reciprocal inhibition in writer's cramp, *Movement Disorders* **10**, 556–61 (1995).
48. J.R. Friedman, C. Klein, J. Leung, H. Woodward, L.J. Ozelius, X.O. Breakefield and M.E. Charness, The GAG deletion of the DYT1 gene is infrequent in musicians with focal dystonia, *Neurology* **55**, 1417–18 (2000).
49. M. Hallett, Is dystonia a sensory disorder? [editorial], *Ann. Neurol.* **38**, 139–40 (1995).
50. W. Bara-Jimenez, P. Shelton, T.D. Sanger and M. Hallett, Sensory discrimination capabilities in patients with focal hand dystonia, *Ann. Neurol.* **47**, 377–80 (2000).
51. W. Bara-Jimenez, P. Shelton and M. Hallett, Spatial discrimination is abnormal in focal hand dystonia, *Neurology* **55**, 1869–73 (2000).
52. R. Kaji, N, Kohara, M. Katayama, T. Kubori, T. Mezaki, H. Shibasaki and J. Kimura, Muscle afferent block by intramuscular injection of lidocaine for the treatment of writer's cramp, *Muscle & Nerve* **18**, 234–5 (1995).
53. R. Kaji, J.C. Rothwell, M. Katayama, T. Ikeda, T. Kubori, N. Kohara, T. Mezaki, H. Shibasaki and J. Kimura, Tonic vibration reflex and muscle afferent block in writer's cramp, *Ann. Neurol.* **38**, 155–62 (1995).

54. R. Kaji, H. Shibasaki and J. Kimura, Writer's cramp: a disorder of motor subroutine? [editorial; comment], *Ann. Neurol.* **38**, 837–8 (1995).
55. K. Rosenkranz, E. Altenmuller, S. Siggelkow and R. Dengler, Alteration of sensorimotor integration in musician's cramp: impaired focusing of proprioception, *Clin. Neurophysiol.* **111**, 2040–5 (2000).
56. N. Murase, R. Kaji, H. Shimazu, M. Katayama-Hirota, A. Ikeda, N. Kohara, J. Kimura, H. Shibasaki and J.C. Rothwell, Abnormal premovement gating of somatosensory input in writer's cramp, *Brain* **123**, 1813–29 (2000).
57. R.A. Grunewald, Y. Yoneda, J.M. Shipman and H.J. Sagar, Idiopathic focal dystonia: a disorder of muscle spindle afferent processing? *Brain* **120**, 2179–85 (1997).
58. Y. Yoneda, S. Rome, H.J. Sagar and R.A. Newald, Abnormal perception of the tonic vibration reflex in idiopathic focal dystonia, *Eur. J. Neurol.* 7, 529–33 (2000).
59. M. Tinazzi, A. Priori, L. Bertolasi, E. Frasson, F. Mauguiere and A. Fiaschi, Abnormal central integration of a dual somatosensory input in dystonia: evidence for sensory overflow, *Brain* **123**, 42–50 (2000).
60. L.W. Tempel and J.S. Perlmutter, Abnormal vibration-induced cerebral blood flow responses in idiopathic dystonia, *Brain* **113**, 691–707 (1990).
61. L.W. Tempel and J.S. Perlmutter, Abnormal cortical responses in patients with writer's cramp [published erratum appears in *Neurology* **44**(12), 2411 (1994)], *Neurology* **43**, 2252–7 (1993).
62. R.J. Feiwell, K.J. Black, L.A. McGee-Minnich, A.Z. Snyder, A.M. MacLeod and J.S. Perlmutter, Diminished regional cerebral blood flow response to vibration in patients with blepharospasm, *Neurology* **52**, 291–7 (1999).
63. W. Bara-Jimenez, M.J. Catalan, M. Hallett and C. Gerloff, Abnormal somatosensory homunculus in dystonia of the hand, *Ann. Neurol.* **44**, 828–31 (1998).
64. K.S. Topp and N.N. Byl, Movement dysfunction following repetitive hand opening and closing: anatomical analysis in owl monkeys, *Movement Disorders* **14**, 295–306 (1999).
65. T. Elbert, V. Candia, E. Altenmuller, H. Rau, A. Sterr, B. Rockstroh, C. Pantev and E. Taub, Alteration of digital representations in somatosensory cortex in focal hand dystonia, *Neuroreport* **9**, 3571–5 (1998).
66. F.A. Lenz and N.N. Byl, Reorganization in the cutaneous core of the human thalamic principal somatic sensory nucleus (ventral caudal) in patients with dystonia, *J. Neurophysiol.* **82**, 3204–12 (1999).
67. H.R. Siebner, C. Auer and B. Conrad, Abnormal increase in the corticomotor output to the affected hand during repetitive transcranial magnetic stimulation of the primary motor cortex in patients with writer's cramp, *Neurosci. Lett.* **262**, 133–6 (1999).

68. K. Ikoma, A. Samii, B. Mercuri, E.M. Wassermann and M. Hallett, Abnormal cortical motor excitability in dystonia, *Neurology* **46**, 1371–6 (1996).
69. M.C. Ridding, G. Sheean, J.C. Rothwell, R. Inzelberg and T. Kujirai, Changes in the balance between motor cortical excitation and inhibition in focal, task specific dystonia, *J. Neurol. Neurosurg. Psychiatry* **59**, 493–8 (1995).
70. H.R. Siebner, J.M. Tormos, A.O. Ceballos-Baumann, C. Auer, M.D. Catala, B. Conrad and A. Pascual-Leone, Low-frequency repetitive transcranial magnetic stimulation of the motor cortex in writer's cramp, *Neurology* **52**, 529–37 (1999).
71. M.L. Byrnes, G.W. Thickbroom, S.A. Wilson, P. Sacco, J.M. Shipman, R. Stell and F.L. Mastaglia, The corticomotor representation of upper limb muscles in writer's cramp and changes following botulinum toxin injection, *Brain* **121**, 977–88 (1998).
72. G. Deuschl, C. Toro, J. Matsumoto and M. Hallett, Movement-related cortical potentials in writer's cramp [see comments], *Ann. Neurol.* **38**, 862–8 (1995).
73. J. Pujol, J. Roset-Llobet, D. Rosines-Cubells, J. Deus, B. Narberhaus, J. Valls-Sole, A. Capdevila and A. Pascual-Leone, Brain cortical activation during guitar-induced hand dystonia studied by functional MRI, *Neuroimage* **12**, 257–67 (2000).
74. A.O. Ceballos-Baumann, G. Sheean, R.E. Passingham, C.D. Marsden and D.J. Brooks, Botulinum toxin does not reverse the cortical dysfunction associated with writer's cramp: a PET study, *Brain* **120**, 571–82 (1997).
75. T. Odergren, S. Stone-Elander and M. Ingvar, Cerebral and cerebellar activation in correlation to the action-induced dystonia in writer's cramp, *Movement Disorders* **13**, 497–508 (1998).
76. V. Ibanez, N. Sadato, B. Karp, M.P. Deiber and M. Hallett, Deficient activation of the motor cortical network in patients with writer's cramp, *Neurology* **53**, 96–105 (1999).
77. A.O. Ceballos-Baumann, R.E. Passingham, T. Warner, E.D. Playford, C.D. Marsden and D.J. Brooks, Overactive prefrontal and underactive motor cortical areas in idiopathic dystonia, *Ann. Neurol.* **37**(3), 363–72 (1995).

Chapter 10

The Cerebral Localisation of Musical Perception and Musical Memory

H. Platel, F. Eustache and J.-C. Baron

Introduction

Does such a thing as a "musical brain"—i.e. with regions devoted to the perception and memory of music and distinct from those thought to specifically underlie language—really exist in humans? Many would think this unlikely, as clearly music does not have the same social and cultural status as language. However, it would be quite difficult from a phylogenetic point of view to determine whether musical abilities stemmed from neural substrates originally devoted to language abilities, or vice versa, as many animal species "sing" but do not "speak".

For well over a century, neuropsychologists have investigated the various components of auditory perception in brain-damaged subjects, and the central disorders of this perception have especially been a topic of considerable interest. The observation of auditory agnosia and amusia (which reflects the selective loss of musical abilities) has been particularly striking. From the original works of Bouillaud on the study of musical abilities in aphasic patients[1] until the middle of the 1960s, the prevalent hypothesis about amusias was that they were a particular form of aphasia. In other words, the loss of musical abilities was attributed to lesions of the same "brain centres" as those involved in language, and recognition of musical sounds was equated with that of verbal sounds. Subsequent neuropsychological studies of brain-damaged subjects gradually dismissed this concept by showing clear-cut double dissociations in deficits of language and music abilities in single patients. Thus, the idea that the processing of musical material in the brain was distinct from that of language gradually became dominant, leading to the design of specific cognitive model.[2,3] However, localization of brain function based on neuropsychology alone is hampered by the frequent occurrence of inconsistencies in findings from patient to patient, which may reflect either individual peculiarities in pre-morbid brain organisation or post-lesion compensatory reorganization, or both.

Experimental psychology, using for example event-related potentials in either healthy or brain-damaged subjects, flourished in the 1960s and added weight to the concept of distinct brain processing for music and language. Based on these studies, it became widely held that the processing of language and music was differentially lateralised, i.e. in the left and right cerebral hemispheres, respectively.[4,5] More recently, however, a number of experimental psychology and neuropsychological studies have gradually led to a more modular concept of music perception which, rather than a mere music/language opposition, addresses the issue of music perception in its overall complexity by considering each of its multiple processes separately.[6–9] Based on these studies, it now appears that at least some of these basic processes have different lateralisation. However, these techniques lack the spatial resolution necessary for understanding the precise organisation of music processing by the brain.

Thanks to the advent of functional neuroimaging about 25 years ago and continuous developments since, it is now possible to map directly brain activity during perceptual and performance tasks in normal subjects.[10] Based on these findings, the last decade has witnessed major breakthroughs in the understanding of the musical brain. This brief overview will focus on the perception and memory of musical material, but the reader interested in other aspects of the musical brain, e.g. learning, singing, and feelings induced by music, is referred to specific papers[11–13] as well as to other chapters of this volume.

Musical Perception: Insights from Functional Neuroimaging

Initial functional imagining studies of the brain's response to non-verbal auditory stimulation were carried out with low sensitivity techniques such as SPECT and FDG-PET. Yet, it was repeatedly shown that, relative to a control condition without auditory stimulation, these stimuli—be they pure tones, musical sequences or environmental sounds—always induced a clear-cut activation of the temporal lobes. For instance, confirming classic electrophysiologic animal studies, it was documented in humans that any type of auditory stimulation activated the posterior–superior temporal lobe in the region of the upper bank of the Sylvian fissure; more precisely, in the primary auditory cortex (Heschl's gyrus or Brodmann's area (BA) 41). For instance, Lassen *et al.*[14] reported an increase in regional cerebral blood flow (rCBF) in the posterior temporal lobe bilaterally when listening to meaningless sounds. In a sound discrimination task, Knopman *et al.*[15] found an increase in rCBF in the left perisylvian region together with a global increase in blood flow in the right hemisphere. Using PET, Lauter *et al.*[16] studied subjects stimulated through the right ear with pure tones from 500 Hz to 4000 Hz, and reported a tonotopic distribution of the responses at the level of the left Heschl's gyrus. Similar to findings in the animal, neuronal activation was topographically dependent on sound frequency, with responses to higher pitch being posterior and medial along Heschl's gyrus, and responses to lower tones being more anterior and lateral This tonotopic organisation of the primary auditory cortex was subsequently confirmed by studies using either magneto-encephalography (MEG)[17] or direct neuronal activity recording using implanted EEG electrodes in epileptic subjects.[18]

Specifically regarding music, several studies have documented that musical experience modifies this tonotopic organisation of the primary auditory cortex; the earlier in life musical experience begins, the stronger the difference with non-musical subjects.[19] Using MEG, Pantev *et al.* also showed that the response of the auditory cortex to both pure tones and complex sounds was clearly stronger in musical than in non-musical subjects. Musicians with perfect pitch (i.e. the ability to recognise and name the fundamental pitch of any heard sound) exhibited stronger auditory cortex responses than people without this innate skill. Using structural MRI, Schlaug *et al.*[20] showed that musicians with perfect pitch even exhibited structural differences, namely greater asymmetry (left larger than right) of the planum temporale than non-musicians or musicians without perfect pitch (see previous chapter). Using PET and a task of harmony judgement, Zatorre *et al.*[21] showed that, at variance with perfect pitch subjects, subjects without perfect pitch exhibited prefrontal cortex activation which may reflect the extra working memory effort needed by non-perfect-pitch subjects to make this musical judgement.

In their pioneer FDG-PET study, Mazziotta *et al.*[22] carried out one of the first functional imaging studies on musical perception. They used material extracted from the Seashore test, which assesses timbre discrimination and pitch memory. During the timbre discrimination task, there was predominant activity over the right hemisphere, especially in the frontal regions. During the pitch memory task, which consisted of discriminating pairs of musical sequences made up of three to five tunes of the same intensity and duration and separated by short silent periods, the brain responses depended on whether or not the subjects were musical. In non-musician subjects, there was an increase in brain glucose metabolism in the right middle and superior temporal gyri, with greater overall activation of the entire right hemisphere relative to the left. However, in semi-professional musicians, who are known to use a more analytical strategy, brain activation was greater in the left hemisphere. It should be mentioned that in this study the strategy used by the subjects was deduced after the brain scanning experiments.

Overall, the vast majority of the functional neuroimaging studies on music and the brain have until now assessed non-musical subjects. However, the PET study of Justine Sergent *et al.*[23] was, and still is, the most remarkable study on musicians to date. In this work, 10 right-handed professional pianists carried out seven different tasks during PET data acquisition, as follows:

(1) Passive fixation of the screen;
(2) Display of a dot and manual response, depending on localisation of the dot;
(3) Passive listening to simple musical scales played on the piano;
(4) Playing musical scales with the right hand while listening to what was played;
(5) Covert reading of a musical score from a J.S. Bach choral presented on the screen;
(6) Covert reading of a musical score from another J.S. Bach choral presented on the screen and listening to its performance played on the piano;
(7) Playing a little-known J.S. Bach partita with the right hand while listening to its performance (main condition).

Comparing the fourth condition to the third revealed activations in the extra-striate visual association cortex, which would therefore specifically underlie the reading of musical scores. Comparing the fifth to the fourth condition revealed activations in bilateral superior temporal regions and the left supra-marginal gyrus (BA 40), which would underlie the mental processing of musical scores. Finally, comparing the main condition to the fifth revealed activations in the left Broca's area and supplementary motor area (SMA), the bilateral pre-cuneus (superior parietal lobule; more so on the left), and the right cerebellum, which would underlie the playing of musical scales. These results highlight cortical regions classically assigned as "association" areas. More specifically, activation of the superior parietal lobule presumably reflects the spatial processing of the musical notations and the transcoding of this spatial information into a visually guided motor performance. Activation of the left Broca's area and SMA presumably reflects the patterning and timing of the motor sequences required for manual execution of the piece.[24] One remarkable observation from these findings is the left-sided predominance of cortical activations during such a high-level music performance task by professional musicians. Drury and Van Hessen[25] recently compared these activations to those found by Petersen *et al.*[26] in a comparable language task (hearing and producing words). This study showed that although there was some overlap of activated areas—suggesting the involvement of a common network of left-hemisphere regions engaged in these linguistic and musical tasks—there was also a clear-cut partial independence of networks, consistent with the double dissociations mentioned above. For instance, Broca's area was engaged in both tasks but the left pre-cuneus only during score reading, and left superior temporal gyrus activation extended more anteriorly when playing music than when reading words.

Also using PET, Robert Zatorre and his group have made considerable contributions to the mapping of the musical brain. In their 1992 study, they reported right inferior frontal activation in a task where the subjects discriminated the pitch of verbal material. This result was obtained by subtracting a condition of passive listening to pairs of vocal sounds from the condition of discrimination of change pitch on the same material.[27]

In 1997, we published an extensive study on the perception by non-musical subjects of the basic components of music, namely pitch, timbre, rhythm and familiarity.[9] This is, as of today, the only study that has simultaneously assessed these four components of musical perception. Our goal was not to reveal the neural networks common to these components, but to address the activations that would be *specific* to each one of them relative to the others. To this end, the same material was presented in all four conditions and consisted of the random arrangement of a tape of 30 musical sequences. For each condition, 50% of the heard sequences were targets to the particular task, i.e. 50% of them presented with a change in pitch, a change in timbre, or an irregular rhythm, and 50% of them could be judged as familiar based on pre-experimental studies on matched young healthy male non-musical subjects. Consistent with our hypothesis, the results (Figure 1) did reveal specific significant activations, which differentiated each condition relative to the others, as follows:

(1) *Familiarity task*: activations were mainly left-sided and involved the anterior part of the superior temporal gyrus and the adjacent inferior frontal gyrus (see below for discussion of these results).

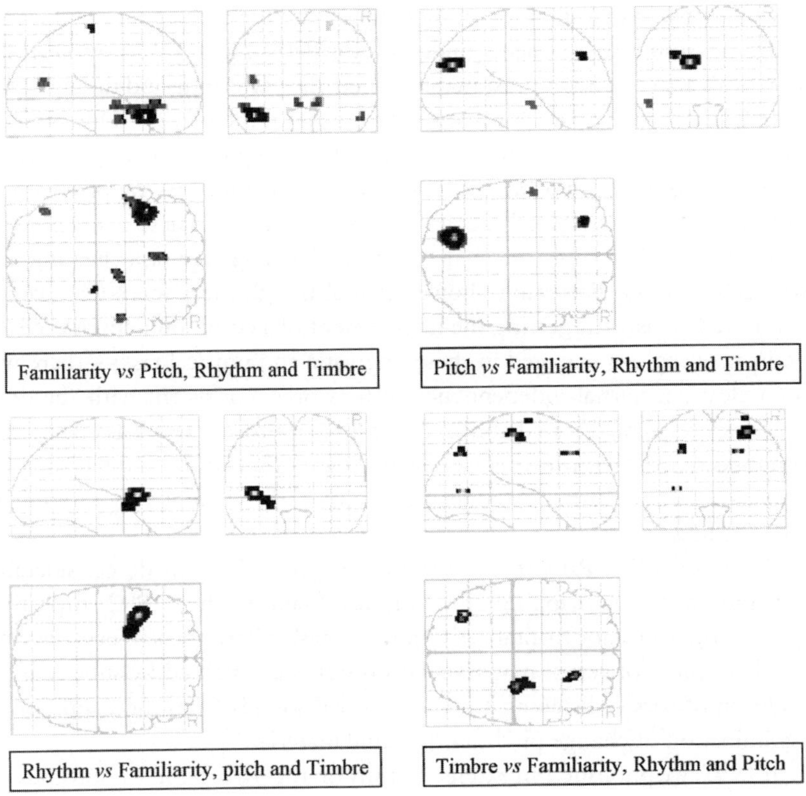

Fig. 1. Activation results of the four main comparisons among pitch, familiarity, timbre and rhythm.[9] The results from the SPM analysis at $p < 0.001$ (uncorrected for multiple comparisons) are displayed according to the classic "glass brain" of Talairach and Tournoux. See text for methodological details and description of the results.

(2) *Rhythm task*: activations were exclusively left-sided and involved Broca's area and the adjacent insula. These findings are in general agreement with the study of Liegeois-Chauvel *et al.*,[7] which showed that temporal cortectomies, whether right, left or bilateral, did not affect rhythm discrimination. Activation of Broca's area may reflect the processing and organisation of sequential auditory stimuli, verbal or otherwise. The adjacent left insula is known to have extensive connections with primary and secondary auditory regions.[9] Anterior left insular activation has been reported by Penhune *et al.*[28] in a task of identification and reproduction of auditory rhythms, and by Wise *et al.*[29] in a task of language articulation.

Thus, the left insula may be an important brain region in the processing of sound material of a sequential character.

(3) *Timbre task*: activations were mainly right-sided and involved the pre-central and middle frontal gyri, but concerned also the left middle occipital gyrus. Of the three psychoacoustic parameters studied, the timbre task was that with the most prominent activations of the right hemisphere, consistent with the experimental and neuropsychological literature.[30]

(4) *Pitch task*: activations adopted an unexpected pattern, involving exclusively the left hemisphere and notably the cuneus/pre-cuneus cortex. The lack of activation of the right hemisphere in this task presumably reflects the nature of our paradigm, which was not designed to reveal activations common to several conditions. The specific activation in the left cuneus/pre-cuneus was thought to reflect engagement of mental imagery in pitch change identification, as suggested by information given by the subjects at debriefing that they had to "visualize the height of the tones" to carry out the task. As detailed above, Sergent *et al.*[23] also found an activation of the left cuneus/pre-cuneus during the reading and playing of musical scores. Consistent with this potential role of the left cuneus/pre-cuneus area in the visual or mental reading of music scores, Horikochi *et al.*[31] reported a case of visual music alexia in a patient with an arterio-venous malformation of the left occipital parasplenial region.

Music Memory: Studies with Functional Neuroimaging

Contrasting with the large number of functional neuroimaging studies that have assessed working, episodic or semantic memory of verbal and visual material,[32,33] very few have dealt with musical material.

One of them is the PET study of Zatorre *et al.*,[34] which supported the idea of a preferential involvement of the right hemisphere in the memorization of non-familiar melodies by non-musical subjects. The paradigm comprised four tasks:

(1) Passive listening of a sequence of noise bursts;
(2) Passive listening of non-familiar melodies made up of eight notes;
(3) Pitch judgement on the first two notes of the melodic sequences of condition 2 above;
(4) Pitch judgement comparing the first to the last note of the same test sequences; only this condition involved memory.

The comparison between condition 3 and condition 2 revealed a significant activation in the right frontal lobe. The comparison between condition 4 and condition 2 disclosed a considerably more complex pattern of cortical and sub-cortical activations, notably involving the frontal and temporal lobes on the right side, and the insular and parietal regions bilaterally. According to the authors, these findings indicate that the simple comparison of pitch involves a neural network which includes the right pre-frontal cortex, whereas the active short-term memory of pitch within a melody engages a much more distributed network, including, amongst other regions, both the frontal and temporal lobes on the right side.

Although it dealt with long-term rather than short-term musical memory, the PET study of Holcomb *et al.*[35] revealed findings similar to those of Zatorre *et al.*[34] In the control task, 12 healthy non-musical subjects passively listened to a series of 60 notes spaced by 2 s, and pressed a button alternately on the right and left sides; in the active task, they were asked to detect two precise notes within the same series of 60 notes, one of high pitch with the instruction to press the right button, and one of low pitch with the instruction to press the left button. These non-musical subjects had to be extensively trained to identify these two notes over the three days preceding the actual PET session. The comparison between the identification task and the passive listening task revealed significant activations in the right inferior and middle frontal gyri, insula, anterior cingulate gyrus, and SMA. The left insula and part of the left cerebellum were also activated. Furthermore, the reaction times were significantly positively correlated with activity in the right middle and inferior frontal gyri (i.e. the longer the identification response time, the greater the functional response), indicating that the neuronal activity in these two regions was in part modulated by the "difficulty" in performing the task. These results therefore suggest that pitch recognition engages preferentially the pre-frontal areas of the right hemisphere.

Although these two studies are consistent with each other and globally agree with the neuropsychological literature regarding the role of the right hemisphere in musical memory, they did not provide any information as to whether there would exist a specific network for musical semantic memory as distinct from verbal memory. Furthermore, they both concerned pitch memory, while episodic memory for melodies has not been investigated so far. In our PET study on the perception of the various components of music referred to above,[9] the familiarity with musical melodies was one of the four components investigated. The specific task and results for this condition are worth being detailed now. Amongst the presented sequences, 50% could be judged as familiar based on pre-experimental studies ("target sequences"). Target sequences were musical excerpts difficult to verbalise, i.e. we excluded songs and used either excerpts from classical music—such as Ravel's *Bolero* or Tchaikovsky's *Nutcracker*—or other known tunes for which neither the title nor the composer would be familiar to French people—such as the American national anthem. All these targets were selected based on extensive pre-experimental tests on a large sample of healthy subjects matched for sex and lack of musical experience to the PET experimental group. The comparison between this task and the three other perceptual tasks of the protocol (namely pitch, timbre and rhythm) revealed specific activations mainly in the left hemisphere and involving the inferior frontal gyrus (BA 47) and the anterior part of the superior temporal gyrus (including BA 22) (Figure 1). These findings highlight the left hemisphere's role in musical familiarity judgement and are consistent with clinical observations showing that left hemisphere damage is associated with impaired music identification of the associative agnosia type.[2,6,8] Interestingly, this left superior temporal region was also activated in Sergent *et al.*'s study of musicians playing scores.[23] Importantly, the activated areas only partially overlapped with areas known to activate during verbal semantic memory tasks, which also involves the left superior temporal gyrus but more posteriorly than with melodies.[26,33] However, a similar region appears to be engaged during listening to stories,[36] which arguably involve some "melody of language". The fact remains that, due to the unusual paradigm used in this study (see above), we cannot exclude the involvement, in our familiarity task, of additional regions similarly activated in the other conditions, including right hemisphere areas.

The recent study by Halpern and Zatorre[37] raises fundamental issues regarding the neuronal substrates of musical memory. In this PET study of mental imagery of familiar melodies, the authors assessed the ability of non-musical subjects to mentally imagine the subsequent notes of both the beginnings of very familiar melodies and tone sequences made up from notes from the familiar melodies. Three conditions were carried out in the following order:

(1) *Control condition*, where the subjects simply listened to non-familiar musical sequences;
(2) *Mental imagery task*, in which the subjects listened to the beginning of familiar melodies and were instructed to mentally imagine the subsequent notes (over a few seconds);

(3) *Music memory condition*, in which the subjects were exposed again to the same non-familiar sequences presented in the first condition, but were asked to replay mentally the entire sequence (mental repetition).

The subjects for the study were highly selected beforehand so as to have strong feelings of familiarity for the chosen musical extracts, and in addition they were re-familiarised with these melodies on the day of the PET session so that they knew exactly at which time they would have to start imagine mentally the subsequent notes. According to the authors, comparing condition 2 with condition 3 should eliminate common processes regarding early auditory analysis, working memory and mental imagery, leaving out of the process of retrieval from semantic memory only. This comparison disclosed activations in the right inferior and middle frontal gyri (BAs 45, 46, 47), in the superior and inferior right temporal gyri (BAs 37, 22), and in the right anterior cingulate and parietal regions (BAs 32, 40). Though less conspicuous than that in the right hemisphere, some activations also involved the left hemisphere, precisely in the middle and inferior frontal gyri (BAs 45/46/9). Although these findings concerning the involvement of the right frontal regions in melody perception are entirely consistent with previous data by the same group,[34] they are in apparent conflict not only with our own findings detailed above[9] but also with the extensive functional imaging literature regarding retrieval from semantic memory of verbal material, which consistently shows a preferential involvement of left hemisphere regions.[33] Halpern and Zatorre interpret their findings in the general framework of the right hemisphere being dominant for the treatment of musical stimuli. They do, however, raise the issue of the possible involvement of episodic memory processes in their mental imagery task of familiar melodies (which served as a control task).

In order to specifically study semantic memory and episodic memory of music, we have carried out a novel PET study.[38] We studied nine right-handed young healthy male subjects with normal hearing and non-musical (according to the classification of Wertheim and Botez).[39] The paradigm included five different conditions: one semantic condition, two episodic conditions and two perceptual control tasks. The paradigm consisted in the presentation of musical extracts specifically prepared for the protocol and selected for their cognitive characteristics based on extensive pre-experimental tests. In the semantic memory task, the subjects were asked to judge if the extract was familiar or non-familiar. Half of the sequences were target melodies selected for their statistically significant familiarity, whilst the remaining 50% were distractors corresponding to non-familiar melodies based on the same criteria.

Two episodic memory tasks were carried out—one with exclusive familiar melodies and the other with non-familiar melodies. In each, the instruction was to recognise the sequences already presented in the semantic task, which was always given before the episodic task and without the subjects knowing that they would be subsequently tested for their memory of the sequences. In the two perceptual control tasks, the instruction was to judge if the last two notes of the melodies were of a similar or different pitch. The comparison between the two memory tasks and the control tasks revealed distinct neural networks (Figure 2). In comparing the episodic task to the control task, bilateral activation of the middle and superior frontal gyri and the pre-cuneus was found, with right-sided predominance. This pattern of network activation is entirely consistent with previous findings regarding episodic retrieval

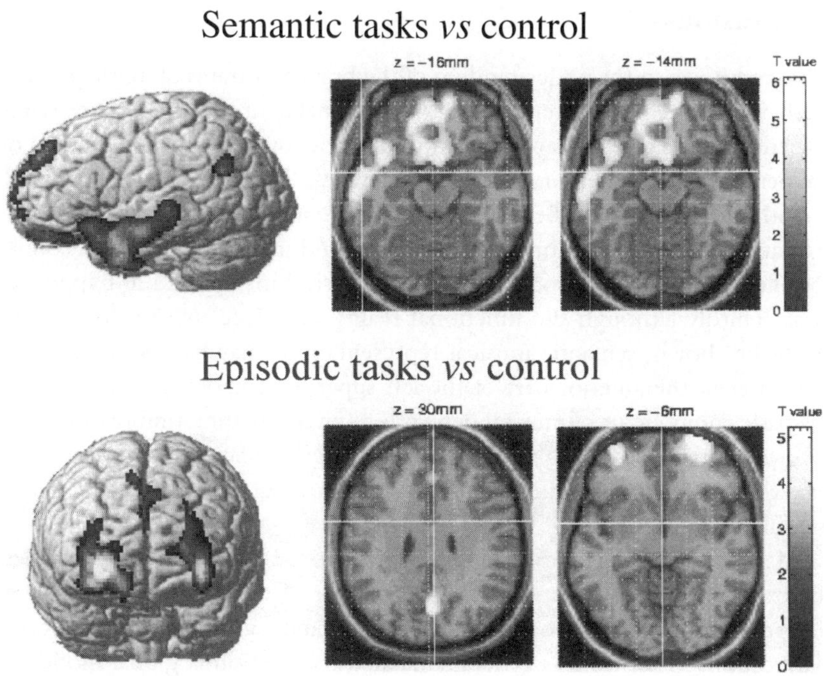

Fig. 2. Activation results of the semantic and episodic musical memory tasks compared to the perceptual control tasks.[38] The results from SPM99 analysis ($p < 0.05$, corrected for multiple comparisons) are displayed on a surface rendering of a standard edited MRI aligned and normalized to Talairach and Tournoux's stereotaxic atlas, with additional transverse cuts focusing on specific clusters. See text for details of the methodology and description of the findings.

of verbal or visual spatial items,[37,40] and therefore does not suggest any specific network for musical memory. The comparison between the semantic memory tasks and the control tasks revealed bilateral activations of the medial frontal regions as well as the left angular gyrus and the anterior part of the left middle and superior temporal gyri. Similar medial frontal activations have been documented in tasks of categorization of semantic association between faces and names,[41] suggesting again non-specificity. However, the activation of the anterior part of the left superior and middle temporal gyri was very similar to our previous findings in judgement of familiarity with musical melodies[9] (see above). These areas may, therefore, possibly specifically subtend semantic musical representations.

Conclusions

Major advances in the understanding of the brain substrates of music processing have been achieved lately thanks to functional neuroimaging. Some tentative conclusions can be drawn following this brief overview, which focused on the perception and memory of musical material. Firstly, distributed networks in both the right and left hemispheres, rather than complete hemispheric specialisation, contribute to musical perception and musical memory. Secondly, specific networks for episodic memory of musical material do not appear to exist. Thirdly although the functional reality of a pure musical lexicon has yet to be shown, semantic musical representations may have specific neural substrates in the anterior part of the left superior temporal gyrus. Fourthly, the basic components of musical perception (pitch, rhythm, timbre) appear to involve bilaterally located brain regions lacking specificity for musical material, which points to some fundamental computational properties of the brain's modular organisation.

Many outstanding questions still remain to be addressed. For instance, the exact relationships between the processing of verbal and musical material, such as between melody processing and language prosody, still require clarification. More work is generally needed to elaborate a global model for music performance, such as accounting for specific skills and assessing the individual strategies. Implicit and autobiographic episodic memory of music are untouched. Finally, the neurofunctional dynamics of these cognitive processes are still essentially unknown.

References

1. J.B. Bouillaud, Sur la faculté du langage articulé, *Bulletin de l'Académie de Médecine* **30**, 752–68 (1865).
2. B. Lechevalier, F. Eustache and Y. Rossa, *Les troubles de la perception de la musique d'origine neurologique* (Masson, Paris, 1985).
3. I. Peretz, Auditory agnosia: a functional analysis. In: S. McAdams and E. Bigand (eds.), *Thinking in Sound: Cognitive Aspects of Human Audition* (Oxford University Press, Oxford, 1993), pp. 199–230.
4. D. Kimura, Some effects of temporal lobe damage on auditory perception, *Can. J. Psychol.* **15**, 156–65 (1961).
5. B. Milner, Laterality effects in audition. In: V.B. Mountcastle (ed.), *Interhemispheric Relations and Cerebral Dominance* (Johns Hopkins University Press, Baltimore, 1962), pp. 244–57.
6. F. Eustache, B. Lechevalier, F. Viader, J. Lambert, Identification and dicrimination disorders in auditory perception: a report on two cases, *Neuropsychologia* **28**, 257–70 (1990).
7. C. Liegois-Chauvel, I. Peretz, M. Babai, V. Laguitton and P. Chauvel, Contribution of different cortical areas in the temporal lobes to music processing, *Brain* **121**, 1853–67 (1998).
8. J. Ayotte, I. Peretz, I. Rousseau, C. Bard, M. Bojanowski, Patterns of music agnosia associated with middle cerebral artery infarcts, *Brain* **23**, 1926–38 (2000).
9. H. Platel, C. Price, J.C. Baron, R. Wise, J. Lambert, R.S.J. Frackowiak, B. Lechevalier and F. Eustache, The structural components of music perception: a functional anatomical study, *Brain* **120**, 229–43 (1997).
10. J.C. Baron, Etude de la neuro-anatomie fonctionnelle de la perception par la tomograpie à positions, *Rev. Neurol. (Paris)* **151**, 511–7 (1995).
11. T. Elbert, C. Pantev, C. Wienbruch, B. Rockstroh and E. Taub, Increased cortical representation of the fingers of the left hand in string players, *Science* **270**, 305–7 (1995).
12. A.J. Blood, R.J. Zatorre, P. Bermudez and A.C. Evans, Emotional responses to pleasant and unpleasant music correlates with activity in paralimbic regions, *Nat. Neurosci.* **2**, 382–7 (1999).
13. D.W. Perry, R.J. Zatorre, M. Petrides, B. Alivisatos, E. Meyer and A. Evans, Localization of cerebral activity during simple singing, *NeuroReport* **10**, 3979–84 (1999).
14. N.A. Lassen, B. Larsen and J.M. Orgogozo, Les localizations corticales vues par la gamma-camera dynamique: une nouvelle approche en neuropsychologie, *L'encéphale* **4**, 233–49 (1978).

15. D. Knopman, A. Rubens, A. Klassen, M. Meyer and N. Niccum, Regional cerebral blood flow patterns during verbal and non-verbal auditory activation, *Brain and Language* **9**, 93–112 (1986).
16. J.L. Lauter, P. Herscovitch, C. Fomby and M.E. Raichle, Tonotopic organization in human auditory cortex revealed by positron emission tomography, *Hearing Research* **20**, 199–205 (1985).
17. C. Pantev, M. Hoke, B. Lütkenhöner and K. Lehnertz, Tonotopic organization of the human auditory cortex: pitch versus frequency representations, *Science* **246**, 486–8 (1989).
18. C. Liegeois-Chauvel, A. Musolino and P. Chauvel, Localization of the primary auditory area in man, *Brain* **114**, 139–53 (1991).
19. C. Pantev, R. Oostenveld, A. Engelien, B. Ross, L.E. Roberts and M. Hoke, Increased auditory cortical representation in musicians, *Nature* **392**, 811–4 (1998).
20. G. Schlaug, L. Jancke, Y. Huang and H. Steinmetz, *In vivo* evidence of structural brain asymmetry in musicians, *Science* **267**, 699–701 (1995).
21. R.J. Zatorre, D.W. Perry, C.A. Beckett, C.F. Westbury and A.C. Evans, Functional anatomy of musical processing in listeners with absolute pitch and relative pitch, *Proc. Natl. Acad. Sci. U.S.A.* **95**, 3172–7 (1998).
22. J.C. Mazziotta, M.E. Phelps, R.E. Carson and D.E. Kuhl, Tomographic mapping of human cerebral metabolishm: auditory stimulation, *Neurology* **32**, 921–37 (1982).
23. J. Sergent, E. Zuck, S. Terriah and B. MacDonald, Distributed neural network underlying musical sight-reading and keyboard performance, *Science* **257**, 106–9 (1992).
24. J. Sergent, Mapping the musician brain, *Hum. Brain Mapp.* **1**, 20–38 (1993).
25. H.A. Drury and D.C. Van Essen, Functional specializations in human cerebral cortex analyzed using the Visible Man Surface-Based Atlas, *Hum. Brain Mapp.* **5**, 233–7 (1997).
26. S.E. Petersen, P.T. Fox, M.I. Posner, M. Mintun and M.E. Raichle, Position emission tomographic studies of the cortical anatomy of single-word processing, *Nature* **331**, 585–8 (1988).
27. R.J. Zatorre, A.C. Evans, E. Meyer and A. Gjedde, Lateralization of phonetic and pitch discrimination in speech processing, *Science* **256**, 846–9 (1992).
28. V.B. Penhune, R.J. Zatorre and A.C. Evans, Cerebellar contributions to motor timing: a PET study of auditory and visual rhythm reproduction, *J. Cogn. Neurosci.* **10**, 752–65 (1998).
29. R.J. Wise, J. Greene, C. Buchel and S.K. Scott, Brain regions involved in articulation, *Lancet* **353**, 1057–61 (1999).
30. P. Auzou, F. Eustache, P. Etevenon, H. Platel, P. Rioux, J. Lambert, B. Lechevalier, E. Zarifian and J.C. Baron, Topographic EEG activations during

timbre and pitch discrimination tasks using musical sounds, *Neuropsychologia* **33**, 25–37 (1994).

31. T. Horikochi, Y. Asari, A. Watanabe, Y. Nagaseki, H. Nukui, H. Sasaki and K. Komiya, Music alexia in a patient with mild pure alexia: disturbed visual perception of nonverbal meaningful figures, *Cortex* **33**, 187–94 (1997).
32. B. Desgranges, J.C. Baron and F. Eustache, The functional neuroanatomy of episodic memory: the role of the frontal lobes, the hippocampal formation, and others aeras, *NeuroImage* **8**, 198–213 (1998).
33. R. Cabeza and L. Nyberg, Imaging cognition II: empirical review of 275 PET and fMRI studies, *J. Cogn. Neurosci.* **12**, 1–47 (2000).
34. R.J. Zattore, A.C. Evans and E. Meyer, Neural mechanisms underlying melodic perception and memory for pitch, *J. Neurosci.* **14**, 1908–19 (1994).
35. H. Holcomb, D. Medoff, P. Caudill, Z. Zhao, A. Lahti, R. Dannals and C. Tamminga, Cerebral blood flow relationships associated with a difficult tone recognition task in trained normal volunteers, *Cerebral Cortex* **8**, 534–42 (1998).
36. B. Mazoyer, S. Dehaene, N. Tzourio, V. Frak, M. Murayama, L. Cohen *et al.*, The cortical representation of speech, *J. Cogn. Neurosci.* **5**, 467–79 (1994).
37. A.R. Halpern and R.J. Zatorre, When that tune runs through your head: a PET investigation of auditory imagery for familiar melodies, *Cerebral Cortex* **9**, 697–704 (1999).
38. H. Platel, J.C. Baron, B. Desgranges, F. Bernard and F. Eustache, Semantic and episodic memory of music are subserved by distinct neural networks, *NeuroImage* **20**, 244–56.
39. N. Wertheim and M.I. Botez, Plan d'investigation des functions musicales, *Encéphale* **48**, 246–54 (1959).
40. F. Bernard, B. Desgrange, H. Platel, J. C. Baron and F. Eustache, Contributions of frontal and medial temporal regions to verbal episodic memory: a PET study, *NeuroReport* **12**, 1737–41 (2001).
41. M.L. Tempini, C. Price, O. Josephs, R. Vandenberghe, S. Cappa, N. Kapur and R.S.J. Frackowiak, The neural systems sustaining face and proper-name processing, *Brain* **121**, 2103–18 (1998).

Chapter 11

Musical Instruments as Metaphors in Brain Science: From René Descartes to John Hughlings Jackson

C.U.M. Smith

Introduction: Metaphors

Metaphors are central to human discourse. Although it has been argued that the sciences should be the realm of plain unembellished speech (*Nullius in verba*), they are nevertheless replete with metaphors and analogies. The neurosciences provide no exceptions to this rule. Metaphors, moreover, are far more than a mere "decoration" or felicitous use of language. Aristotle in *Poetics* (1459a) writes that "... the greatest thing by far is to be master of metaphor. It is one thing that cannot be learnt from others; it is also a sign of genius, since good metaphor implies an intuitive perception of similarities in the dissimilar." "The mind of man," writes the 19th century physicist John Tyndall,[1] "may be compared to a musical instrument, with a certain range of notes, beyond which in both directions we have an infinitude of silence." This, like poetry, says more than can be easily expressed in didactic prose. Giambattista Vico writes that metaphors perform a "uniquely revelatory function" and, furthermore, that "every metaphor is a fable in brief".[2] Thomas Kuhn agrees. "Consistency with an accepted underlying metaphor," he writes in *Structure of Scientific Revolutions*,[3] "goes far towards determining what will and what will not be accepted as an explanation." Mark Johnson[4] goes so far as to say that "metaphor is... a conceptual and experiential process that structures our world".

Students of literature have expended much time and ink in an endeavour to understand the function of metaphor. Max Black,[5] for instance, calls the metaphor word the focus and argues that it summons up a system of associated commonplaces. To call a man a wolf, he points out, causes "the system of commonplaces" associated with "wolf" to become attached to "man". The notion of "wolf" organises our view of man. I.A. Richards[6] coined the terms "tenor" and "vehicle" for two thoughts which interact together and work with each other. Julian Jaynes in his well-known book, *The Origins of Consciousness in the Breakdown of the Bicameral Mind*, invented the terms "metaphrand") for that which is illuminated) and "metaphrier" (for that which does the illuminating), whilst Lakoff[7] uses the term "target" and "source".

Although, as Aristotle says, mastery of metaphor is the greatest thing, there is, as always, a downside. It is not only that metaphors may mislead, skewing our attention in unproductive directions, but also that they may harden into what Douglas Berggren[8] calls "myth". Berggren defines myth as "believed absurdity." Perhaps this is what Vesalius encountered as a student at the Castle School in Brussels when he was forced to add a drawing of the medieval three-cell psychology to his anatomical notes. Perhaps this is what our students encounter today when they learn that brain is to mind what computer hardware is to computer software.[9] Berggren adds that the danger is that the target (metaphrand) is mistaken for, or equated with, the source (metaphrier); when, in other words, the metaphrier becomes the literal truth about the subject. "It is the familiar, or inherited and submerged, metaphor," he goes on, "which is the most dangerous."

Descartes: The Church Organ

It may be that we can trace the first use of musical instruments as metaphors for the brain, or, in this case, the mind back to classical antiquity. It will be recalled that Plato (*Phaedo*) includes amongst the group of friends around the deathbed of Socrates a pythagorean philosopher, Simmias, who suggests that the soul is the harmony of the body. Socrates is, of course, dismissive of this metaphor, recognising that it goes against the whole of his philosophy of anamnesis. More than 2000 years later, at the beginning of the modern era of philosophy, we find René Descartes, regarded by many as the instigator of scientific neurophysiology, also making use of metaphors from musical instruments to illuminate the workings of the nervous system.

Descartes was very well versed in music and musicology. His very first literary composition was *Musicae Compendium*,[10] a New Year's Day present to his great friend Isaac Beeckman. In this manuscript Descartes sets out theories of musical composition and includes a large amount on the psychophysics of music backed up by numerous experiments on instruments such as lutes, flutes, etc. *Musicae Compendium* remained in manuscript until shortly after the philosopher's death in 1650 and was translated into English in 1653 and French in 1658.

Descartes' use of musical instruments as metaphors in neurophysiology arrived later, when he came to write his *Treatise of Man* (*l'Homme*) in the late 1620s and early 1630s. It will be recalled that his major metaphor in *Treatise* was taken from the water-powered statues constructed by the Francini brothers in the grottoes at St Germaine-en-Laye, just outside Paris. However, he also makes use of church organs as important metaphriers to illuminate the working of his mechanistic neurophysiology. This is unsurprising for, as we shall see below, ecclesiastical organs were often by far the most advanced mechanisms of their day.

It will be remembered that the Cartesian neurophysiology sees the "activated" blood fuming off from the dark fire in the heart ascending via the carotids to the ventricles of the brain (Figure 1). As it passes through the innumerable vessels in the marrow of the brain the "animal spirits", a very subtle fluid, are filtered out. This makes its way into the cerebral ventricles, whose walls are studded with innumerable valves opening into tubular nerves leading to the body's muscles. When these valves open, the animal spirits, under pressure in the ventricles, escape down the hollow tubular nerves to inflate the muscles. This is the neurophysiology which Descartes illuminates by way of his church-organ metaphor.

"If you have ever had," he writes in *L'Homme* (p. 166), "the curiosity to examine the organs in our churches, you will know how the bellows push air into certain receptacles—'wind-chests'. And you will know how the air passes from there into one or other of the pipes depending on the different ways in which the organist moves his fingers." Descartes then goes on to apply this metaphrier to illuminate his neurophysiology. The heart, he says, may be likened to the organ's bellows; the brain's ventricles to the "wind-chest"; external objects to the organist's fingers which press certain keys and cause the air in the wind-chest to flow into certain pipes.

It is interesting to note that the early 17th century was a period during which much attention was given to the construction of organs, including water-powered organs. The latter instruments were, of course, nothing new in the Renaissance. The earliest records of water-powered organs stretch back to the Alexandrians in the third century BC. The best-known case is that of Ctesibus (*c.* 250 BC), who left a fragmentary account of an organ where water provided constant pressure on the wind-chest. Hydraulically powered organs

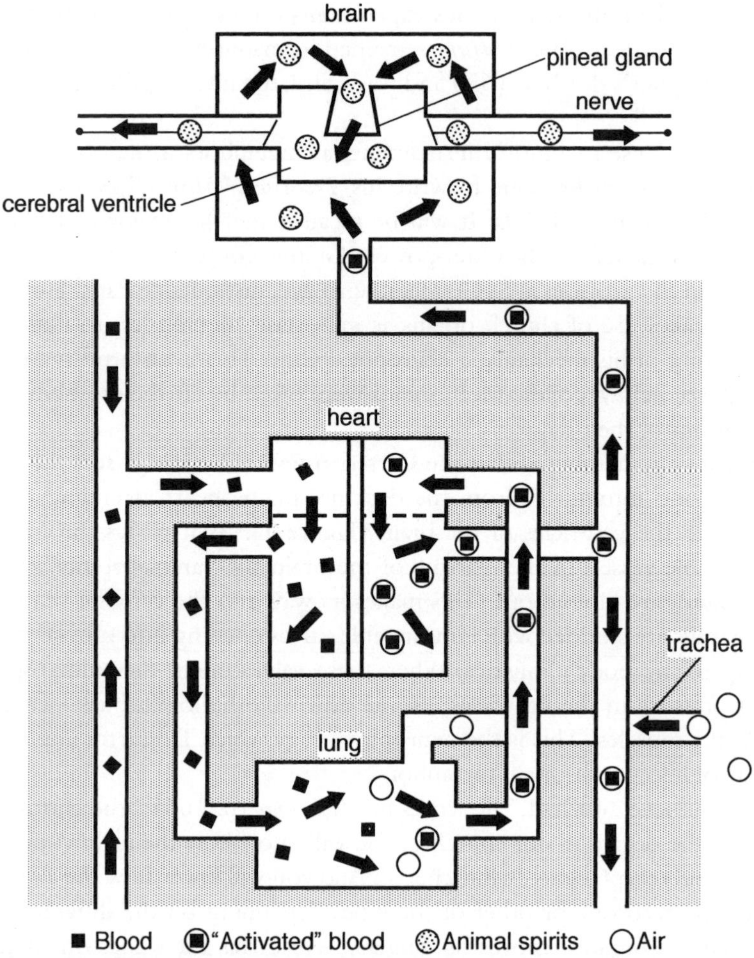

Fig. 1. Cartesian neurophysiology. Explanation in text. (Modified from Smith.[31])

were of course a great boon to the servants of the Church. An account written in the 10th century AD tells of an instrument with 26 bellows worked by 70 sweating monks, and in the mid-14th century the organ at Halberstadt was powered by 20 bellows worked by 10 labourers. It is hardly surprising, then, that during the 16th century numerous water-powered organs began to be constructed. At the end of the century, in 1596, the year of Descartes' birth, Luca Blasi built a hydraulically powered organ for the Quirinale in Rome.

It was this organ that was reconstructed by perhaps the most famous of all builders of water-powered organs, Athanasius Kircher (1602–1680), with the help of Matteo Marione in 1647–8. It will be remembered that Descartes visited Italy (Venice and Rome) in the years 1623–4. This was before Kircher's reconstruction of the Quirinale organ but during the existence of Blasi's instrument. It is difficult to believe that Descartes, fascinated by all new inventions, did not pay a visit. If he did he would have found a valuable hint for the neurophysiology he was to construct on his return to France and the Netherlands.

Organs had from the earliest times been masterpieces of engineering. Figure 2 is an illustration from the first volume of Kircher's treatise. It gives an idea of the craftsmanship involved.

Kircher's Quirinale organ used a technique employed by iron foundries in Italy as early as the mid-16th century. It involved pouring water down a long tube so that it mixed with air, forming a vortex: another phenomenon which much occupied Descartes. At the bottom of the tube the air and water are separated in a special chamber, the "Aeolian chamber", and the air is led away to pressure up the wind-chest and, as Figure 3 shows, the escaping water drives bellows via a water-wheel.

It is not difficult to see how these general ideas about the mixture and then separation of fluids might have influenced Descartes' imagiination when he came to construct his neurophysiology (Figure 1).

Kircher's famous book, *Musurgia Universalis*,[12] published in 1650, provides an exhaustive compendium of early 17th century musicology. He describes and illustrates the huge ingenuity which was devoted to the construction of organs and other instruments. Some organs used the flow of water to turn a paddle wheel connected to a drum, which in turn controlled the flow of air into the organ pipes and hence the melody (Figure 4).

Finally, *Musurgia Universalis* describes how such early automated organs could be, to use a modern term, "programmed", and even how to build a device to compose music: the *arca musarithmica*. Kircher's illustration of an automated organ is shown in Figure 5. The water-powered cylinder turns. The tune represented by a series of indentations on its surface actuates the keyboard. At one side four smiths beat an anvil: a reference to Pythagoras, who (as one legend has it) first discovered harmonics by listening outside a blacksmith's forge.

There is no record that Descartes ever met Athanasius Kircher, and the *Musurgia* was published in the year Descartes died. Nevertheless Kircher was active in many scientific fields in the mid-17th century. Indeed, the breadth of his genius has led to a comparison with Leonardo. His work was noted and discussed by both Boyle and Leibniz.

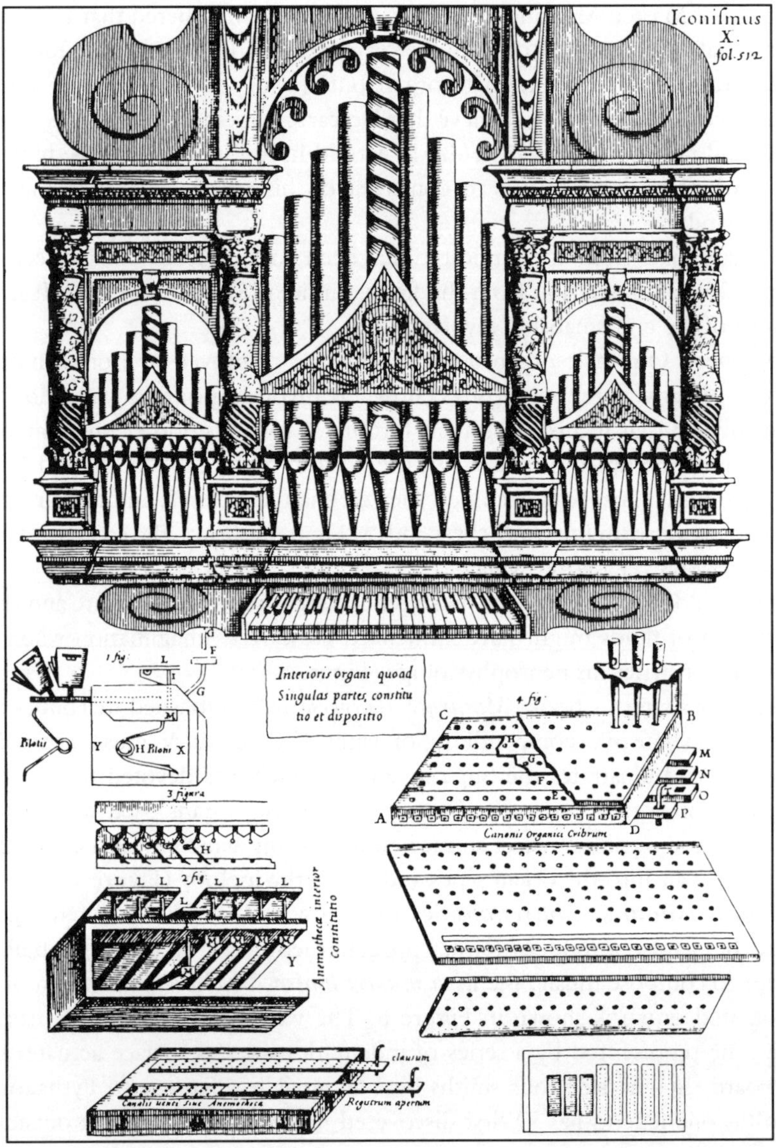

Fig. 2. Seventeenth century organ to show the intricacy of construction.[12]

Descartes extracts some of what, following Max Black, we might call the "commonplaces" of organs to illuminate other features of his brain model. He points out that "the harmony of an organ does not depend on the externally visible arrangement of the pipes or on the shape of the sound-chests

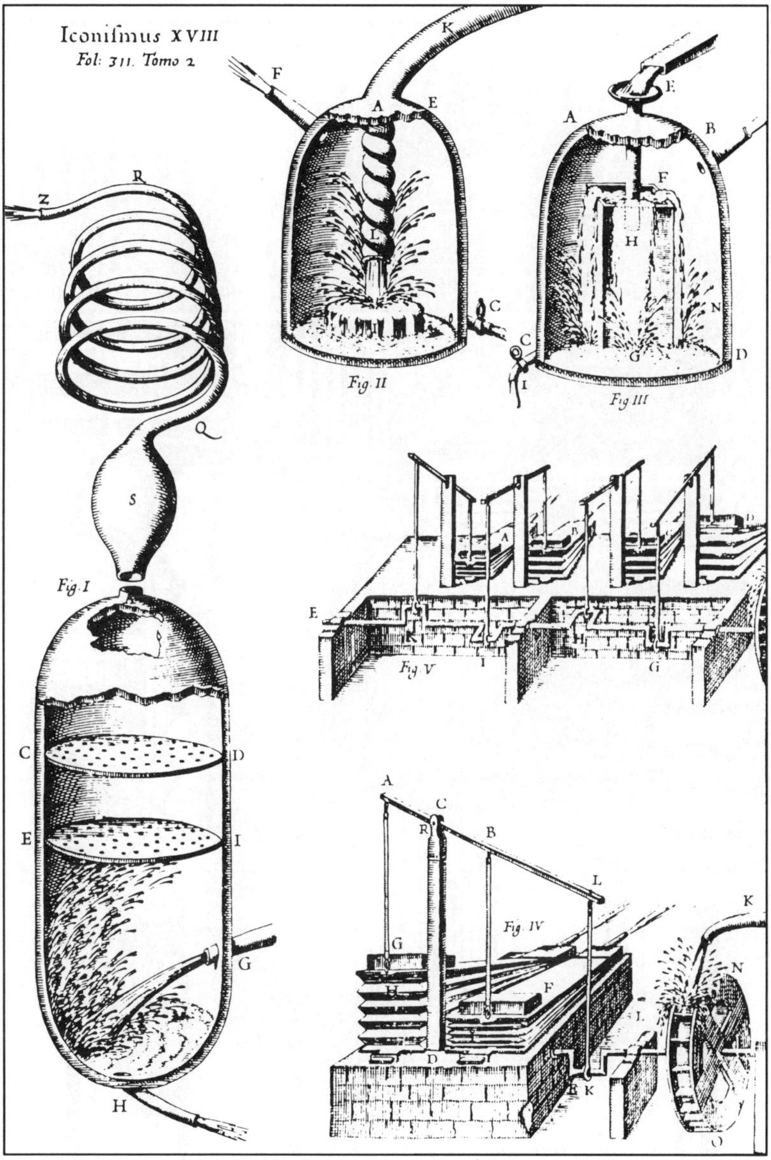

Fig. 3. A variety of aeolian chambers and pumps.[12]

or other parts, but solely on three factors: the air which comes from the bellows, the pipes which make the sound and the distribution of the air in the pipes". Similarly, he says, with the neurophysiology. It does not depend on the external shape of the visible parts which anatomists distinguish in

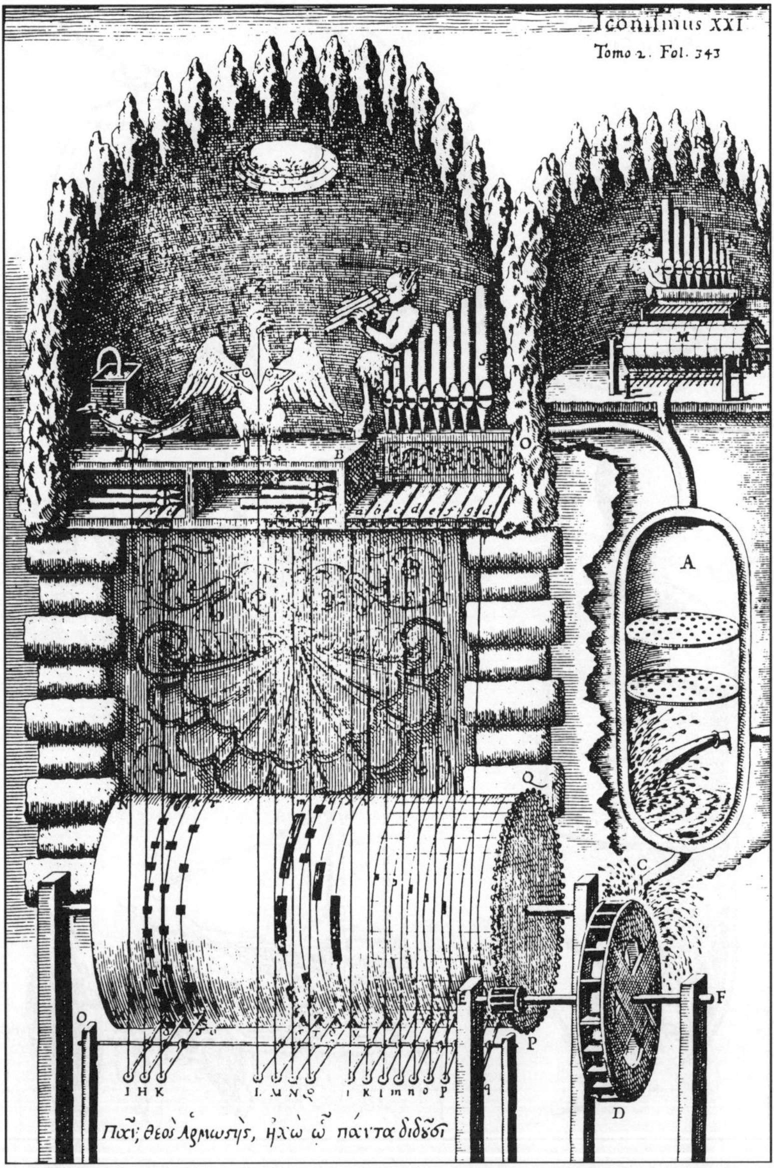

Fig. 4. Aeolian chamber serving the dual purpose of driving a water wheel and pressurising wind chests. The water wheel controls not only the organ's keyboard but also Pan, in his grotto, playing his pipes, accompanied by a cuckoo and a crow, whilst, in a smaller grotto, Echo replies.[12]

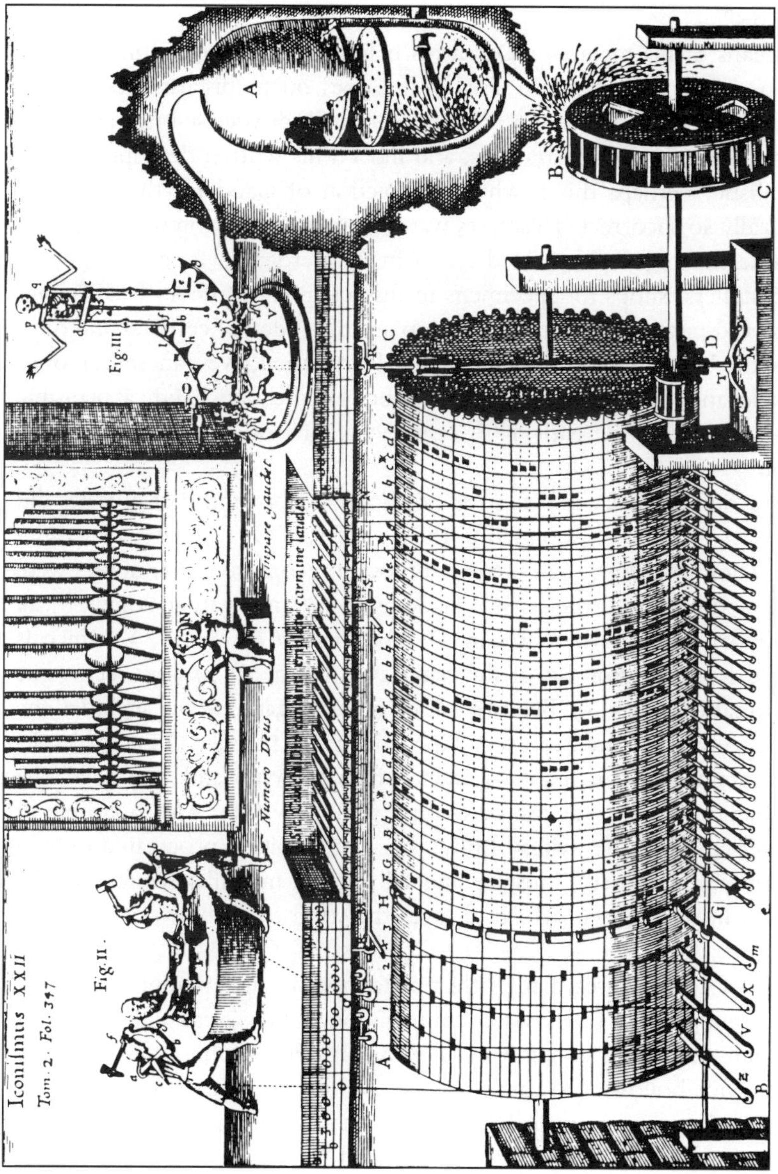

Fig. 5. Mechanism controlling an organ's keyboard and, to the left, four smiths with differently weighted hammers beating out a harmony.[12]

the substance of the brain, or on the shape of the ventricles, but solely on three factors: "the spirits which come from the heart, the pores of the brain through which they pass, and the ways in which the spirits are distributed in these pores".

By means of his metaphor Descartes believes he has been able to focus attention on the essentials. In *Treatise* he goes on to discuss these essentials. As is clear from his account, these do not include precise brain anatomy. Perhaps this is why his illustrations, and indeed his written descriptions, are so unrealistic. Perhaps this is why his depiction of gland H (the pineal) is anatomically so incorrect. Descartes was not afraid of anatomising. Indeed, he became the object of some derision in Amsterdam, where he regularly visited butchers' shops for specimens to dissect. But his theory in *l'Homme* evidently did not require him to develop an exact idea of cerebral anatomy. He was no Vesalius, no Thomas Willis. Here, then, we can see at once the upside and the downside of metaphor: on the one hand, a plausible theory—at least for the early 17th century; on the other a misdirection of attention.

The recognition that nerves were not hollow tubes and that muscles did not contract by inflation soon led to the downfall of Cartesian-type iatromechanics. Thomas Willis (1621–1675), although recognising that nerves were not hollow tubes, nevertheless still made use of of an organ analogy: "... all this medullar Trunk," he writes in *The Anatomy of the Brain*,[13] "which is continued from the bottom of the brain even to the *Os sacrum* seems like the Pneumatick Chest, or Bellows, of a pair of Organs, which includes the blast or breath destinated to every Pipe; for in like manner the animal spirits are contained in this marrowy tract, which blow up and actuate all the Nerves hanging thereto as the occasion serves" (p. 124). And, a couple of pages later (p. 126), he writes of how the animal spirits (procreated only in the "brain and Cerebel") "inspire and fill full the medullar trunk: like the Chest of a musical Organ which receives the wind to be blown into all the pipes".

Willis, of course, uses many other metaphors in his attempt to decribe the functioning of the brain: water courses, ponds, tides, seas, light rays, etc. The "organ" metaphor certainly did not match well with his conviction that nerves are not hollow: "no cavity can be seen in them, no not by the help of spectacles or a microscope" (p. 127). Is this an instance of Berggren's "believed absurdity"? As the facts of brain anatomy became better known, it became more and more difficult to make use of wind-instrument analogies. In the next century attention shifted to strings.

David Hartley: Stringed Instruments

In 1745/1749 David Hartley devised an iatromechanics based on vibration in solid nerves. The source of his theory was a suggestion published by Isaac Newton in *Principia Mathematica* and *Optics*. Hartley's general theory was destined to be highly influential.[14] It has often been regarded as the foundation work in psychophysiology.[15,16]

At the centre of the theory is a metaphor derived from a musical instrument: a stringed instrument such as a violin or cello. Hartley uses the metaphor to illuminate the physical basis of memory, crucial to his associationist psychology. "The tone of a musical string," he writes, "always leans toward the state into which it was last put."[17] If a string is tautened and then relaxed to its former state, he says, its tone will be somewhat higher than formerly. If this procedure is carried out on numerous occasions, the string comes to have a permanently higher pitch than it had originally. This is because the vibration of a string depends on both its tension and its unit mass. Stretching a string thins it and hence reduces its unit mass, and in consequence increases its period of vibration.

Hartley uses this phenomenon as a metaphor for the physical basis of memory. The medullary substance of the brain, according to his theory, is in a constant vibratory state. Repeated exposure to a particular vibration, caused by a particular stimulus, alters its molecular structure (his phrase) so that it is predisposed to vibrate in that mode. Hartley's neurophysiological ideas are, in fact, just as speculative as those of Descartes a century before. Like those of Descartes, they were soon discarded, although the association psychology, for which they formed the physical basis, lived on. His use of a metaphor from a musical instrument in this case illuminates his basic idea of the brain's functioning. He sees the physical basis of mentality as a hugely complex vibration in the medullary substance of the brain. This concept was carried through into some of the most influential pychophysiology of the 19th century.

Herbert Spencer: Piano and Piano-mecanique

Herbert Spencer published the first edition of *Principles of Psychology* in 1855 and a greatly expanded second edition in two volumes in 1870 and 1872 (published as parts IV and V of *Synthetic Philosophy*).[18] John Hughlings Jackson was strongly influenced by the second edition.[19] Spencer's psychophysiology is complex and, as befits the philosopher of evolution, pervaded by evolutionary ideas. I have written about it at length elsewhere.[20] However, it is relevant to note here that amongst his many metaphors, musical instruments, especially the pianoforte and the recently invented piano-mécanique, are especially prominent. In fact Spencer was not the first to make use of the pianoforte metaphor. In *Elements of Physiology* Johannes Müller[21] writes that "the fibres of all the motor, cerebral and spinal nerves may be imagined as spread out in the medulla oblongata and exposed to the will like the keys of the pianoforte".

Spencer, however, makes a far more extensive use of this metaphor. There are three significant instances. First he seeks to show that the many-splendoured subjectivity we all live through is in fact built from combinations and permutations of "atomic", or, to use his own term, "unit" feelings. Nothing very revolutionary about this, of course. Mental atomism was common amongst the British empiricist philosophers of the 18th century. Spencer, however, uses a musical analogy to explain his theory. He writes that "there is at least one kind of feeling which, as ordinarily experienced, seems elementary that is definitely not elementary." He is referring to musical tones. He points out that below about 10 Hz a tone is usually experienced as a succession of individual "blows" or "taps". As the frequency is increased, however, the sensation changes to that of a continuous tone, whose quality changes as the frequency changes. The tone's harshness or sweetness, liquidity or clearness, depends furthermore on combinations of frequencies. It is of course unfortunate, or perhaps fortunate, for Spencer (we remember what Huxley said about beautiful theories and ugly facts) that he was unaware of Helmholtz' 1863 "place" theory of auditory physiology. For Spencer concludes that the experiencing of musical tones is paradigmatic. It shows how "an enormous number of qualitatively contrasted kinds of consciousness that severally seem elementary, prove to be composed of one simple kind of consciousness (a sudden 'happening' or 'shock'), combined and recombined with itself in multitudinous ways."[22]

What are the neurophysiological correlatives of these "unit feelings"? In both the first and the second edition of *Principles of Psychology*, Spencer is writing decades before the establishment of the neuron doctrine and almost a century before Hodgkin and Huxley showed us the nature of nerve impulses or action potentials. So his ideas now seem antiquated. His candidate for the neurophysiological correlative is "the intermittent wave of the nerve current".[23] But are there enough of these neurophysiological units to correlate with the multitudinous different qualities and modes of feeling which we live through in our everyday lives? Is the neurohistology rich enough? Here Spencer brings in his second musical metaphor. If the keys of a piano are struck separately, he says, about 100 different notes may be sounded. But consider, he goes on, the number of different chords which may be obtained when more than one key is struck at once. This number he computes to be in excess of 10^{30}. Similarly in the brain: "A limited number of cells and fibres becomes the seat of a relatively unlimited number of perceptions."[24]

Spencer's final musical metaphor is even more intriguing. In some ways it is reminiscent of Descartes. Just as Descartes had been impressed with the mechanical artefacts at St Germaine-en-Laye, so Spencer was influenced by another marvel of contemporary technology: the Victorian musical box.

"Every one," he says,[25] "has watched the revolving barrel of a musical box... and every one sees that the set of pins (on the barrel) arranged in a special way, represents, in a sense, the harmonised melody produced." It is easy, he continues, "to conceive of an arrangement permitting indefinite multiplication of such pin sets". Indeed, just such an instrument, Debain's piano-mécanique, was exhibited at the Crystal Palace in 1851.

Instead of a barrel, the pins were set upon a flat sheet which passed down into the instrument between two rollers. Any number of such sheets—Spencer calls them "tune boards"—can, in principle, be manufactured. Athanasius Kircher, in the first half of the 17th century, would have been delighted, and probably unsurprised, by this idea. Descartes missed a trick, perhaps because his main concern was to establish that mechanistic brain theory was not a mere absurdity. The cerebrum and the cerebellum, Spencer believed, may be likened to "vast magazines of such tune-boards, duly classified and adjusted for being brought into instant action".[26] These tune-boards have been elaborated over aeons of evolutionary time and are ready to be triggered into action when appropriate stimuli occur.

Spencer's example is the approach of an enemy. There is no time here to describe his quite elaborate theory.[20] In essence the tune-board is activated and plays upon unit feelings whose physical aspects are located in the medulla. The use of a metaphor from a musical instrument is clear enough. He concludes this section of *Psychology* as follows: "In the language of our illustration, we may say that the superior nervous centres in playing upon the inferior ones, bring out not only specific chords and cadences of feelings, but, in so doing, arouse reverberating echoes of all kindred chords and cadences that have been struck during an immeasurable past—producing a great volume of indefinite tones harmonising with definite tones."[18]

John Hughlings Jackson's concept of "barrel-organism" bears striking resemblance to Spencer's concept of "tune-boards". Although Jackson references the concept to W.T. Gairdner, it is hard to believe that so ardent a Spencerian could not have been influenced by the quite extensive treatment given in the latter's *Psychology*. However this may be, Jackson, following Gairdner, uses it as metaphor for repeated automatic action and/or speech after brain injury. This automatism often repeats that which was taking place immediately before the injury. Jackson relates the sad case of a young clergyman who suffered a brain injury as he was about to get married and for the rest of his life, until the age of 80, "talked of nothing but his approaching wedding".[27] He also refers to a clerk engaged in constructing a catalogue who, after a paralytic stroke, could only say, over and over again, "list complete". The barrel organ, in these cases, is playing on even though the ghostly organ-grinder is no more.

Conclusion

This rapid survey of the use of musical instruments as metaphors in brain science shows that it recurs again and again from the Pythagoreans in classical antiquity through to the 19th century with Johannes Müller, Herbert Spencer and Hughlings Jackson. In some cases, for instance Herbert Spencer's reference to Debain's piano-mécanique, the metaphor directs the scientist's attention towards the detailed microstructure and in this sense prefigures to some extent our contemporary ruling metaphor, the computer. In other, and to my mind more interesting cases, which include Spencer's use of piano chords, the metaphor directs our attention upwards to the total outcome of the brain's operations.

In this regard, we might return to a variant of Descartes' wind instrument metaphor. We might liken the totality of the brain's activity to the note sounded by a flute when different stops are closed. This metaphor, it seems to me, counters one of the dangers of contemporary neuroimaging. The fascinating pictures from fMRI, MEG, etc., with their centres for this and regions for that, often seem to suggest that it is sufficient for these localities to "light up" for the perception or thought to occur.

Llinas,[28] amongst others, has emphasised that we should not forget the "silent" areas, the "silent" neurons, in the cerebrum. A metaphor from the sound generated by a flute or oboe or other stopped wind instrument helps to emphasise this. It helps to emphasise that "silent" neurons are as important as "active" neurons in forming the cerebral pattern associated with consciousness. William James, that most influential of neuropsychologists, writes that the major principle of his psychology is that "the consciousness which is itself an integral thing not made of parts 'corresponds' to the entire activity of the brain, whatever that may be at the moment".[29]

In our final metaphor, then, it is the total vibration of the instrument which provides the note, not the particular stop or stops which are covered. It is the total activity pattern of the brain, not just the particular regions which "light up" in the fMRI or MEG, which corresponds to the perceptual or other consciousness. Friedrich Nietzsche, that 19th century master of metaphor, provides a final figure, once again emphasising totality rather than detailed mechanism. Furthermore, he completes the range of instruments used as metaphors. Instead of wind or string instruments, he goes to the orchestra's final resource: percussion. He likens the activity of the brain when a thought or perception occurs to the intricate pattern of a Chladni figure formed by sand when a tightly stretched membrane vibrates.[30]

References

1. J. Tyndall, *Fragments of Science*, 8th ed., Vol. 2, pp. 53–74, *Matter and Force* (Longmans, Green & Co., London, 1892).
2. G. Vico, *Scienza Nuova* (1744), transl. T.H. Begrin and M.H. Fisch (Cornell University Press, Ithaca, 1940), Chap. 2.
3. T. Kuhn, *The Structure of Scientific Revolutions* (Chicago University Press, 1962).
4. M. Johnson, Why metaphor matters to philosophy, *Metaphor and Symbolic Activity* **10**, 157–62 (1995).
5. M. Black, Metaphor, *Proceedings of the Aristotelian Society* **55**, 273–94 (1955).
6. I.A. Richards, *The Philosophy of Rhetoric* (Oxford University Press, London, 1936).
7. G. Lakoff, The contemporary theory of metaphor. In: A. Ortony (ed.), *Metaphor and Thought* (Cambridge University Press, 1997), 2nd ed., pp. 202–51.
8. D. Berggren, The use and abuse of metaphor, 1 & 2, *Review of Metaphysics* **16**, 237–58, 450–72 (1962).
9. V. Kennedy, The computational metaphor of mind: more bugs in the program, *Metaphor and Symbolic Activity* **14**, 281–92 (1999).
10. R. Descartes, *Musicae Compendium* (1618), transl. Walter Robert, with introduction and notes by Charles Kent (American Institute of Musicology, 1961).
11. R. Descartes, *Traité de l'Homme* (Paris, 1633/1662); transl. T.S. Hall, *Treatise of Man* (Harvard University Press, Cambridge, Massachusetts, 1972).
12. A. Kircher, *Musurgia Universalis* (Roma, 1650), edited with a foreword by Ulf Scharlau (Georg Olms Verlag, Hildesheim/New York, 1970).
13. T. Willis, *The Anatomy of the Brain and the Description and Use of the Nerves in the remaining medical works of that Famous and Renowned Physician, Dr Thomas Willis* (1664). English transl. in 1681 by S. Pordage, London; ed. W. Feindel (McGill University Press, Montreal, 1965).

14. C.U.M. Smith, David Hartley's Newtonian neuropsychology, *J. Hist. Behav. Sci.* **23**, 123–36 (1987).
15. G.S. Brett, *A History of Psychology* (George Allen and Unwin, London, 1921), Vol. 2.
16. R.M. Young, *Mind, Brain and Adaptation in the Nineteenth Century* (Cambridge University Press, Cambridge, 1979), p. 97.
17. D. Hartley, *Observations on Man, His Frame, His Duty and His Expectations* (Thomas Tegg, London, 1749), p. 254.
18. H. Spencer, *Principles of Psychology*, 2nd. ed. (Williams and Norgate, London), Vol. 1 (1870); Vol. 2 (1872).
19. C.U.M. Smith, Evolution and the problem of mind: Part 2, John Hughlings Jackson, *J. Hist. Biol*. **15**, 241–62 (1982).
20. C.U.M. Smith, Evolution and the problem of mind: Part 1, Herbert Spencer, *J. Hist. Biol.* **15**, 55–88 (1982).
21. J. Müller, *Elements of Physiology* (Taylor and Walton, London, 1842).
22. H. Spencer, *ibid.*, vol. 1, p. 150.
23. *Ibid.*, p. 562.
24. *Ibid.*, p. 563.
25. *Ibid.*, p. 566.
26. *Ibid.*, p. 567.
27. J.H. Jackson, On affections of speech from disease of the brain. In J. Taylor (ed.), *Selected Writings of John Hughlings Jackson* (Hodder and Stoughton, London, 1932), Vol. 2, pp. 184–212.
28. R. Llinas and D. Paré, The brain as a closed system modulated by the senses. In: R. Llinas and P.S. Churchland, *The Mind–Brain Continuum* (MIT Press, Cambridge, MA, and London, 1996).
29. W. James, *The Principles of Psychology* (1890), reprinted (Dover, New York, 1950), Vol. 1, p. 177.
30. F. Nietzsche, The Philosopher. In: D. Breazeale (ed.), *Philosophy and Truth: Selection from Nietzsche's Notebooks of the Early 1870s* (Humanities, New Jersey, 1979).
31. C.U.M. Smith, *The Problem of Life* (Macmillan, London, 1976).

Chapter 12

The Music of Madness: Franklin's Armonica and the Vulnerable Nervous System

Stanley Finger and David A. Gallo

The armonica (or glass armonica) was invented by Benjamin Franklin in 1761 as a way to simplify the playing of musical glasses. Franz Anton Mesmer purchased one of his instruments. Leopold and Wolfgang Mozart heard Mesmer play it, and Wolfgang was among several major composers (including Gluck, Beethoven, and Donizetti) who wrote compositions or parts for it. Nevertheless, the armonica quickly garnered a sinister reputation. First, it was looked upon as a health hazard, the belief being that armonica players either went crazy, became physically ill, or even died from its unearthly sounds. Second, its music was used to promote images of madness, ghosts, and the crypt. And third, Mesmer used the instrument during his seances, ostensibly to promote healing by enhancing the flow of animal magnetism through the nerves. Although Franklin played the armonica and remained of sound mind throughout his own long life, he might have diminished the popularity of his own instrument by being extremely critical of Mesmer and his theories in his letters and in his committee's formal report of 1784 to the King of France.

Benjamin Franklin

Benjamin Franklin (1706–1790; Figure 1) is usually regarded as one of the greatest minds of the 18th century.[1–4] The reputation he garnered as a logical thinker, a skilled communicator, and a Renaissance man is even more remarkable when one realizes that many Europeans looked upon his homeland, the American colonies, as a vast cultural wasteland at the time.

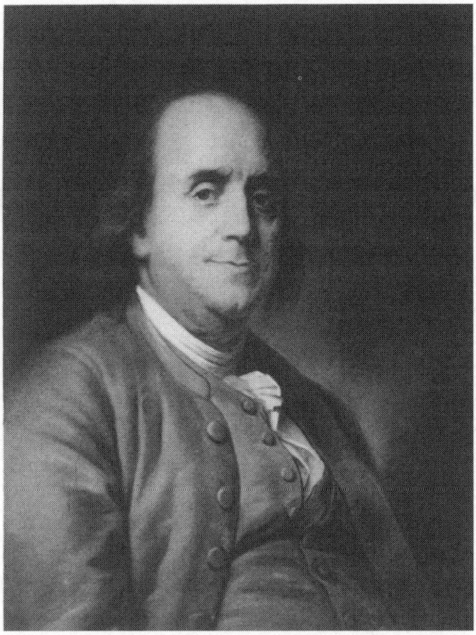

Fig. 1. Benjamin Franklin (1706–1790) as painted by Joseph-Sifrède Duplessis.

Franklin's parents came from England, and he was born in 1706 in Boston, Massachusetts. His father, Josiah, was a candle maker of good judgment who instilled a love of music in the boy and taught him to read. Reading led his son to the printing trade, writing, and publishing, first in Boston and then in Philadelphia. Through hard work, smart acquisitions, and good fortune, the man who told his countrymen how to become "healthy, wealthy, and wise" in *Poor Richard's Almanack*[5] left the printing business in 1748. By this time Franklin had also established the American Philosophical Society, outlined a plan for establishing the University of Pennsylvania, served as a colonial postmaster, taught himself several foreign languages, and was actively promoting social, political, and educational causes. Not to be overlooked is the fact that he had become increasingly involved with invention and electrical science.

In 1746, three years after witnessing an Edinburgh-trained physician (Archibald Spencer) perform some electrical experiments, and six years after inventing a new iron stove, Franklin began to experiment with electricity.[1] He first replicated some experiments from *Gentleman's Magazine* with a charged glass tube that produced sparks. Both the equipment and the magazine article were given to him by Peter Collinson, a friend who would remain a valuable correspondent on electrical matters (see letter to Collinson, September 1753[6]). Franklin then began to ask local glassblowers to make equipment for him, borrowed additional pieces of apparatus from others (e.g. Thomas Penn, 1702–1775), and even purchased all of Spencer's instruments. By 1748 he was deeply involved with understanding electrical phenomena.

Franklin's sustained efforts, especially with atmospheric electricity, resulted in an 80-page pamphlet, *Experiments and Observations on Electricity,* which appeared in 1751.[7] It was translated into French a year later and then went into other editions. In it Franklin showed the "sameness" of lightning and artificial electricity and introduced his new theory of opposing (plus and minus) charges. On its pages he also described how to "capture" lightning from the clouds with rods. In yet another section of the publication, the practical man, who would establish the first American fire insurance company, recommended pointed iron lightning rods as the best means of protecting buildings from Nature's wrath.

Franklin's pamphlet secured his reputation as a scientist during what he described in his autobiography as the "Age of Experiments." By 1753 the largely self-educated man who loved to tinker was widely recognized as the greatest authority on electricity, much to the chagrin of the Abbé (Jean-Antoine) Nollet (1700–1770), a leading French scientist who liked to think of himself as the authority on such matters.

Although his most important discoveries and inventions had now been made, Franklin enjoyed corresponding with great men of science and medicine about electricity and related phenomena (e.g. heat, light, sound, magnetism) throughout the rest of his long life. For example, in a letter dated December 21, 1757, he informed John Pringle (1707–1782), who had asked his opinion on the matter, that electrotherapy was considerably less than it was made out to be as a means of treating paralyses. Franklin explained that he had tried it on "a number of paralytics" without significant, lasting success. Although he witnessed some instances of temporary improvement, he was skeptical of the cause. He reasoned to Pringle, who would later become President of the Royal Society (1772–1778), that such effects could well have been produced by the physical demands of traveling or "by the hope of success."[6] Franklin would draw on what he knew about the power of suggestion almost three decades later, when asked to evaluate Franz Anton Mesmer's (1734–1815) medical "science."

Franklin was so respected for his "natural philosophy" of electricity that he was awarded the Sir Godfrey Copley Medal from the Royal Society in 1753.

In the same year he also received honorary Masters of Arts degrees from the "College of Cambridge" (Harvard) and Yale College. Other degrees from other institutions followed, including a Doctor of Civil Law from Oxford in 1762 (hence "Dr Franklin"). He was also made an honorary member of many European scientific societies, including London's famed Royal Society, to which he was formally admitted in 1757.[8]

Franklin devoted himself more to politics and public service after 1753, doing what he could to unite the colonies. Among his achievements on the home front were helping to draft the "Declaration of Independence" of 1776 and serving in the Continental Congress. His aspiration was to have Americans think of themselves first and foremost as Americans, rather than as residents of a particular colony, be it his own Pennsylvania or Virginia or New York.

Franklin served as the chief diplomat from the colonies to Europe prior to the American Revolution. Although he found London cold and rainy, it was his primary base for 16 years. Late in 1776, when the colonists began to rebel against the British, he was sent to France, where he had earlier been elected to the Academy of Sciences (in 1772). His mission was to secure economic and military assistance for the Americans. Not only was his diplomacy successful, but the educated, plain-spoken Pennsylvanian became something of a cult hero, personifying a rare but admirable sort of "nobility" from the New World. Although he requested a replacement in 1783 (he was then 77 and suffering from bladder stones and gout), he retained both his post and his residence in France until 1785.

Before returning to Philadelphia, where he completed the last sections of his autobiography in 1789 and died a year later, Franklin served on a committee appointed by King Louis XVI (1754–1793). Its job was to evaluate a mysterious force called "animal magnetism," which Franz Anton Mesmer contended he could manipulate to help the sick and disabled. The choice of Franklin to serve on the committee made perfect sense, for several reasons. First, he was a recognized outsider; an independent scientist who was greatly respected. Second, Mesmer's animal magnetism and Franklin's electricity were thought by some (including Mesmer) to have common features. And third, Franklin was the inventor of the armonica (also known as the glass armonica), an innovative but expensive instrument owned and mastered by Mesmer. Claiming it could enhance the flow of animal spirits, Mesmer occasionally played Franklin's instrument during his séances.

With this in mind, let us now turn to the history of Franklin's musical instrument, which acquired a bad reputation not only because of its association with Mesmer, but also because of a growing belief that playing the instrument, or even listening to it, could be dangerous to a person's health. In telling the story of how Franklin invented the armonica, how it acquired its ominous reputation, and what Franklin and Mesmer thought about each other, we are compelled to repeat some facts that appeared in a recent article by the present authors.[9] In this contribution, however, we provide more background information and documentation, while presenting the story more from Franklin's perspective.

Musical Glasses

It has long been known that tapping cups, bowls, or jars of various sizes or filled with varying amounts of water or wine can produce different musical sounds. Glass or ceramic instruments based on this principle were played in Persia and China in the 13th century. Since glass appeared about 4500 years ago, there are reasons to suspect that glass instruments have an even longer history.[10]

There is a reference to musical glasses in Franchino Gafori's (Gaffurius; 1451–1522) *Theoria musicae*,[11] which was published in Milan in 1492. He provides an illustration of one individual tapping glasses filled with different amounts of liquid, while another matches the sounds by tapping bells of different sizes. Western European books from the 1600s also describe "wine music" made by filling sets of glasses with varying amounts of fluid.[12] At that time, musical glasses were treated largely like toys or novelties, and they were played at social gatherings.

During the 1700s, sets of glasses became popular as concert instruments. The literature abounds with references to the "verrillon" (from *verre*, the French word for "glass"), an instrument that could be accompanied by violins, basses, and other instruments. The verrillon was really just a table on which many wine glasses filled with different amounts of liquid were set. The musician's job was to strike specific glasses with a stick (sometimes muffled) to elicit desired notes.

One individual who achieved fame playing musical glasses was Richard Pockrich (*c*. 1690–1759; sometimes spelled "Puckridge" or "Puckeridge"), a free-spirited Irishman. Among other things, he was a brewer, inventor, adventurer, politician, and starry-eyed scientist. As a musician he made money in 1743 and 1744 performing concerts in Dublin on his "angelick organ," which was essentially a verrillon. Although he first tapped his glasses, he later showed that he could make music by rubbing his moistened fingers around their rims.

By turning to fingertip friction, he produced new, more celestial sounds, which could be sustained for longer periods of time.

Soon performers of musical glasses were playing throughout Europe. One such person was the young German composer Christoph Willibald Gluck (1714–1787). In the spring of 1746, he played a concerto at the Haymarket Theatre in London with a *Glasspiel* of 26 glasses. We are told that the glasses were "tuned with spring water, accompanied with the whole band, being a new instrument of his own invention, upon which he performs whatever may be done on a violin or harpsichord."[13]

In 1761, Miss Ann Ford (1737–1824),[14] who might have been a pupil of Pockrich and had become one of the leading performers on musical glasses, published a pamphlet on how to play the glasses "in a few days, if not a few hours" with controlled pressure from moistened fingers. In 1766, and perhaps even more telling of how popular music glasses had become, we find Oliver Goldsmith (*c.* 1730–1774)[15] writing about them in *The Vicar of Wakefield.* To quote: "The two ladies threw my girls quite into the shade, for they would talk of nothing but high life, and high-lived company; with other fashionable topics, such as pictures, taste, Shakespeare, and the musical glasses" (1895 edition, p. 60).

From the same time period, special mention must be made of Edmund Hussey Delaval (1729–1814) of the University of Cambridge. Delaval, who experimented with chemistry and electricity, was an amateur music glass performer, but he played well and probably had the most complete set of musical glasses at the time. In a letter penned by Thomas Gray (1716–1771) to a gentleman friend named Brown on 28 March 1760, we read:

> "We heard Delaval the other night play upon the water glasses, & I was astonish'd. No instrument that I know has so celestial a tone. I thought it was a Cherubim in a box."[16]

Benjamin Franklin was in England at the time and had even attended George Frederick Handel's (1685–1759) last performance (he conducted the *Messiah*). From his letters we know that he also went to hear Delaval play. Franklin knew Delaval prior to this time. In fact, he thought so highly of him as an electrical scientist that he had become the first of his nominees for membership in the Royal Society of London:

> "Edward Delaval M.A. and Fellow of Pembroke Hall in Cambridge, being personally known to us, and desirous of being elected into the Royal Society, we recommend him as a Gentleman extremely well qualify'd to become a valuable member." (Francis Blake, B. Franklin, and B. Wilson, 17 May.[8])

In his lifetime, Franklin nominated at least 37 members to the Royal Society.[8] Most experimented with electricity. But it was hearing Delaval play the glasses so beautifully, and not his physical science, that inspired Franklin to invent the armonica.

The Armonica

One of Franklin's correspondents was Giambatista Beccaria (1716–1781), a priest and professor of physics in Turin, Italy. In 1753 Beccaria wrote a book on artificial electricity[17] that supported Franklin's own theories. Just before he left Europe in 1762, Franklin wrote a letter to Beccaria as a sort of farewell.[6] It was dated 13 July and in it he told his friend about his new musical instrument.

Franklin explained: "Mr Puckeridge, a gentleman from Ireland, was the first who thought about playing tunes, formed from these [drinking glass] tones... by passing his fingers round their brims." But, he continued, "Mr E. Delaval, a most ingenious member of our Royal Society, made one [a glass instrument] in imitation of it, with a better choice and form of glasses, which was the first I saw or heard." Franklin went on:

> "Being charmed with the sweetness of its tones, and the music he produced from it, I wished only to see the glasses disposed in a more convenient form, and brought together in a narrower compass, so as to admit a greater number of tones, and all within reach of hand to a person sitting before the instrument, which I accomplished, after various intermediate trials, and less commodious forms, both of glasses and construction, in the following manner."

The rest of his letter describes how he invented a new instrument, one that was easier to play and possessed better sound quality. His device used 23 soda-lime bowls (glasses without stems) of different sizes that were blown and tuned by an experienced glassblower. The glassblower drilled a hole through the center of each chosen bowl and the bowls were assembled on an iron spindle from largest (nine inches in diameter) to smallest (three inches in diameter). A small piece of cork between the bowls prevented them from touching.

The spindle was placed horizontally in a wooden case. An attachment to a foot treadle like that used for a spinning wheel permitted the sitting player to spin the bowls at a given speed. As a further aid to the musician, glasses corresponding to different notes had their rims marked and painted in different colors. A shallow trough of water was later added to keep the rims of the glasses moist, but it is not clear whether this was Franklin's idea. In his original description, Franklin wrote only that the fingers should be washed and then kept moistened with a sponge and clean water.

Figure 2 shows an early engraving of the armonica. To play the instrument, the musician simply touched his or her hands to the rims of the glasses while they were spinning. Because the musician's hands no longer had to circle the rims, more than two bowls could be played at the same time, even with a single hand. Another advantage of the new instrument was that the glasses did not have to be tuned, which had been a time-consuming process when evaporative liquids were used.

Franklin's original instrument was completed in 1761. This dating is consistent with a letter dated April 1761, in which Thomas Penn complained to the Governor of Pennsylvania, James Hamilton (1710–1783), that Franklin was spending entirely too much of his time in England on "philosophical matters and on musical performances on glasses".[18] Franklin, of course, did not agree. On 2 March 1763 he wrote to Cadwallader Colden (1688–1776): "While in England, *after my chief Business was over*, I amus'd myself, with contriving and bringing to a considerable Degree of Perfection, a new musical instrument, which has afforded me and my Friends a good deal of Pleasure"[19] (italics added).

Franklin called his invention the "armonica," the name coming from the Italian word for "harmony." As he put it at the end of his 1762 letter to

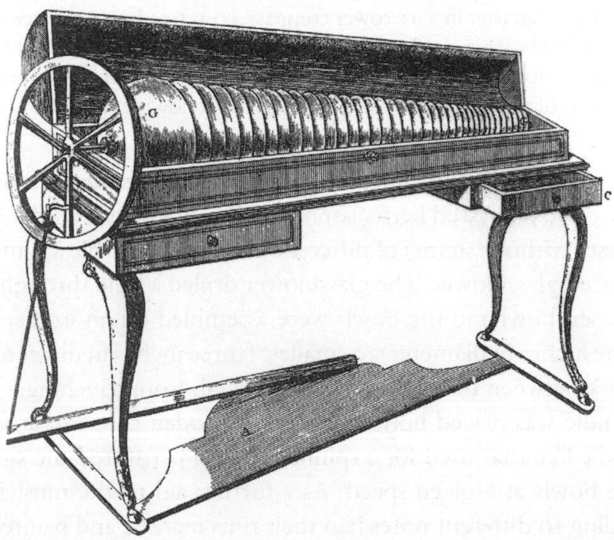

Fig. 2. An 18th century engraving of the Franklin armonicas.[19]

Beccaria: "In honour of your musical language, I have borrowed from it the name of this instrument, calling it the Armonica." In 1771 Beccaria thanked the American "in the name of Italy."[20] He published his letter in the preface to his revised book on artificial electricity a year later.[21] Franklin, in turn, helped to promote the English translation of the new volume, which provided even more support for his own electrical theories.[22]

Almost immediately, however, some individuals (especially in Germany) called his instrument an "harmonica." The addition of the letter "h" led some people to believe, erroneously, that Franklin had actually invented the mouth organ. The mouth harmonica was, in fact, not invented until 1829, and it was first called the "aeolina" by the firm of Wheatstone, its London manufacturer.[19] A more closely related instrument, but again one not invented by Franklin, is the glass harp, which employs glasses arranged vertically.

The Armonica Catches on in America

The armonica was hailed as the first popular musical instrument invented by an American.[10] By the end of 1762 it was being built commercially by Charles James of Purpool Lane, near Gray's Inn, London. In an advertisement in *Jackson's Oxford Journal*, dated 29 May 1762, James, who Franklin soon found to be "negligent," wrote that he had been employed to manufacture the instrument by an "ingenious and well known inventor."[19] After James suddenly died, the firm of Hughes and Co. at the Cockpit Glasshouse in London took over the manufacturing.[19]

The armonica first sold for 40 guineas. England, however, was not the only country to manufacture Franklin's new musical instrument. Soon hundreds were also streaming out of workshops in Germany.

The armonica clearly revolutionized the playing of musical glasses. Its notes seemed to come from nowhere in particular and then linger in the air. Its sounds were ethereal, mystical, otherworldly, and even ghostlike. Simply put, there was nothing quite like it.

Franklin, who also played the harp, violin, viola da gamba, and guitar, enjoyed playing his new instrument for his own enjoyment and for small groups of guests. He liked rather simple melodies and unadorned Scotch airs, and he even composed songs for it.

In *The Autobiography of Leigh Hunt*[23] there is a lovely passage about Franklin and his armonica. The event must have taken place in 1762, right after Franklin returned to America. To quote from Hunt (1784–1859), an

English critic, poet, journalist, and friend of many important literary figures (e.g. Keats, Shelley, Lamb): "I have heard Dr Franklin invented the Harmonica, he concealed it from his wife till the instrument was fit to play; and then woke her with it one night, when she took it to be the music of angels."[23]

Shortly after his wife Deborah (1708–1774) was introduced to armonica music in the aforementioned way, Franklin saw fit to use his instrument to ease the strain of a meeting with Mrs Ann Graeme. This woman's daughter had just been jilted by his son William (1731–1813), and she was not pleased by how her Elizabeth had been treated.

To Franklin's delight, concerts in the colonies began to include parts for the glass armonica.[24] Robert "King" Carter (1728–1804), a music lover of immense wealth, bought one in 1764 that was probably played at the Raleigh Tavern in Williamsburg on 2 May 1765. George Washington (1732–1799) was among those in the audience.

In addition, some of those who heard Franklin play his harmonica wrote verses for him, about him, and about the instrument. One such person was Nathaniel Evans (1742–1767) of Philadelphia. Among the lines he composed in 1763 we find: "Th' Armonica shall join the sacred choir, Fresh transports kindle, and new joys inspire."[19]

For a while, nothing seemed to give Franklin more pleasure than his armonica. He personally designed the "blue room" on the third floor of his Philadelphia house with a musical theme, and it was here that he kept and played his armonica when home.[24] The armonica, however, did not always stay home. It was designed so it could easily be taken on trips, and Franklin did not hesitate to take it with him when he went back to Europe.

The Armonica in Europe

Marianne Davies (1744 – *c.* 1816) was the first of several European musicians who took armonica playing to a decidedly higher level. She was already known in England as a professional singer and for her skillful playing of the flute and harpsichord when she obtained her armonica, probably from Franklin himself. Davies first began to play it publicly early in 1762, sometimes with her sister Cecilia (*c.* 1756–1836) singing to the music. An announcement appearing in the *Bristol Journal*, dated 12 January, 1762, reads:

> "The celebrated glassy-chord was invented by Mr Franklin of Philadelphia; who has greatly improved the musical glasses, and formed them into a compleat (*sic*) instrument to accompany the voice; capable of a thorough bass,

> and never out of tune. Miss Davies from London, was able to perform in the month of January, several favourite airs, English, Scotch, and Italian on the Glassy chord accompanied occasionally with the voice and German flute."

Davies gave concerts in major British cities before taking her armonica to the continent. She was cheered in Italy and France, and may have been even more popular in Germany, where Franklin became "as famous among German musicians for his harmonica as among German electricians for his lightning rod."[4] Recognizing the draw of the instrument, Davies later begged Franklin not to teach other musicians how to play it. Her request was made in 1783, long after the armonica made its debut, and was based on economics. Franklin did not grant her wish.

In 1767, Davies played in Vienna, where she quickly became a favorite of the royal court. Gluck was then chapel-master. It was probably in the Austrian capital that Leopold Mozart (1719–1787), his young son Wolfgang (1756–1791), and Mesmer heard the armonica for the first time. We know that the Mozarts were in Vienna during the winter of 1767–68 attempting to get one of Wolfgang's early operas (*La Finta Simplice*) performed. Years later, in a letter from Leopold Mozart to his wife dated 21 September 1771, we read: "You will surely remember Miss Davies with her harmonica."[10]

As for Mesmer (Figure 3), he was born in Inganz (Swabia), a part of Germany near Lake Constance (Konstanz), in 1734. He first studied philosophy and theology at the Dillingen Seminary in Bavaria. He then enrolled at the University of Ingolstadt in Bavaria and finally the University of Vienna, eventually graduating in medicine in 1766.[25] In 1768, he married Maria Anna von Posch (Bosch), a woman of considerable wealth. The couple settled into a large mansion in Vienna.

Mesmer became friendly with Leopold Mozart at that time. He soon commissioned Wolfgang to write *Bastien und Bastienne*, which was first performed in his private theater late in 1768.[25] (Leopold had previously failed in his attempt to get his son's *La Finta Simplice* performed.)

Wolfgang was appreciative and he later made a witty reference to Mesmer in *Cosi Fan Tutte*, his comic opera of 1790.[26] A chambermaid disguised as a doctor approaches two "dying" men waving an iron wand, while singing in Italian:

> "This is the magnet,
> That mesmeric stone,
> Which originated in Germany
> And then became so famous in France."

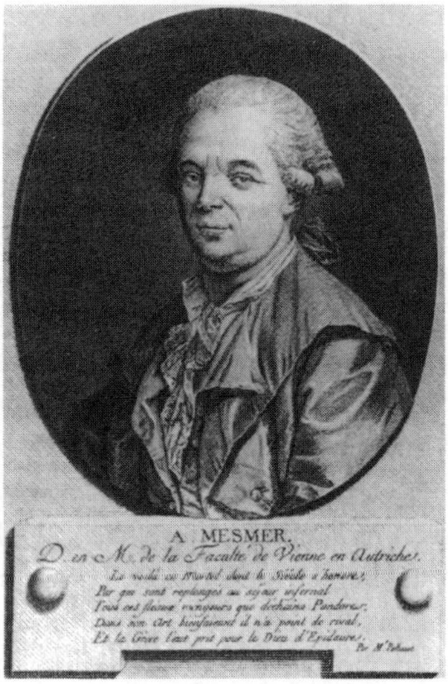

Fig. 3. Franz Anton Mesmer (1734–1815).

After the music conveys an image of magnetism flowing into their bodies, and a few convulsions, the once-dying men raise their heads and the words "freed from death" are sung with great joy.

The Mozarts and Mesmer also saw each other during the 1770s. Two letters from Leopold Mozart to his wife in 1773 reveal that Mesmer adored his armonica and loved to play it for his guests.[25] The first is dated 21 July and again makes mention of Marianne Davies:

> "The Mesmers are all well and in good form as usual. Herr von Mesmer, at whose house we lunched on Monday, played to us on Miss Davies's Harmonica or glass instrument and played very well. It cost him about 50 ducats and is very beautifully made. . . . We dined with them on Saturday and also on Monday."[26]

The second letter was sent on 12 August. Leopold wrote with great pride that Wolfgang, then 16, was allowed to play on Mesmer's beloved instrument. He also let it drop that he would like to have one of his own:

> "Do you know that Herr von Mesmer plays Miss Davies's harmonica unusually well? He is the only person in Vienna who has learnt it and he possesses a much finer instrument than Miss Davies does. Wolfgang too has played upon it. How I should like to have one!"[10]

Nevertheless, Wolfgang was not ready to write compositions for the armonica in 1773. The situation changed after he heard Marianne Kirchgässner (1769–1808) play it 18 years later. Kirchgässner was a successful but blind concert musician who claimed that anything played on the harpsichord could also be played on the armonica. In 1791 she played the armonica in Vienna. Mozart was so inspired that he composed *Adagio and Rondo for Glass Harmonica, Flute, Oboe, Viola and Cello* (k617) and *Adagio Solo for the Glass Harmonica* (k356) just for her.[27] He might even have started a third work, but fell ill and died before the year ended.[10]

During the closing decades of the 1700s and into the 1800s, many other composers wrote musical pieces for the armonica. More than 300 original compositions were composed for it.[28] Ludwig van Beethoven (1770–1827), for example, selected the armonica to accompany spoken words in his *Leonora Prohaska*. Financial constraints, however, prevented the work for narrator and armonica from being performed as intended.

The armonica was also appreciated by many famous people from other walks of life. One was Johann Wolfgang Goethe (1749–1832), the Romantic poet and *Naturphilosophe*, who had a strong interest in aesthetics.[10] Another was Marie Antoinette (1755–1793), who was Viennese by birth and studied the armonica under Marianne Davies before becoming Queen of France. Thomas Jefferson (1743–1826), who arrived in Paris on 9 August 1784 to replace Franklin as American representative, was a third such person. The chief architect of the "Declaration of Independence" and third American president even thought about ordering one that was six octaves long from London (three octaves was then the maximum size produced), but in the end decided to let the matter drop.

Bad Vibrations?

The armonica, obviously loved by some, was soon feared and avoided by others. Franklin, who enjoyed playing his own armonica, knew that musical glasses had long had a strange and even sinister history—one laced with all sorts of claims about special and perhaps even supernatural powers. As noted, he knew about Pockrich, the Irish verrillon player. The following tale about the power of Pockrich's musical glasses was published in 1759, the same year in which the musician and his instrument perished in a fire:

> "Mr Pockrich, in his brewery near Island-bridge, happening one day to be seized by bailiffs, thus addressed them: 'Gentleman, I am your prisoner, but

> before I do myself the honour to attend you, give me leave as an humble performer of musick, to entertain you with a tune.' . . . In the meantime, he flourishes a prelude on the glasses, and afterwards displays his skill thro' all the pleasing turns and variations of the Black Joke. The monsters, charm'd with the magic of his sounds, for some time stand at gaze. At length, recovering (*sic*) their trance, thus accost the Captain: 'Sir, upon your parole of honour to keep the secret, we give you your liberty.' 'Tis well, playing upon the glasses is not more common: if it were, I believe our trade would find little employment.' "[29]

But even before there was a Pockridge, there was a belief that glass music could affect both mind and body. One need only consult Georg Philipp Harsdorfer's (1607–1658) reissue of David Schwenter's (1585–1636) *Deliciae physicomathematicae*. In the Nürnberg edition of 1677 one finds an experiment with four glasses filled either with brandy, wine, water, or salt water (or oil). Based on ancient traditions, the sounds were associated with the four bodily humors and the four basic emotions. Among other things, it was stated that the sounds could affect the thickness of the blood.[10]

Although coming from a different perspective, Franklin did not deny that the music from his instrument could have strange effects on some people. He was convinced, however, that these effects were due to the power of suggestion, and that a skillful healer could use suggestion to his advantage. To his credit, Franklin had successfully "treated" Princess Izabella Czartoryska (1746–1835), the wife of a Polish diplomat who seemed to be suffering from depression, and he did it with the aid of the armonica.

In a memoir written in 1772, the 26-year-old princess wrote about her encounter with the 66-year-old American:

> "I was ill, in a state of melancholia, and writing my testament and farewell letters. Wishing to distract me, my husband explained to me who Franklin was and to what he owed his fame. . . . Franklin had a noble face with an expression of engaging kindness. Surprised by my immobility, he took my hands and gazed at me saying: *pauvre jeune femme*. He then opened a harmonium, sat down and played long. The music made a strong impression on me and tears began flowing from my eyes. Then Franklin sat by my side and looking with compassion said, 'Madam, you are cured.' Indeed that moment was a reaction to my melancholia. Franklin offered to teach me how to play the harmonium—I accepted without hesitation, hence he gave me twelve lessons."[30]

Still, many people in Franklin's lifetime and into the opening decades of the 19th century remained more than a little fearful of the armonica. Although claims were made that it could be used to cure, it still seemed to have sinister effects. As put in one historical article:

> "According to Röllig, its social effects were such as no other instrument whatever has produced. Its tones could reconcile quarreling friends; restore fainting men to consciousness; make women faint; send a dog into convulsions; make a sleeping girl wake screaming through a chord of the diminished seventh, and even cause the death of one very young."[10]

The named authority at the beginning of this quotation is Karl Leopold Röllig of Hamburg, who was probably born in 1735 and died in 1804. Röllig wrote a treatise on the armonica in 1787[31] and tried to modify the instrument for keyboard playing.

Some of the fears stemmed from what happened to those who had played the instrument. Marianne Kirchgässner, whose armonica performance had so inspired Mozart, died a horrible death that "was attributed to deterioration of her nerves caused by the unusually piercing vibrations of the instrument."[27] Mozart himself died within months after starting to compose pieces for the armonica. And Marianne Davies had become bedridden for more than a year and eventually succumbed to health problems, which she specifically attributed to the armonica.

In addition, there was the deliberate use of the armonica to convey feelings of madness and conjure images of the supernatural. The latter is best exemplified by Étienne-Gaspard Robertson's (1763–1831) *fantasmagorie* ("phantasmagoria"), constructed in Paris in 1798.[32,33] By skillfully using magic lantern projections on invisible screens or smoke in a darkened room, Robertson, a Belgian-born student of optics, made ghosts and mysterious luminous shapes arise from crypts. He also produced nightmarish moving scenes of witches, the dead, and the supernatural before horrified onlookers (Figure 4). He told his frightened audience that this was what they had to look forward to, and then terrified them even more by illuminating the skeleton of a young woman on a pedestal. While this was going on, the eeriest, most unearthly sounds that the glass armonica could produce permeated through the closed auditorium, enhancing the chilling effects.

The fact that Mesmer's elaborate theories about a mysterious force called animal magnetism were discredited late in the 18th century only made things worse. On the one hand, some people looked upon Mesmer as more than a fraud or a charlatan—they saw him as unbalanced or crazy. On the other, Mesmer used the armonica in his practice in part because he maintained its

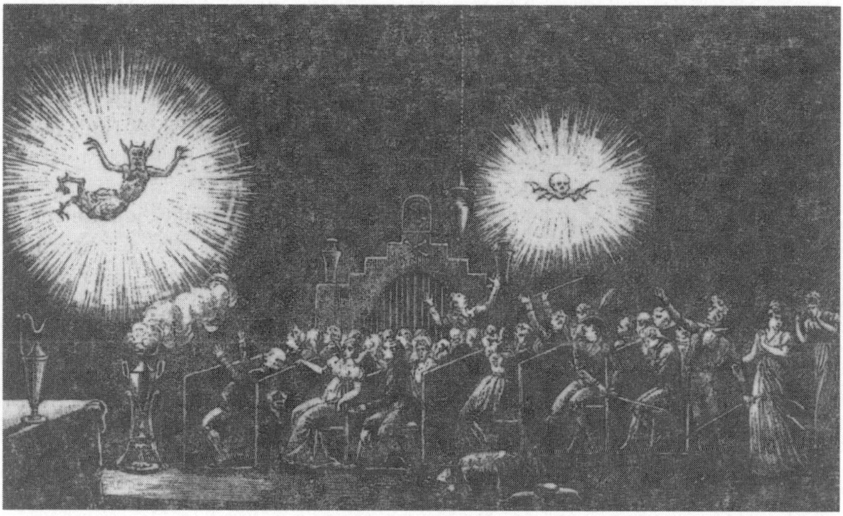

Fig. 4. Magic lantern images of the supernatural created by Robertson, who enhanced the effect of his illusions with armonica music. He produced his frightening *fantasmagorie* shows in Paris around 1800.[32]

music could affect the flow of the animal magnetism, and hence affect the health of the individual.

In response to these fears, some communities banned the instrument, while a few inventors, encouraged by Thomas Jefferson, among others, tried to reduce physical contact with it. As noted, one such person was Röllig, who worked on constructing a keyboard; other inventors tried bows.[24]

Small wonder that Domenico Donizetti (1797–1848) chose to include a part for the glass armonica in his immensely popular opera *Lucia di Lammermoor.* The part for it was in the opera's famous mad scene, the crowning highlight of the work. Unfortunately, Donizetti was unable to find a good armonica player in 1836, when the work was produced. As a result, he was forced to rewrite the armonica part for some flutes.

Mesmerism and the Armonica

The controversy that surrounded Mesmer began with his medical dissertation of 1766:[34] "*Dissertatio Physico-Medica de Planetarum Influx in Corpus Humanum*" ("The Influence of the Planets on the Human Body"). Not only was its subject matter questionable, but records show that he stole many of "his" seminal ideas from others. One such person was Paracelsus (Philippus Aureolus Theophrastus Bombastus von Hohenheim, 1493–1541), who wrote about planetary influences during the Renaissance. Another was Richard Mead (1673–1754),[35] whose book of 1704 translates as *On the Influence of the Sun and Moon upon Human Bodies and the Diseases Arising Therefrom*.[25]

Mesmer used the term "animal gravity" in his earlier writings, but in 1775 changed it to "animal magnetism." His basic contention was that animal gravity/magnetism is an imperceptible fluid that can be found throughout the cosmos. Every object in the universe can influence every other object because of it. The stars, sun, planets, and moon can affect it, and it can affect the nerves and body.

Mesmer's 27 principles of animal magnetism can be found in "*Mémoire de F. A. Mesmer, Docteur en Médecine, sur ses Découvertes*."[36] Here he explains that this subtle but powerful fluid had, under different circumstances, also been called "gravity," "fire," "light," "magnetism," and, of special interest to Franklin, "electricity."

One also reads that disruption of the normal flow of this fluid through the body can account for illness. But there is hope—a skilled physician can learn to locate the blockages and, by applying magnetism, re-establish the flux and provide cures. In contrast to what most other popular healers, such as Jean-Joseph Gassner (1727–1779), were claiming at the time, Mesmer left theology out of his system.

During the 1770s, Franziska ("Franzl") Oesterlin resided with the Mesmers while she coped with violent bouts of hysteria. By applying magnets to her body to control the "ebb and flow" of her symptoms (an idea borrowed from Father Maximilian Hell; 1720–1792), Mesmer explained that he had successfully treated her hysteria. In his own words:

> "It was on July 28, 1774, that my patient having suffered another of her attacks, I placed three magnets on her, one on the stomach and one on each leg. Almost immediately she began to show severe symptoms. She felt painful volatile currents moving within her body. After a confused effort to find a direction, they flowed downward to her extremities. Alleviation followed and lasted for six hours. A repetition of the attack on the following day caused me to repeat the experiment, with the same success."[26,36]

Soon Mesmer came to the realization that the curative agent was not the magnets themselves, but his own special gift. He was blessed with an ability to "magnetize" by animal magnetism. This revelation led him to abandon metal magnets, although he still used objects that he had "magnetized."

Anxious to demonstrate his special powers to the establishment, Mesmer contacted Jan Ingenhousz (1730–1799), the Dutch-born physician who, among other things, had experimented with electricity.[26] Like Delaval before him, Franklin had nominated Ingenhousz for membership in the Royal Society (in 1769). Now serving as court physician in Vienna, Ingenhousz was not in the least impressed with these demonstrations. He denounced Mesmer and his theory and became one of his harshest critics.

Ingenhousz, who remained in contact with Franklin, penned his feeling about Mesmer to his American friend on 5 October 1778. Franklin was then serving as the American Commissioner to France. Ingenhousz warned Franklin that the pernicious Mesmer was now trying to establish himself in the French capital:

> "I hear from Fontana the Vienna conjuror Dr Mesmer is at Paris, that he has been presented to the Royal academy, that he still pretends a magnetical effluvium streams from his finger and enters the body of any person without being obstructed by walls or any other obstacles, and that such stuff, too insipid for to get belief by any old woman, is believed by your friend Mr Le Roy, who protects him and will recommend him in London, where he has a mind to exercise his magnetical effluvia."[37]

Mesmer had, in fact, been pushed out of Vienna. The precipitating event was his well-publicized but failed attempt to find a permanent cure for the blindness of Maria Theresia von Paradis (Paradies, 1759–1824), who happened to be the goddaughter of the Empress of Austria. She was a very talented and extremely popular pianist, organist, singer, and composer, and it is believed that she suffered from psychogenic blindness since childhood. She was a friend of the Mozarts and Wolfgang wrote *Concerto in B-Flat* (k456) specifically for her.[38] In 1777, after it appeared that Mesmer had ruined both the nerves and the technique of the woman, the empress demanded an end to "all this nonsense."

Mesmer took his armonica with him to Paris, but not his wife, the couple no longer having much to do with each other.[26] In 1778, shortly after arriving in the French capital, he set up his practice in a room at the Place Vendôme. When it became clear that more space was needed, he moved his practice to Créteil, then just outside the city.

He also found a well-placed assistant in Paris, which was important because he never received official approval to practice medicine, as required of foreigners. Charles-Nicolas Deslon (also D'Eslon or d'Eslon; 1750–1786), who performed many functions for him, was then a member of the Faculté de

Médecine. He was also physician to Compte d'Artois (1757–1836), the brother of Louis XVI and a future French king (Charles X).

At the height of Mesmer's popularity, his dimly lit seance room contained several large wooden tubs, or *baquets*, which were filled with water and perhaps iron or glass powders, and magnetized (Figure 5). Jointed iron bars jutted out over the lids and rims of the tubs. Mesmer would enter the room wearing long flowing garments and instruct his patients to touch the bars to the parts of their bodies that were afflicted, and he would also touch each of them with his hand or a wand. With groups between 20 and 30, he tied a rope around those at the *baquet* and extended the unknotted part of the rope to others further away. He also had each person hold a neighbor's thumb as still another way to allow the magnetic force to flow from one person to another.

It was critical for a patient to be brought into a "crisis." This was Mesmer's term for an intense emotional change that often manifested itself as a fit or a fainting spell. The crisis could be so overpowering that patients sometimes had to be taken to padded rooms until they recovered.[25,26]

Mesmer, himself tall, imposing, and charismatic, recognized that his own appearance and demeanor could enhance the effects of his treatment. So could his beautiful flowing lilac robe, rituals, mirrors, lighting, and testimonials. The

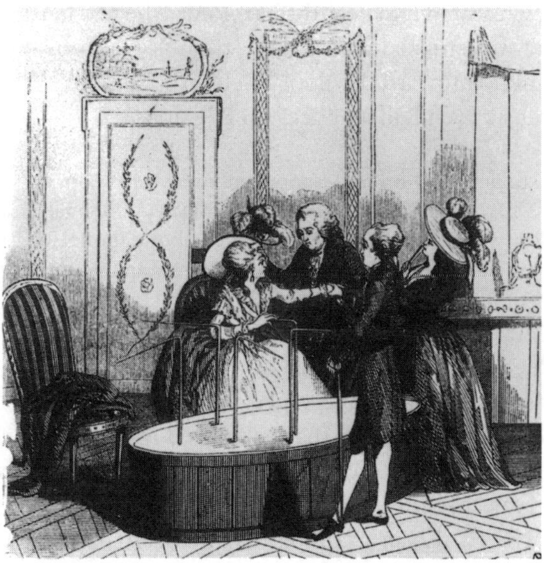

Fig. 5. An 18th century engraving of a *baquet* with magnetized rods being held by women seeking a cure.

same was true for the eerie music coming from behind the curtains covered with astrological symbols. It came from an armonica or (second best) a piano. As put by music historian King[10]: "In these cures hypnotism undoubtably played a large part, and there seems little doubt that Mesmer used his mastery of the highly emotional tones of the harmonica to induce a receptive state in his patients."

From Mesmer's perspective, the armonica music that permeated the room did more than just create an ambiance or set the mood. He maintained that the presence of certain types of music could ease the flow of animal magnetism into the ailing person's body. Proposition 16 in "*Mémoire de F. A. Mesmer, Docteur en Médecine, sur ses Découvertes*"[36] states very clearly that animal magnetism can be communicated, propagated, and reinforced by sounds. In short, Mesmer looked upon armonica music as a part of the cure; it was more than just relaxing or a pleasant adjunct to what he was doing.

The following story illustrates the power of the music. Sometime between 1778 and 1779 an army surgeon was taken to Mesmer's clinic suffering from gout. Mesmer began by pressing his own finger against a part of the body that hurt. This produced a tingling sort of pain that followed his finger as he moved it around the man's body. He then played the armonica, which threw the man into crisis. A witness to the event described what transpired in a letter: "Mr Mesmer then seated him near the harmonica; he had hardly begun to play when my friend was affected emotionally, trembled, lost his breath, changed color, and felt pulled toward the floor" (letter of Le Roux[25]).

Mesmer's music even had an effect on D'Eslon:

> "Mesmer experimented on him—apparently not very seriously—by playing on the glass harmonica or the piano and conveying animal magnetism to him. D'Eslon was obliged to beg for mercy about the music, presumably because of the discomfort caused by the charge of animal magnetism which it carried."[25]

In a way, the armonica also served as a therapy for Mesmer, relaxing him and lifting his spirits, at work and especially at home. In 1779, he played it for Gluck, who was so impressed that he advised Mesmer to improvise rather than continue using sheet music.[10] Mesmer took Gluck's suggestion to heart.

Later that year, Mesmer invited Franklin and his lady friend Madame Brillon (1744–1824), also an accomplished musician, to his house to hear him perform.[39,40] The details of what transpired remain unclear, although a letter written by Madame Brillon would suggest that Mesmer was more interested in discussing "electrical fluid" with Franklin than he was in playing the armonica for his guests.[40] Indeed, Mesmer felt that his animal magnetism and Franklin's electricity had more than a little in common. He also believed that both he and Franklin had discovered fundamental truths, were authorities on these powerful fluids, and wanted to use their new knowledge to benefit all mankind.

Mesmer, however, probably underestimated Franklin's skepticism about his magnetic force. Franklin, who took Ingenhousz's warning seriously, left Mesmer's house unconverted. Until proven otherwise, many of Mesmer's claims seemed explainable by suggestion alone.

In a letter written a month later, Mesmer invited Franklin back to witness some cures. His hope was that the respected American could "discover for himself the advantages of animal magnetism."[40] It is unclear whether or not they met this second time.

Franklin's ever-increasing skepticism can be appreciated from another letter. With reference to iron rods and patient expectancies, he explained:

> "I cannot but fear that the expectation of great advantage from this new method of treating disease will prove a delusion. That delusion may, however, and in some cases be of use while it lasts. There are in every great, rich city, a number of persons who are never in health, because they are fond of medicines. . . . If these people can be persuaded to forbear their drugs, in expectation of being cured by only the physician's finger, or an iron rod pointing at them, they may possibly find good effects, though they mistake the cause."[2]

Mesmer's professional situation was now deteriorating at an increasingly rapid rate. On the one hand, the French Academy of Sciences rejected what he had written and the Royal Society of Medicine refused to allow him to present his ideas to its membership.[26] On the other, the working relationship he had with Deslon had become so strained that Deslon left to start his own clinic.

Nevertheless, Mesmer did gain some needed support and additional income at that time. One particularly welcome source of both was the Societies of Harmony.[41] To Franklin's chagrin, one of its members was his rebellious grandson, William Temple Franklin (1760–1823). But much better known was the Marquis de Lafayette (1757–1834), who was commissioned by Mesmer to introduce animal magnetism to America. In this context, the French hero of the American Revolutionary War wrote favorably about Mesmerism to George Washington on 14 May 1784:

> "A German doctor named Mesmer, having made the greatest discovery about animal magnetism, has trained some pupils, among whom your humble servant is considered the most enthusiastic. . . . Before leaving I will obtain

permission to let you into Mesmer's secret, which, you can count on it, is a great philosophical discovery."[42]

Washington was polite but chose not to get involved with Mesmerism.[40] His mind was not changed when Lafayette personally handed him a letter from Mesmer on 25 November 1784.[43] Unlike Washington, Franklin and Jefferson openly expressed their decidedly negative thoughts about Mesmer and his pseudoscience. For Franklin, everything that had to be said had just appeared in his published report to the King of France.

The Franklin Commission

While Lafayette was trying to make medical inroads with George Washington, issues about Mesmer, his theory, and his claims of success were boiling over in France. King Louis XVI, whose wife Marie Antoinette had embraced the theory, was advised that mesmerism demanded a proper evaluation. He responded by setting up a formal commission to investigate it.[44,45] The commission was headed (in name at least) by Franklin. It included four other members of the Académie Royale des Sciences (le Roy, Bailly, Lavoisier, and de Borie) plus four prominent physicians of the Faculté de Paris (Borie, Sallin, d'Arcet, and Guillotin; after Borie died, Majault replaced him). This was not, however, the only commission to examine mesmerism at this time.[46] With the king's approval, the Société Royale de Médecine set up its own commission and issued its own report. In addition, the king sanctioned a "secret" inquiry that had more to do with morals and whether Mesmer was taking sexual advantage of women.

The influential "*Rapport des Commissaires*,"[47] bearing Franklin's name first, was issued five months later, in August of 1784. It quickly sold 20 000 copies.[39] It is generally thought, however, that Antoine Lavoisier (1743–1794), the discover of oxygen who, along with Louis XVI and Marie Antoinette, was guillotined during the French Revolution, was the key figure behind the document.

In the introduction to the English translation of 1785 we are informed that "M. Mesmer refused to have any communication with these gentlemen; but M. Deslon, the most considerable of his pupils, consented to disclose to them his principles, and assist them in their enquiries."[48]

The report itself begins by familiarizing the reader with Mesmer and his theory of animal magnetism. It then describes how the commissioners set out to observe the effects of animal magnetism. They witnessed a seance conducted by Deslon in this context. It is noted that Deslon's *baquet* room did not have an armonica, Mesmer's musical instrument of choice. But the reader is told that "a piano forté is placed in one corner of the apartment, and different airs are played with various degrees of rapidity," and also informed that, according to Deslon, "the magnetism is transmitted by the sounds to the surrounding patients."

Interestingly, when the commissioners held an electrometer to the *baquet*, the needle did not give any hint of a magnetic or electrical force. Nevertheless, the seance did affect the patients, some of whom convulsed before the others, often triggering chain reactions with their neighbors. As for the music, ". . . it has been observed, that the changing of the key and the time, in the airs played upon the piano forté, had an effect upon the patients; so that a quicker motion agitates them more, and renews the vivacity of their convulsions."

With these observable facts before them, the commissioners turned to the thornier issue of accounting for what they had observed. They knew that curing a patient did not prove that animal magnetism existed. Expectations, suggestion, and other factors could play roles. Hence, they next turned to clever experiments on themselves and others to shed light on that which had been observed.

What followed might be thought of as the first use of the methods of modern experimental psychology to investigate mental phenomena and the workings of the human mind. Even by today's standards, the experiments and logic employed by the commissioners are exemplary.[49] Because he was in his late 70s and suffering from gout and painful kidney stones, some of the trick experiments were conducted at Franklin's residence in Passy, then a lovely town a few miles outside Paris. As the scientists and physicians saw it, it was important for the now ailing patriarch of good science, as well as the titular head of the commission, to see things firsthand. Franklin took advantage of the opportunity and even designed, performed, and served as a subject in some of these experiments.

It was found that Franklin, the other commissioners, and his staff could not be magnetized. In contrast, a few of the lower-class, uneducated, sick patients chosen by Deslon, all of whom expected a cure, "experienced sensations" and sometimes went into crisis. This finding led to more experiments "to determine to what degree the power of the imagination can influence our sensations."

One of the experiments that Franklin witnessed involved a 12-year-old boy hand-picked by Deslon because he was so susceptible to animal magnetism. Deslon was asked to magnetize just one apricot tree from the bunch of apricot trees in Franklin's garden. Deslon did this and augmented the magnetism by hiding in the orchard and pointing his cane at the selected tree. The boy was then brought into the orchard, where he was told that one tree (not identified) was magnetized. He was then instructed to embrace the trees in the manner requested by Deslon. As he went from tree to tree, his sweating, perspiring, coughing, and headache increased, until he fainted at the fourth tree. The magnetized tree, however, stood 24–38 feet away.

Other experiments at Passy produced similar results. One involved a susceptible woman who had been blindfolded and led to believe that Deslon was in the room magnetizing her, when he was not. She shuttered and felt pain within 3 min, and went into crisis shortly thereafter. Another experiment had Deslon supposedly magnetizing a susceptible patient from behind a door when he was not present, again with positive effects. When the reverse experiment was conducted, with Deslon really trying to magnetize the woman without her knowing it, nothing happened.

The inescapable conclusion from these and other experiments was that every effect attributed to animal magnetism could be accounted for by suggestion and imagination. The instructions, the costumes, the rituals, the design of the *baquet*, and the type of music played, all helped to produce the desired effect on certain patients—those who believed in the practitioner's powers and wanted to get better.

This unanimous opinion drew different reactions from the two most ardent supporters of animal magnetism, Mesmer and Deslon. Looking first at Deslon, at the end of the Franklin Commission Report, we read:

> "M. d'Eslon is not much adverse to the admission of these principles. He declared in our session held at the house of Dr Franklin the 19th of June, that he thought he might lay it down as a fact that the imagination had the greatest share in the effects of the animal magnetism. . . . He remarked to the commissioners that the imagination thus directed to the relief of suffering humanity, would be a most valuable means in the hands of the medical profession, and persuaded of the reality of the power of the imagination, he invited the commission to embrace the opportunity which his practice afforded to study its procedure and its effects."

Unfortunately, Deslon did not have the opportunity to use the power of the imagination to cure sick souls. He died without warning right after the report was issued. It was rumored that he was being magnetized at the time.

Mesmer, in contrast, did not accept the report, period. He was especially bothered by the fact that the commissioners had relied on his "incompetent," fired assistant to test his theory of animal magnetism. Mesmer's objections, however, were ignored by his critics, including those responsible for the health of the populace. Frustrated, he left Paris for England and Italy, and eventually settled in Switzerland, where he lived in relative obscurity. In 1815, while on his deathbed, he instructed a priest to play the armonica one last time for him.[26]

After the commissioners issued their report, the aged Franklin wrote a letter to Ingenhousz regarding how gullible people can be about unsubstantiated medical claims. He also commented on the riches that can be accrued by unscrupulous healers. He lamented:

> "Mesmer continues here and has still some Adherents and some Practice. It is surprising how much Credulity still subsists in the World. I suppose all the Physicians in France put together have not made so much Money during the Time he has been here, as he has done."[48,50]

Exactly 50 years earlier, when he was just 29, the young colonist of great common sense had written: "He is the best physician who knows the worthlessness of the most medicines." This was among his entries in *Poor Richard's Almanack.*

Resurrection

Fearful that its sounds could wake the dead, believing that it could affect nervous physiology and mental status, banned in some towns, used to create supernatural images, and not helped by the decidedly negative Mesmer association, the armonica declined in popularity throughout the 19th century.[10,28,51] To say that the armonica died, however, would be overstating the point. It had merely lost its allure.

Looking back, it has been suggested that the use of leaded glass might have given the bad health myth a foundation in rational medicine.[28] The evidence for lead poisoning, however, is scanty at best. What is easier to understand in terms of the armonica's precipitous decline are two more earthly factors: its expense and changes in taste.

Not only was Franklin's instrument costly to buy, it was difficult for the average musician to maintain. The glass was so brittle that it could be broken during transport, by the human voice, or even by the instrument's own notes. Getting perfectly matched replacement glasses was a time-consuming, frustrating, and expensive process. Especially for a person on a concert tour, glass breakage could cause great anxiety.

As for changing tastes, once the Romantic revolution brought forth a bolder and richer kind of orchestral music for large concert halls, there was less demand for certain instruments, especially those that would have been played by soloists or small ensembles. Glass instruments, with their soft ethereal notes, found themselves on the wrong side of the curve as the demand for powerful orchestral pieces increased.[28]

Like Lazarus, who rose from the dead, the armonica managed to be resurrected, but not until 1956. The occasion was the 250th anniversary of Franklin's birth (it was also Mozart's 200th birthday), and celebrations were organized by the Franklin Society of Philadelphia with the support of hundreds of other societies. One of the participating organizations was the American Academy of Arts and Sciences, and it sponsored the building of a replica that master organist E. Power Biggs (1906–1977) could play with a keyboard.[52]

Master glassblower Gerhard Finkenbeiner of Waltham, Massachusetts constructed a better instrument in 1981, again with a few changes. One was the use of semiconductor-grade fused quartz glass as opposed to the more brittle soda-lime glass, and another was the addition of a silent motor to drive the spindle.[51] His armonica did not employ a keyboard.

Today there is a glass music society, a periodical called *Glass Music World*,[13,28,51,53,54] armonica websites, and even a book for children about the instrument. And now, more than 200 years after Franklin's commission took the wind out of Mesmer's sails, we are again seeing a rise in allegations about the ability of the armonica to affect body and mind.

So can armonica music affect the nervous system? And is the armonica really the instrument of madness? Those who believe so are now able to add another "fact" to their lists. As told by a reporter for the *Boston Globe*, armonica builder Gerhard Finkenbeiner seemed not himself as he unexpectedly took off from Norwood Memorial Airport, New England in his Piper Cherokee airplane on 9 May 1999.[55] The meticulous German immigrant whose musical instrument was used by the Metropolitan Opera and in the movie *Interview with a Vampire* did not, contrary to habit, file a flight plan. He has not been heard from since.

Acknowledgments

This research was supported by a Faculty Research Grant from Washington University to the first author.

References

1. A.O. Aldridge, *Benjamin Franklin: Philosopher and Man* (J.B. Lippincott and Co., Philadelphia, 1965).

2. B. Franklin, *The Life of Benjamin Franklin, Written by Himself. New First Edition from Original Manuscripts and from His Printed Correspondence and Other Writings, by John Bigelow* (rev. 2nd ed.), Vol. III (Lippincott, Philadelphia, PA, 1881), pp. 258–9.
3. L.W. Larabee, R.L. Ketcham, H.C. Boatfield and H.H. Fineman (eds.), *The Autobiography of Benjamin Franklin* (Yale University Press, New Haven, 1964).
4. C. Van Doren, *Benjamin Franklin* (Viking, New York, 1938), p. 299.
5. B. Franklin, *Poor Richard's Almanack* (Blackwell, Lake Oswego, OR, 1732) (reprinted 1987), p. 45.
6. B. Franklin, *Experiments and Observations on Electricity*. . ., 5th ed. (F. Newberry, London, 1774), pp. 119–35, 367–9, 437–42.
7. B. Franklin, *Experiments and Observations on Electricity* . . . (E. Cave, London, 1751).
8. L.W. Labaree (ed.), *The Papers of Benjamin Franklin: April 8, 1758 Through December 31, 1759,* Vol. 8 (Yale University Press, New Haven, 1965), p. 356.
9. D.A. Gallo and S. Finger, The power of a musical instrument: Franklin, the Mozarts, Mesmer, and the glass armonica, *Hist. Psychol.* **3**, 326–43 (2000).
10. A.H. King, The musical glasses and the glass harmonica. Paper extracted from the Proc. R. Music. Assn., Session LXXII, London, 1946, pp. 99, 109–111, 114.
11. F. Gafori, *Theoria Musicae* (Milan, 1492).
12. G.P. Harsdorfer, *Deliciae Physico-Mathematicae* (Nürnberg, 1677).
13. T.D. Rossing, Acoustics of the glass harmonica, *J. Acoust. Soc. Amer.* **95**, 1106–11 (1994).
14. A. Ford, *Instructions for the Playing of the Musical Glasses* (London, 1761).
15. O. Goldsmith, *The Vicar of Wakefield: A Tale* (Eugene Swiney, London). Reprinted in 1895 by Houghton Mifflin Co., Boston, 1771.
16. P. Toynbee and L. Whibley (eds.), *Correspondence of Thomas Gray, Vol. II. 1756–1765* (Clarendon, Oxford, 1935).
17. G. Beccaria, *Dell' Elettricismo Artificiale*... (Nella Stampa di F.A. Campana, Turin, 1753).
18. E. Wright, *Benjamin Franklin: His Life as He Wrote It* (Harvard University Press, Cambridge, MA, 1990), p. 159.
19. L.W. Labaree (ed.), *The Papers of Benjamin Franklin: January 1, 1762 Through December 31, 1763,* Vol. 10 (Yale University Press, New Haven, 1966), pp. 118, 180–2, 204.
20. L.W. Labaree (ed.), *The Papers of Benjamin Franklin: January 1, 1771 Through December 31, 1771,* Vol. 18 (Yale University Press, New Haven, 1974).
21. G. Beccaria, *Elettrismo Artificiale* (Nella Stampa Reale, Turin, 1772).
22. G. Beccaria, *A Treatise upon Artificial Electricity*... (J. Nourse, London, 1776.).
23. L. Hunt, *The Autobiography of Leigh Hunt, with Reminiscences of Friends and Contemporaries* (Harper, New York, 1850).
24. O.G. Sonneck, Benjamin Franklin's relation to music, *Music* **19**, 1–14 (1900).

25. F.A. Pattie, *Mesmer and Animal Magnetism* (Edmonston, New York, 1994), pp. 73, 103.
26. V. Buranelli, *The Wizard from Vienna: Franz Anton Mesmer* (Coward, McCann & Geoghegan, New York, 1975), pp. 56, 62.
27. C.F. Pohl and K.M. Pisarowitz, Kirchgessner, Marianne. In: S. Sadie (ed.), *The New Grove Dictionary of Music & Musicians*, Vol. 10 (Macmillan, London, 1995), p. 74.
28. V. Meyer and K.J. Allen, Benjamin Franklin and the glass armonica, *Endeavour* **12**, 185–8 (1988).
29. B. Newburgh, *Essays Poetical Moral and Critical* (Alex M'Culloh, Dublin, 1759).
30. Z.J. Lipowski, Benjamin Franklin as a psychotherapist: a forerunner of brief psychotherapy, *Per. Biol. Med.* **27**, 361–6 (1984).
31. K.L. Röllig, *Über die Harmonika: ein Fragment* (Berlin, 1787).
32. É.-G. Robertson, *Mémoires: Récréatifs, Scientifiques, et Anecdotiques d'un Physicien-Aéronaute* (Chez l'Auteur et à la Librairie de Wurtz, Paris, 1831–33). Reissued with présentation by Philippe Blon, Langres, France, Café Clima, 1985.
33. T. Castle, *The Female Thermometer: Eighteenth-Century Culture and the Invention of the Uncanny* (Oxford University Press, New York, 1995).
34. F.A. Mesmer, *Fredericus Antonius Mesmer de Planetarum Influxu in Corpus Humanum. Dissertatio Physico-Medica* (Typis Ghelenanis, Cindobonae, 1776).
35. R. Mead, *De Imperio Solis ac Lacunae in Corpora Humana, et Morbis Oriundis* (Raphaelis Smith, London, 1704).
36. F.A. Mesmer, *Mémoire de F. A. Mesmer, Docteur en Médecine, sur ses Découvertes* (Chez Fuchs, Paris, 1799). Translated as *Memoir of F.A. Mesmer on His Discoveries* (Eden, Mt Vernon, NY, 1957).
37. C.A. Lopez (ed.), *The Papers of Benjamin Franklin: July 1 Through October 31, 1778*, Vol. 27 (Yale University Press, New Haven, 1988), p. 506.
38. R. Angermueller, Paradies, Maria Theresa von. In: S. Sadie (ed.), *The New Grove Dictionary of Music & Musicians*, Vol. 14 (Macmillan, London, 1995), p. 175.
39. C.A. Lopez, Franklin and Mesmer: an encounter, *Yale J. Biol. Med.* **66**, 325–31 (1993).
40. K.M. McConkey and C. Perry, Benjamin Franklin and mesmerism, *Int. J. Clin. Exp. Hypn.* **33**, 122–30 (1985).
41. M.A. Gravitz, Mesmerism and masonry: early historical interactions, *Amer. J. Clin. Hypn.* **39**, 266–70 (1997).
42. R.C. Fuller, *Mesmerism and the American Cure of Souls* (University of Pennsylvania Press, Philadelphia, PA, 1982), p. 16.
43. E.E. Hale and E.E. Hale, Jr, *Franklin in France* (Roberts Brothers, Boston, 1888), p. 309.
44. A. Gauld, *A History of Hypnotism* (Cambridge University Press, Cambridge, 1992).

45. A.R. Howard, A historical note on animal magnetism, *Amer. Psychol.* **30,** 863 (1975).
46. D.M. Whalmsley, *Anton Mesmer* (Robert Hale, London, 1967).
47. B. Franklin, Majault, Le Roy, Sallin, Bailly, D'Arcet, De Borie, Guillotin, and Lavoisier, *Rapport des Commissaires Chargés par le Roi de l'Examen du Magnétisme Animal* (Chez les Marchands de Nouveautés, Paris, 1784).
48. B. Franklin, Majault, Le Roy, Sallin, Bailly, D'Arcet, De Borie, Guillotin, and Lavoisier, *Report of Dr Benjamin Franklin, and Other Commissioners, Charged by the King of France, with the Examination of Animal Magnetism, as Now Practiced at Paris. Translated from the French with an Historical Introduction.* London, printed for J. Johnston, No. 72, St Paul's Churchyard. (This report can also be found in: M.M. Tinterow, *Foundations of Hypnosis* (Charles C Thomas, Springfield, IL, 1970, 1785), pp. 82–128.)
49. S.J. Gould, The chain of reason vs. the chain of thumbs, *Nat. Hist.* 7, 12–21 (1989).
50. A.H. Smyth (ed.), *The Writings of Ben Franklin: Collected and Edited with a Life and Introduction*, Vol. 9 (Macmillan, New York, 1906).
51. G. Finkenbeiner and V. Meyer, The glass harmonica: a return from obscurity, *Leonardo* **20**, 139–42 (1987).
52. B.E. Owen, *E. Power Biggs: Concert Organist* (Indiana University Press, Bloomington, IN, 1987).
53. B. Stevens, *Ben Franklin's Glass Armonica* (Carolrhoda, Minneapolis, 1983).
54. W.W. Zeitler, William Wilde Zeitler: original music for the glass armonica ("By far the most extensive website about the glass armonica on the Internet."); wwzeitler@glassarmonica.com (2001).
55. T. Robertson, Waltham man's disappearance baffling, *Bost. Globe* B-1 (1999).

Chapter 13

The Mozart Effect

John R. Hughes and John J. Fino

Introduction

The Mozart effect refers to an enhancement of performance or a change in neurophysiological activity associated with listening to Mozart music. The effect has been found in subsequently improved performance on spatial IQ test results of 8–9 points by 36 undergraduates and in increased scores on spatial–temporal reasoning,[1] increased EEG coherence,[2] increased correlations of neurophysiological activity on the temporal and left frontal areas,[3] increased spatial–temporal reasoning after piano lessons in preschool children,[4] changes in amplitude of alpha rhythm and increased interhemispheric coherence,[5] and finally in changes in EEG power and coherence, especially on the right temporal area.[6] The goal of this chapter is to present four related studies: (1) The Mozart effect on epileptiform activity, (2) evidence for a chronic change of this effect, (3) the distinctive aspects of Mozart music as a clue to brain coding, and (4) characteristics of the melodic line of Mozart music, compared to other well-known composers.

I. The Mozart Effect on Epileptiform Activity

Method

EEGs were recorded on 18-channel instruments, either paper writing or digital units with both referential and bipolar montages, utilizing the standard International 10–20 System of Electrode Placement. The 29 patients (ages 3–47) for this study were chosen if they had very many, usually repetitive,

(1) focal discharges (periodic lateralized epileptiform discharges), or (2) bursts of generalized spike and wave complexes in waking or in comatose states. Avoided were patients with these discharges only in the sleep tracing, since a constant state of awareness or alertness (or a lack thereof) was maintained as much as possible throughout the test. The numbers of focal discharges or the durations of generalized bursts were counted. In the case of status epilepticus the duration of the ictal events was measured over a given period of time. The numbers of discharges or durations of bursts were counted during five different states (each usually for 10 min): (1) before, (2) during Mozart music, (3) after, (4) during control music (old-time pop piano tunes), and (5) afterward. Statistical differences were determined by t-tests, Fisher's exact test and the F-test for variability. The Mozart music was *Sonata for Two Pianos in D Major* (K.448), as performed by Murray Perahia and Radu Lupu, especially since most of the previous studies on the Mozart effect have used this selection.

Brain maps were generated by selecting >30 epochs of 2 s of artifact-free EEG, performing a fast Fourier transform (FFT) and plotting amplitude, absolute and percent power as a function of frequency. Frequency ranges included the standard bands of delta (1–3.5 Hz), theta (4–7.5), alpha (8–12.5), beta 1 (13–18) and beta 2 (19–25), but also were changed to more specific ranges. Significant differences in any two maps were determined by considering one as a database, dividing it into 30 different epochs, determining the mean (X) and standard deviation (SD) for every point on the map. A computer program then compared the X amplitude and SD of the comparison file with the database file. For every point on the brain map, the computer program then plotted the number of SDs from the X of the database file.

Results

Statistically significant results during the Mozart music were found in 23 of 29 instances (79%). An example is seen in Figure I.1, showing a status epilepticus in a 47-year-old male, unconscious, with periodic ictal activity maximal on the frontal areas, usually lasting 16–80 s. Before the Mozart music 62.0% of the time ictal patterns were seen, during the music this value decreased to 21.2% and afterward 50.0% . Although variability of effect was, at times, striking from one patient to another, similar results between patients were also seen. Figure I.2 shows two different patients, both in a generalized status epilepticus, one (V.D.) with bilateral spike and wave complexes at 2/s and the other (M.R.) at 3/s. In both patients, continuous bilateral spike and wave complexes were seen during 90–100% of the time before and during the first

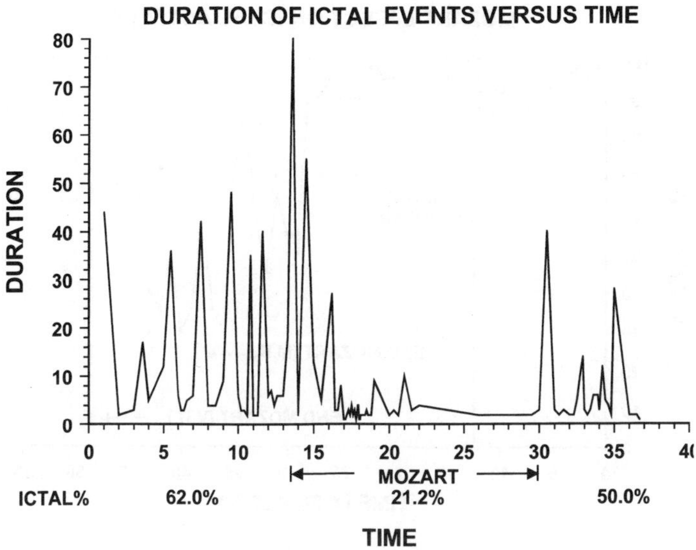

Fig. I.1. Decrease in duration of ictal episodes with Mozart music. The duration of ictal episodes (in seconds) is seen on the vertical axis, and time (every 20 s) on the horizontal axis. Pre-Mozart is seen on the left, during Mozart in the middle and post-Mozart on the right. The % is the time in that period with ictal rhythms.

300 s of the Mozart music. Then for both at 300 s after the onset of the music a sudden decrease in these complexes occurred to around 50%, followed by variable amounts. Sudden changes like that seen in Figure I.2 were also noted at 40 (3 pts), 60 (1 pt) and 80 (1 pt) s after the onset of the Mozart music.

Not only did the rate or frequency of the focal discharges usually decrease in number during the Mozart music; Figure I.3 shows the decrease in the amplitude of these discharges. Means of the amplitude were 81 μV (before) to 66 μV (during) to 73 μV (after the music). Means of the rate or frequency of the discharges (per 20 s) were 13.2 to 10.1 to 13.6 before, during and after the music. The latter changes were significant ($p < 0.05$).

The Allegro begins the Sonata, followed by an 8 s pause and then the Andante begins. At times, the Allegro eliminated the epileptiform activity just before the pause, as seen in Figure I.4(a), but during the pause without music, the activity would at times return, as in Figure I.4(b). In Figure I.5 a similar effect is seen when the music reduced the average number of bifrontal discharges from 13 to 0–7, but at the pause the number increased to even more at 18, followed by another marked decrease, a second increase and finally

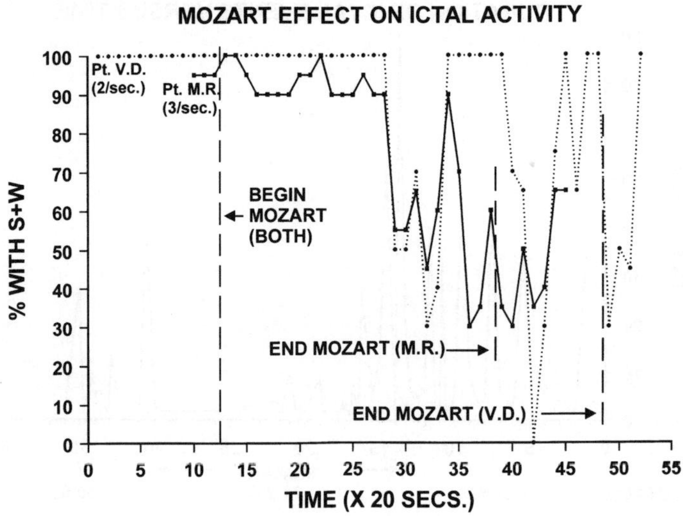

Fig. I.2. Sudden change in absence status epilepticus for two patients at 300 s after the onset of the music. The percentage (%) of time with spike and wave complexes is seen on the vertical axis, and time (each 20 s) on the horizontal axis. Patient V.D., with 2/s complexes, is seen with dotted lines; patient M.R., with 3/s complexes, is seen with solid lines. Both show a sudden decrease in ictal bursts after 300 s of music. The end of the music is designated for each patient by vertical dashed lines.

another decrease. Other than during the obvious pause without music, sudden and variable changes in the frequency of the discharges could not be easily correlated with noticeable changes in the characteristic of the music.

In Figure I.6 (top right for patient C.T.), PLEDs on the *left* anterior-midtemporal area decreased from 167 to 50 during the music, but the *right* posterior temporal area showed no significant change, from 112 to 94. However, the curves for another patient (P.R.) in the same figure showed no change on the *left* temporal discharge, but a marked decrease was seen on the *right* temporal area, from 20 to 0, followed by a rise to higher values. The control music produced no change in either the left or the right temporal discharges. In another trial of the control music, Figure I.7 shows more details of the absence of any change from either the left or the right temporal discharges.

Figure I.8 shows the FFT of the activity from all 21 electrodes before the Mozart music and demonstrates various peaks that seem nearly eliminated during the music, later to return after the music. The specific changes that likely explain the decreases in the peaks were seen, mainly on the central areas.

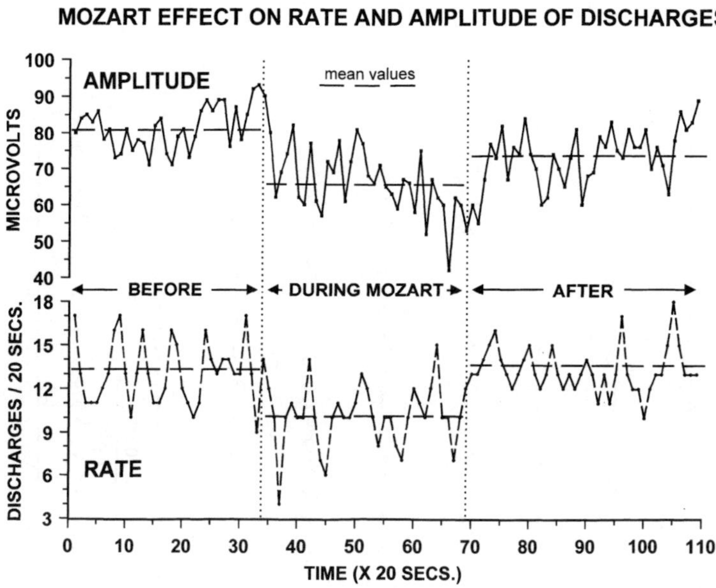

Fig. I.3. Decrease in amplitude (top) and rate (bottom) of discharges during Mozart music. On the vertical axis, amplitude is seen (top) in microvolts and rate of frequency per 20 s (bottom). On the horizontal axis, time (per 20 s) is seen. Horizontal dashed lines represent the mean values.

The specific values in the background theta were 32 (left) and 33 (right) before the music, significantly decreased to 18 during the music, and 31 and 32 afterward. The decrease in the alpha range from 11 and 13 (before) to 8 (during), then back to 12 (after) was not statistically significant. One other change appeared in the background and this was a significant *increase* of delta waves on the frontal midline region from 38 (before) to 47 (during) to 36 (after). Yet another similar change was seen during actual ictal activity in the same patient. In the delta range the values on the frontal midline were 39 (before), significantly increased to 55 (during), and back to 35 (after).

Discussion

The major discussion point of the Mozart effect is to explain why such an effect might occur. The answer likely lies within the superorganization of the microanatomy of the cerebral cortex. Mountcastle[7] was the first investigator to provide evidence for the impressive neocortical organization that exists

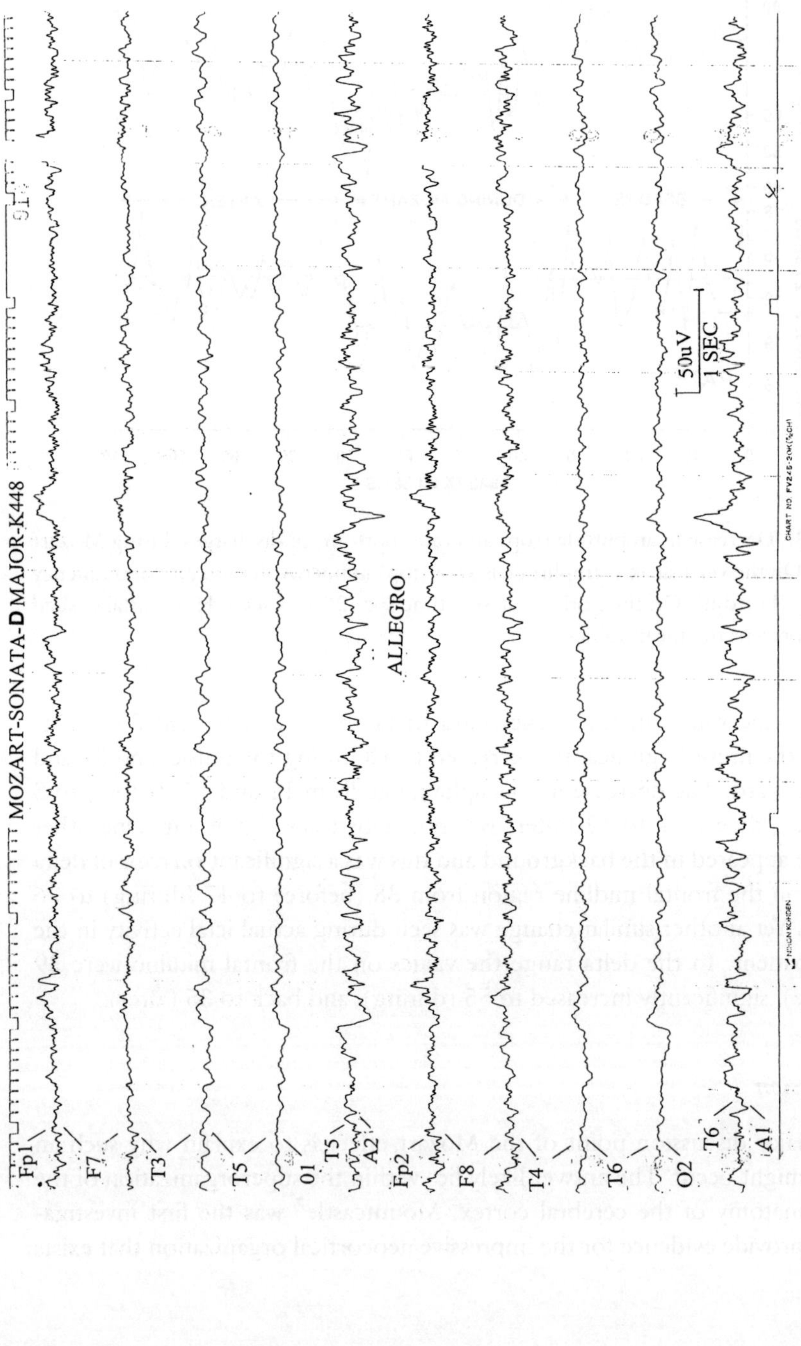

Fig. I.4(a). Allegro of the Mozart music (K.448) without discharges. Note the montage on the left and the time and voltage calibrations (bottom).

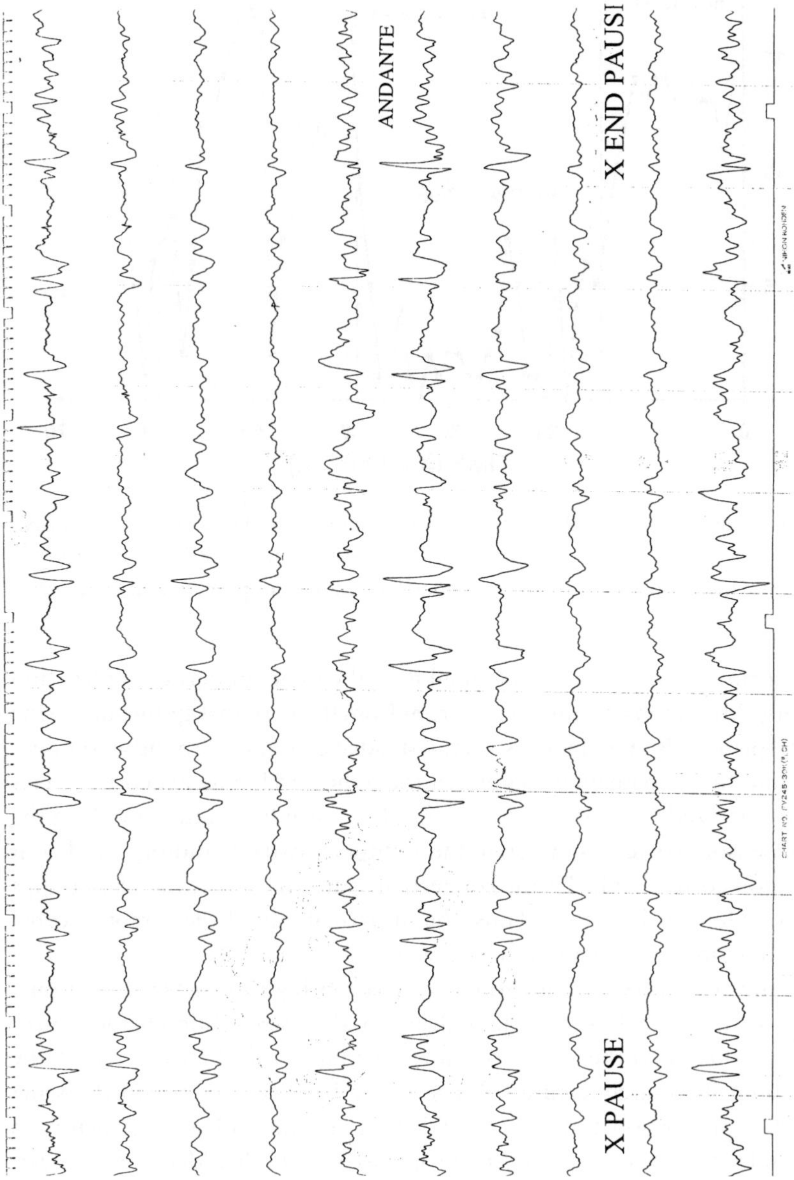

Fig. I.4(b). Increase in discharges during the Pause and then decrease with the Andante. Same montage as in (a).

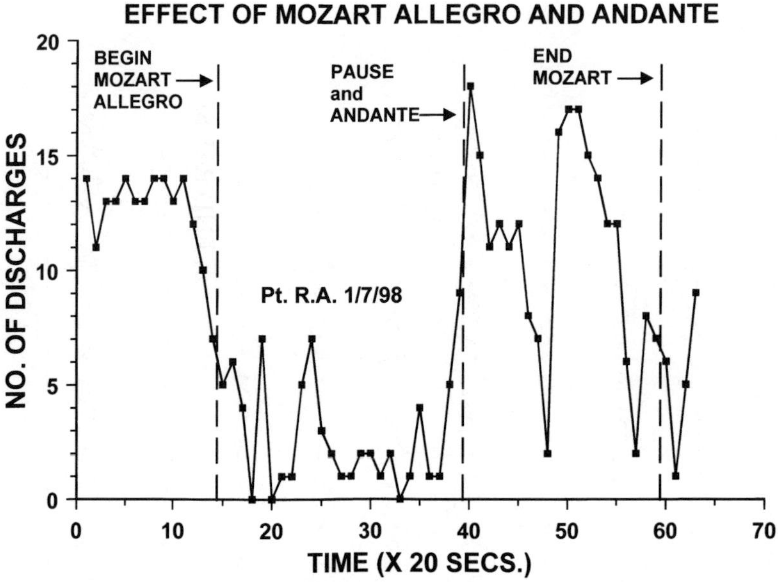

Fig. I.5. Effect of Allegro, Pause, and Andante on number of discharges. Vertical axis is number of discharges (per 20 s), and horizontal axis is time (each 20 s). The Allegro, Pause, Andante, and end of the Mozart music are indicated by vertical dashed lines.

in the form of columns of cells that all have the same properties of place and modality. Migration of immature neurons from the germinal epithelium to the cortical plate ends up in highly structured radial columns, forming an ontogenetic unit, the fundamental building block in the developing neocortex.[8] This highly organized columnar arrangement of cells can be found not only in the somatosensory cortex,[7] but also in the auditory,[9] visual,[10] motor,[11] and even association cortex.[12] Finally, the connectivity patterns of cortical relationships are also columnar in nature. Thus, the microanatomy of the cerebral cortex can be described as very highly organized.

The music of Mozart can also be described as highly organized. Not only the beauty of the melody but the brilliance of the orchestration has led musicologists to refer to the *science* of Mozart's music, and the word repeatedly used about it is "architecture."[14] The music has been built with the same instinct of proportion and the same fidelity to elemental laws of structure as are found in famous cathedrals. Anderson[14] also claims that Mozart in expressing himself in words was in reality thinking in terms of music. At times, words and names were written backward and phrases reversed, and in his music he

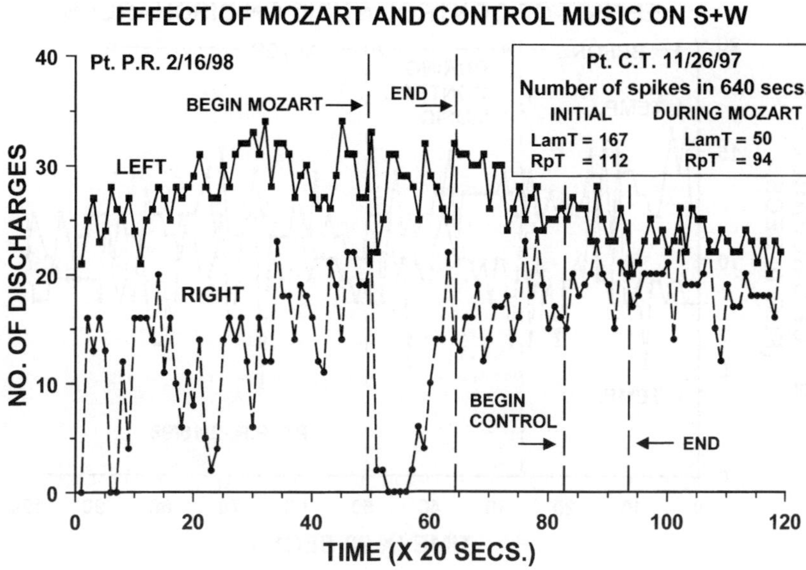

Fig. I.6. Effect of Mozart music on bitemporal PLEDs. On the top right, in patient C.T., a significant decrease is seen on the left but not on the right temporal area. The curves for patient P.R. show a clear decrease on the right, but not on the left temporal area. Number of discharges (per 20 s) appears on the vertical axis, and time (per 20 s) on the horizontal axis.

would use a minor key, play all kinds of tricks with it, reversing it, turning it into a major key, etc. Thus, the architecture of Mozart's music is brilliantly complex, but also highly organized. The superorganization of the cerebral cortex would seem to resonate with the superior architecture of Mozart's music to *normalize* any suboptimal functioning of the cortex. It might be overextending the hypotheses to consider that this music could produce a supernormal performance beyond the intrinsic capability of any given cortex, but at least we can hypothesize that any suboptimal functioning might well be optimized by this music to allow a maximal performance for any given individual.

Shaw and his colleagues[1,2,4,15–17] have written extensively about the columnar arrangement of the cortex as the basis for the Mozart effect, especially using the "trion" model (a mathematical realization of Mountcastle's principles) for the coding of musical structure and other higher brain functions. This same group of investigators[17] even predicted that a reversal of an epileptic state could be accomplished by patterned electrical stimulation which was suggested by their trion model calculations. Our results would confirm such

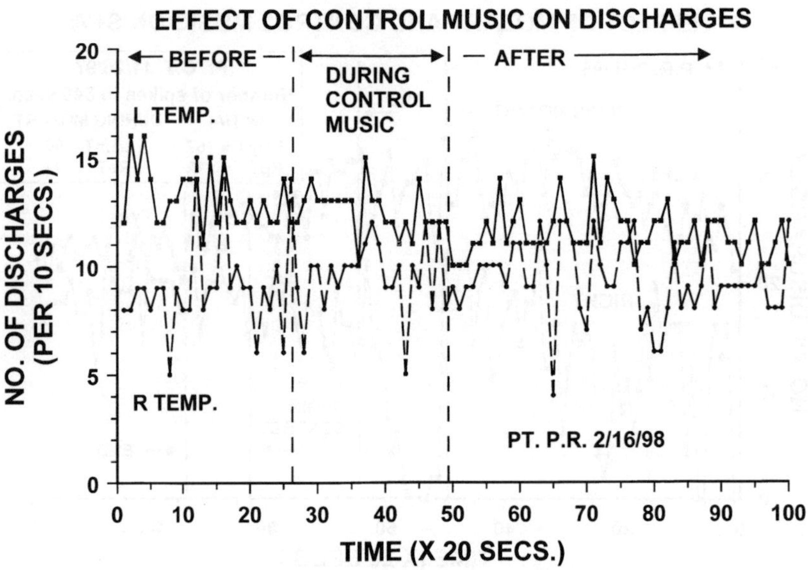

Fig. I.7. Lack of change in discharge during control music. The number of discharges (per 10 s) is seen on the vertical axis, and time (per 20 s) appears on the horizontal axis. The number of discharges on the left (above) and right temporal areas (below) are shown in the two curves, as are the times before, during and after the music (dashed vertical lines).

a reversal and imply that Mozart music would provide the equivalent of *patterned* electrical stimulation. Our results may be similar to the newly described phenomenon of "quenching," an increase in the seizure threshold and an inhibition of seizure development from 1 Hz stimulation of the amygdala for 15 min.[18]

The effect of the Mozart K.448 Sonata cannot be simply viewed as the result of changing the state of awareness or a reflection of some deep appreciation of this music. Some patients were in coma and others were in status epilepticus without any outward signs of reactivity. Furthermore, the control music did not produce any significant changes. Therefore, the Mozart effect is viewed as direct or primary on the cerebral cortex and not secondary to an alerting stimulation or to an intervening emotional state.

At times, the post-Mozart period with silence showed evidence of a continuing effect of the music by the fewer discharges after the music than during the pre-Mozart periods. Examples can be seen in Figures I.1 and I.2. Thus, a carryover effect is noted. Examples from other studies include the results

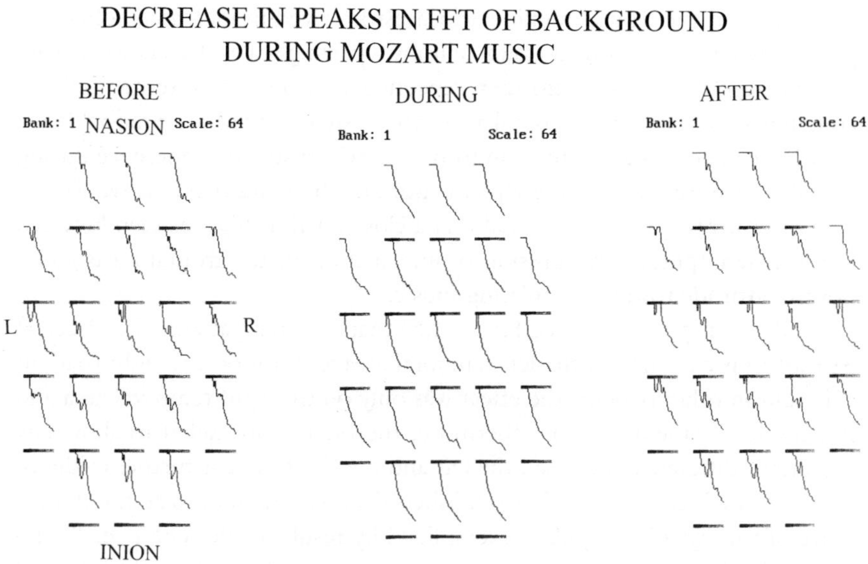

Fig. I.8. Decrease in peaks in the FFT of background activity during Mozart music. On the left are the results before the music, in the middle during the music and on the right after the music. The nasion (above), inion (below), left and right sides are designated, and the FFT for each electrode is represented. The horizontal lines below each FFT show the frequency range of 1–25 Hz.

of Rauscher *et al.*,[1] in which increased spatial–temporal reasoning appeared much better on day 2 than on day 1. Another example from the same group showed effects in preschool children that indicate "long-term modifications in the underlying neural circuitry". Finally, Sarnthein *et al.*,[2] showed increased coherence values not only during Mozart music but also after the music.

The brain maps showed a *decrease* in theta and alpha activity on the central areas and an increase in delta activity on the mid-frontal areas. Petsche *et al.*[6] has shown with Mozart music a decrease in power on all areas, but especially a decrease in theta on the *central* areas and also the anterior quadrant, similar to our findings. Their decrease in alpha was mainly on the temporal areas and our findings of the changes in alpha activity on the central areas were not statistically significant. The results of Gunther *et al.*[19] of a decrease in brain activation on the temporal and parietal areas during music perception are also consistent with our decreases in activity, as is their lower alpha activity associated with improvement in spatial testing. Our *increase* in delta activity on the frontal and midline areas is consistent with the results of Petsche *et al.*,[20] who reported the frontal midline area most involved in increased coherence patterns when a professional violin-cellist was playing scales. Earlier work from the same group[21] is also consistent, reporting an increase in interhemispheric coupling, especially on the frontal areas while listening to Mozart music. Iwaki *et al.*[5] also reported an increase in frontal interhemispheric coherence during stimulating music, but in the alpha band, not the delta band, as we found. The latter investigators concluded that a close relationship was seen between the interhemispheric transmission of information to the frontal areas and a positive attitude toward stimulating music.

Evidence is presented (see Figure I.6) that in some patients the effect of Mozart music is only on the left temporal area and not on the right (patient CT), but in other patients the effect was only on the right temporal area and not the left (patient PR). Furthermore, the brain maps failed to show any significant differences between the left and the right side, as further evidence of bilateral effects. Some other published data would emphasize the importance of the *right* hemisphere, exemplified by results of Petsche *et al.*,[6] who reported a decrease in theta power anteriorly, especially on the right side, and a frequency change in the beta band, almost restricted to the right side. Other work[22] has emphasized EEG changes on the right hemisphere, especially at the anterior and posterior poles when discriminating for pitch and timbre. On the other hand, the *left* hemisphere has been emphasized in the report of Weiser and Walter,[23] who described a performing organist with a seizure from the right temporal lobe with the result of imprecise movements of the associated left hand, but with faultless right hand movements, likely from the left hemisphere and compensating for errors of the left hand. Finally, Bever and Chiarello[24] concluded that the *left* hemisphere is dominant for analytic processing of musical sounds and the *right* hemisphere for holistic processing, based on the finding that musicians recognize simple melodies better in the right ear, but naive listeners show the reverse finding.

Summary

The Mozart effect, using the *Piano Sonata in D Major* (K.448), was examined in patients with seizures. In 23 of 29 instances, significant decreases in epileptiform activity were noted from patients even in coma, with status epilepticus or with periodic lateralized epileptiform discharges (PLEDs). The effect may be immediate or require 40–300 s to manifest itself. The change in the amount of ictal activity in one patient in coma was from 62% before the music to 21% during the Mozart music. Amplitudes of these discharges also have been decreased. Examples of PLEDs on both temporal areas are shown in which the effect was only on the left temporal area but in other patients only on the right temporal area. Brain maps during the music showed that theta and alpha activity *decreased* on the central areas, while delta waves increased on the frontal midline areas. The basis of this effect is likely that the superorganization of the cerebral cortex with its highly structured radial columns seen throughout both hemispheres may resonate with the superior architecture of Mozart's music.

References

1. F.H. Rauscher, G.L. Shaw and K.N. Ky, Listening to Mozart enhances spatial-temporal reasoning: towards a neurophysiological basis, *Neurosci. Lett.* **185**, 44–7 (1995).
2. J. Sarnthein, A. von Stein, P. Rappelsberg, H. Petsche, F.H. Rauscher and G.L. Shaw, Persistent patterns of brain activity: an EEG coherence study of the positive effect of music on spatial-temporal reasoning, *Neurol. Res.* **19**, 107–16 (1997).
3. B.E. Rideout and C.M. Laubach, EEG correlates of enhanced spatial performance following exposure to music, *Percept. Motor Skills* **82**, 427–32 (1996).
4. F.H. Rauscher, G.L. Shaw, L.J. Levine, E.L. Wright, W.R. Dennis and R.I. Newcomb, Music training causes long-term enhancement of preschool children's spatial-temporal reasoning, *Neurol. Res.* **19**, 2–8 (1997).
5. T. Iwaki, M. Hayashi and T. Hori, Changes in alpha band EEG activity in the frontal area after stimulation with music of different affective content, *Percept. Motor Skills* **84**(2), 515–26 (1997).
6. H. Petsche, H. Pockberger and P. Rappelsberger, EEG topography and mental performance. In: F.H. Duffy (ed.), *Topographic Mapping of Brain Electrical Activity* (Butterworths, Boston, 1986), pp. 63–98.
7. V.B. Mountcastle, Modality and topographic properties of single neurons of cat's somatic sensory cortex, *J. Neurophysiol.* **20**, 408–34 (1957).
8. P. Rakic, Specification of cerebral cortical areas, *Science* **241**, 170–6 (1988).
9. M.M. Merzenich, S.A. Colwell and R.A. Andersen, Auditory forebrain organization: thalamocortical and corticothalamic connections in the cat. In: C.N. Woolsey (ed.), *Cortical Sensory Organization*, Vol. 3 (Humana, Clifton, New Jersey, 1982), pp. 43–57.
10. D.H. Hubel and T.N. Wiesel, Functional architecture of macaque monkey visual cortex. *Proc. R. Soc. London B Biol. Sci.* **198**, 1–59 (1977).
11. G. Meyer, Forms and spatial arrangement of neurons in the primary motor cortex of man, *J. Comp. Neurol.* **262**, 402–28 (1987).
12. V.B. Mountcastle, J.C. Lynch, A. Georgopoulos, H. Sakata and C. Acuna, Posterior partial association cortex of the monkey; command function for operations within extrapersonal space, *J. Neurophysiol.* **38**, 871–908 (1975).

13. V.B. Mountcastle, The columnar organization of the neocortex, *Brain* **120**, 701–22 (1997).
14. E. Anderson, *The Letters of Mozart and His Family* (W.W. Norton, New York, 1985).
15. X. Leng, G.L. Shaw and E.L. Wright, Coding of musical structure and trion model of cortex, *Music Perception* **8**(1), 9–62 (1990).
16. M.N. Bodner, Y.D. Zhou, G.L. Shaw and J.M. Fuster, Symmetric temporal patterns in cortical spike trains during performance of a short term memory task, *Neurol. Res.* **19**, 509–14 (1997).
17. X. Leng, J.V. McGrann and G.L. Shaw, Reversal of epileptic state by patterned electrical stimulation suggested by trion model calculations, *Neurol. Res.* **14**, 57–61 (1992).
18. S.R.B. Weiss, X.-L. Li, E.C. Noguera *et al.*, Quenching: persistent alterations in seizure and after discharge threshold following low-frequency stimulation. In: M.E. Corcoran and S.L. Moshe (eds.), *Kindling* 5 (Plenum, New York, 1998), pp. 101–20.
19. W. Gunther, N. Muller, W. Trapp, C. Haag, A. Rutz and A. Straube, Quantitative EEG analysis during motor function and music perception in Tourette's syndrome, *Eur. Arch. Psychiatry Clin. Neurosci.* **246**(14), 197–202 (1996).
20. H. Petsche, A. von Stein and O. Filg, EEG aspects of mentally playing an instrument, *Brain Res. Cogn.* **3**(2), 115–23 (1996).
21. H. Petsche, The EEG—a cryptogram? In: S. Zschocke and E.J. Speckmann (eds.), *Basic Mechanisms of the EEG* (Birkhauser, Boston, 1993), pp. 13–27.
22. P. Auzou, F. Eustache, P. Etevenon *et al.*, Topographic EEG activations during timbre and pitch discrimination tasks using musical sounds, *Neuropsychologia* **33**(1), 25–37 (1995).
23. H.G. Wieser and R. Walter, Untroubled musical judgment of a performing organist during epileptic seizure of the right temporal lobe, *Neuropsychologia* **35**(1), 45–51 (1997).
24. T.G. Bever and R.J. Chiarello, Cerebral dominance in musicians and nonmusicians, *Science* **185**, 536–9 (1974).

II. Is There a Chronic Change of the Mozart Effect on Epileptiform Activity? A Case Study

Introduction

The previous section shows the results of the Mozart effect on patients with epilepsy, demonstrating that Mozart music (K.448) was usually associated with an acute decrease in the amount of epileptiform activity, both ictal and interictal and both generalized and focal in origin. The goal of this study on one patient was to see if a chronic effect could be found, by repeatedly exposing the patient to the music during wakefulness over a 24 h period. Both clinical seizures and epileptiform activity were assessed.

Method

EEGs were originally recorded in this patient on 18-channel instruments, utilizing the standard International 10–20 System of Electrode Placement. For this study on the chronic effect, an 8-channel ambulatory EEG instrument was used with electrodes on $F_{3,4}$, $C_{3,4}$, $F_{7,8}$, $T_{3,4}$, and $T_{5,6}$ positions. The recording was begun at 0900 on 15 October 1998 and continued for 24 h. Since previous records (5) had shown both many bilateral spike and wave complexes at 1–2/s (Lennox–Gastaut syndrome) and many focal discharges on the right posterior temporal area (T_6), the number of seconds with the generalized discharges and separately with the focal discharges was counted over the 24 h period.

The number of seizures (drop attacks) was also counted by the mother and also by the teacher while the child attended school. The typical pattern of attacks throughout the day was determined by reviewing the previous 45 days, counting the number of attacks within three time periods (0900–1400, 1400–1800, and 1800–2200 h) during the waking periods of the patient.

Every hour on the hour for 10 min during wakefulness over a 24 h period, Mozart music was played (*Sonata for Two Pianos in D Major*—K.448, as performed by Murray Perahia and Radu Lupu). The music was continued at the school attended by the patient.

The patient was an 8-year-old female who had had an arteriovenous malformation on the right posterior temporal area. A neurosurgical operation had been performed 2 years earlier to remove the malformation since many seizures had occurred. For the past 2 years many focal EEG discharges on the right posterior temporal area and also many bilateral spike and wave complexes at 1–2/s had been seen. Many combinations of antiepileptic drugs had been given and at the time of this recording the patient was taking Topamax and Klonopin. The study was done at a time when the patient's seizures had clearly increased over the usual number.

Results

Figure II.1 shows that the number of clinical seizures on 15 October 1998 decreased from 9 to 7 to 1 over 3 periods of wakefulness. This decrease from

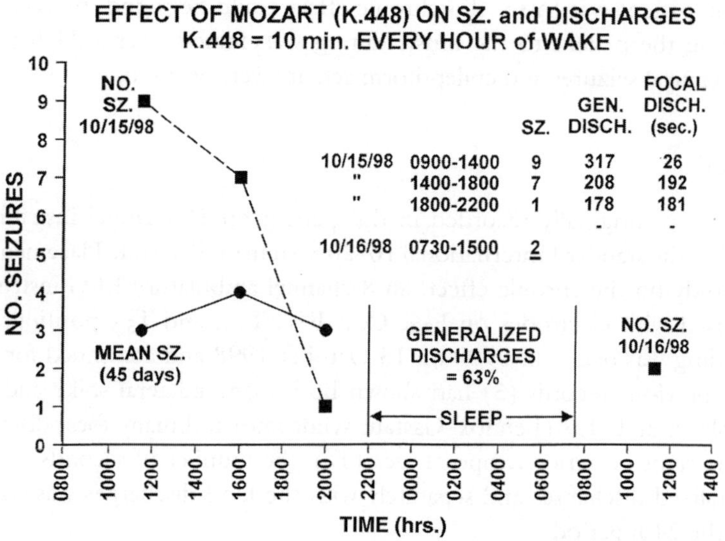

Fig. II.1. The effect of Mozart music on clinical seizures and EEG discharges over 30 h from 0800 (15 October 1998) to 1400 the next day (16 October 1998) is shown on the horizontal axis. The number of seizures is shown on the vertical axis decreasing from 9 to 7 to 1 and 2 on 16 October 1998. The mean number of seizures from the 45 days before is also shown. The number of generalized and focal epileptiform discharges is shown on the upper right. See text for details.

0900 AM to 2200 PM contrasts with the typical pattern over the day, usually showing a steady number (3–4) from 0900 to 1400, also from 1400 to 1800, and finally from 1800 to 2200 h. The number of attacks on the next day (16 October 1998) was 2 from 0730 to 1500 h, in contrast with the 9 on the previous day over the similar time period. The figure also shows the number of seconds with generalized and with focal discharges over the 24 h period. Throughout 15 October 1998 the number of seconds with bilateral spike and wave complexes at 1–2/s, responsible for the patient's drop attacks, decreased from 317 to 208 to 178. The number of seconds with focal discharges did not change in any orderly way. During sleep from 2200 PM to 0800 AM on the next day, for 63% of the time, generalized discharges appeared, usually resembling electrical status epilepticus of sleep (ESES), seen nearly continuously for long periods but followed by relatively normal activity also appearing for long periods.

Discussion

The major finding in this patient was that a chronic change of the Mozart effect did appear. From presenting the music every hour for 10 min during wakefulness, the number of clinical attacks significantly decreased and the number of related generalized discharges also decreased. Furthermore, on the next day the number of attacks decreased, compared to the number during the same time period on the previous day. This decrease in clinical attacks throughout the first day was uncharacteristic since other data on the patient showed a relatively steady number of seizures that usually appeared throughout the day, although at the time of the recording the number of attacks had generally increased for the previous week.

One unexpected result was that, even though clinical and electrographic improvement had appeared, the majority (63%) of the sleep record showed ESES. A tentative conclusion would be that the latter pattern does not have a direct relationship with the number of clinical attacks before or after the night with ESES. Thus, a patient may show improvement in the number of clinical attacks, both the night before and during the next day, and still show the ESES pattern. This latter pattern is known to "look much worse than the patient" with its nearly continuous generalized spike and wave complexes in sleep, but without any *obvious* clinical attacks, either during the day or night. One common finding in children with ESES is that they have a diminished capacity to learn.[2] Although out patient was unexpectedly found to be bright and intelligent, further inquiry has shown that the patient has a clearly diminished cognitive status now, compared to a year ago, as would be expected with the Lennox–Gastaut syndrome.[3]

Further studies are required to see how often such a chronic change of the Mozart effect might be found, as appeared in this patient.

Summary

This report shows that a patient with the Lennox–Gastaut syndrome had fewer clinical seizures and also fewer generalized bilateral spike and wave complexes over a 24 h period while exposed to Mozart music (K.448) for 10 min every hour during wakefulness.

Acknowledgment

The authors wish to thank Gordon Shaw, Ph.D., for his support.

References

1. J.R. Hughes, Y. Daaboul, J.J. Fino and G.L. Shaw, The "Mozart Effect" on epileptiform activity, *Clin. Electroencephalogr.* **29**(3), 109–11 (1998).
2. G. Patry, S. Lyagoubi and C.A. Tassinari, Subclinical "electrical status epilepticus" induced by sleep in children, *Arch. Neurol.* **24**, 242–52 (1971).
3. E. Niedermeyer, The Lennox–Gastaut syndrome; a severe type of childhood epilepsy *DZ. Nervenheilk.* **195**, 263–83 (1969).

III. Distinctive Aspects of the Music—A Clue to Brain Coding

Introduction

Considerable evidence[1–4] now exists to support the Mozart effect, which refers to an enhancement of various types of performance while listening to Mozart music. The previous section showed a report on the acute decrease in clinical seizures and EEG epileptiform activity during music of this composer (K.448),[5] and later[6] demonstrated that a *chronic* change could also be seen from hourly exposures of this music over a 24 h period of time. The Mozart effect has been the topic of a book,[7] has generated discussions throughout the world, and has resulted in many popular recordings, especially used by families that have concentrated on the mental development of their children. One important question now is: What are the distinctive aspects of Mozart music that account for all of these many beneficial effects? If discovered, these same distinctive characteristics should lead us to conclusions regarding the kinds of stimuli that resonate well within the cerebral cortex to explain these effects. Thus, these special features of Mozart music should inform us *about the brain, its coding, and the way it responds favorably to certain stimuli*.

Method and Apparatus

Index of periodicity

In order to study the many aspects of different musical selections and their internal complexity, the use of the computer became essential. Figure III.1 outlines the method for quantifying the music to determine any distinctive feature and for determining one aspect that became apparent, namely periodicity.

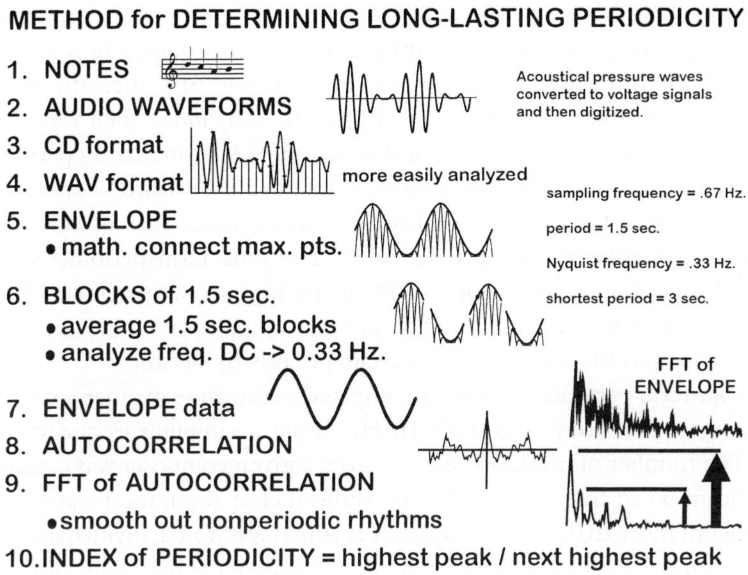

Fig. III.1. Method for determining long-lasting periodicities. See text for details. Long-lasting periodicities were from 15 to 120 s; a similar technique was used for short-lasting periodicities (0.25–10 Hz).

The musical notes were first converted into audio waveforms, i.e. acoustical pressure waves converted into voltage signals and digitized. The CD format was converted into a WAV format, which could be more easily analyzed. The maximal points were mathematically connected to create an Envelope with a sampling frequency of 0.67 Hz (period = 1.5 s) and thus with a Nyquist frequency of 0.33 Hz (shortest period = 3 s). Blocks of 1.5 s were averaged and frequencies from DC to 0.33 Hz were analyzed. These data were then converted into an Envelope, showing relative amplitude over time. Then a fast Fourier transform (FFT) of the Envelope provided a write-out of the relative amplitude of all periodicities from 3 s to 120 s. The next procedure was an autocorrelogram of these data to see better the major periodicities. Finally, the FFT of the autocorrelogram most clearly showed the relative amplitude of the major periodicities, smoothing out the nonperiodic rhythms.

A Periodicity Index was chosen to represent the *degree* of periodicity; this index was the ratio of the highest peak to the next-highest (×10). Thus, if a musical selection was extremely periodic and consistently showed a dominant peak of activity every 30 s, the 30 s value would be highest, set at the value of 100 and the next-highest peak would be minimal (e.g. 20) so that the index would be $100/20 = 5(\times 10) = 50$. The highest value of these periodicities was always assigned the value of 100 and when other competing periodicities without one dominant peak were also evident (e.g. 50), then the index in this case would be $100/50 = 2(\times 10) = 20$. This index then represented the degree to which a certain musical selection had a dominating periodicity, rather than a number of periodic changes that could be heard or appreciated. Long-lasting or long-term periodicities included those that occurred every 3–120 s throughout a musical selection. The long-term periodicities were divided into those with major (>50% of the highest) and minor (25–49%) peaks. For each musical selection the numbers of major and minor peaks were counted, as was the incidence of a certain periodicity of time.

Short-term periodicities were investigated in the same manner, except that the range under study was 0.25–10 Hz, using a sampling frequency of 20 Hz. The number of musical selections from a given composer was counted as significant when the autocorrelogram showed clear rhythmical features. The number of those that were the highest (at 100%) was noted, divided into those at <1/s and >1/s. Subharmonics and harmonics of the dominant short-term periodicities were also counted, including the second harmonic. Using the system devised by the Acoustical Society of America and endorsed by the USA Standards Association, middle C was represented as C_4 at 262 Hz.[8]

Results

Long-lasting periodicities

Figure III.2 (bottom), as an example of the type of analysis used, shows the musical envelope of a Mendelssohn selection (*Gondolier's Song*), with four periodic changes over the 2.2 min of this song. The top of the figure shows that the main periodicity was, as expected, at 30 s. All peaks, >50% (major) and 25–49% (minor), were counted for this and all other selections and the data are seen in Table III.1. This table shows that the largest number of major peaks was found in Mozart music and both major and minor peaks appeared significantly more often in the music of Mozart and the two Bachs, compared to the 164 selections from the 55 other composers. This same table shows the time of the periodic change that most often occurred. The period of 30 s was most often used by Mozart, 50 s by J.C. Bach, 60 and 90 s by the other composers, and 120 s by J.S. Bach. This table shows the most common periodic changes, but other periods were found in the selections of all composers.

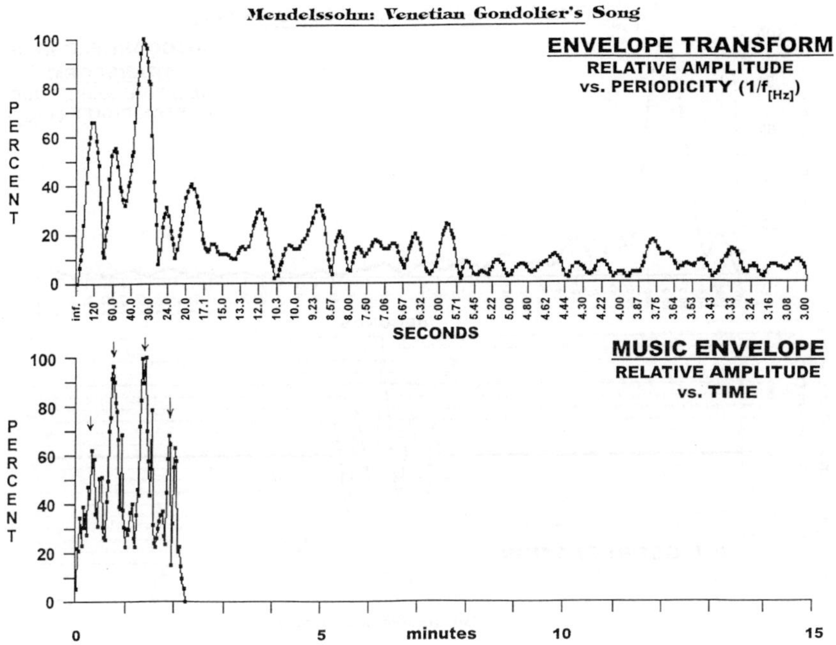

Fig. III.2. Music Envelope (bottom) and Envelope Transform of Mendelssohn's *Venetian Gondolier's Song*. The bottom shows time (min) on the horizontal axis and relative amplitude (%) of power on the vertical axis, demonstrating a prominent peak at 30 s.

Table III.1. Long-lasting periodicity (15–120 s). Different composers.

		Number of Major/ Minor Peaks		Time of Period (s) Incidence (%)				
Composer	No.	Major (>50%)	Minor (25–49%)	30	50	60	90	120
Mozart	(81)	9.2*	6.4†	8	11	14	21	31
J.C. Bach	(67)	9.0*	7.7†	3	14	9	25	38
J.S. Bach	(38)	0.7*	6.8†	2	0	10	14	49
55 others	(164)	6.0	4.8	4	12	16	25	23

*$p < 0.00002$; †$p < 0.0001$.

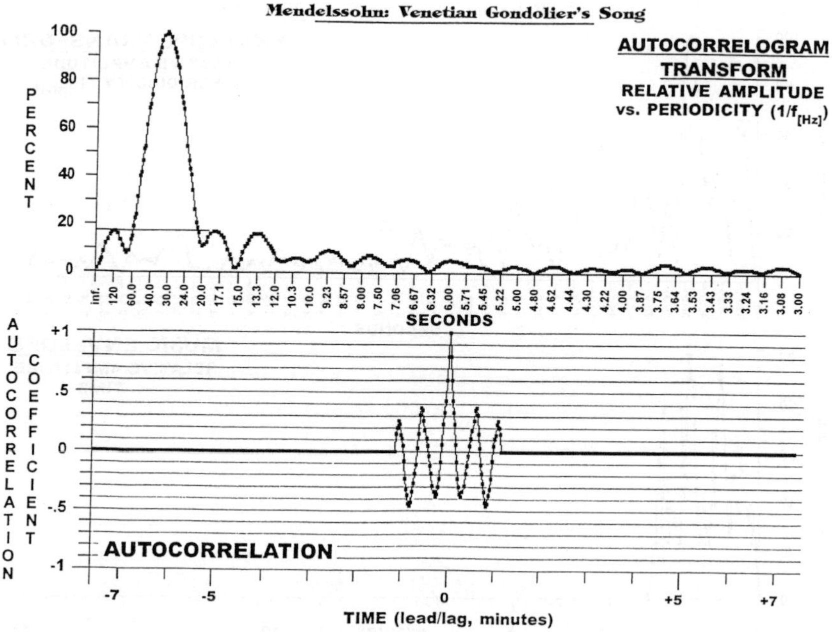

Fig. III. 3. Autocorrelation (bottom) and Autocorrelation Transform (top) of Mendelssohn's *Gondolier's Song*. The horizontal axis (bottom) shows the lead/lag in minutes around zero (0) time to determine the clear periodicity, and the vertical axis shows the autocorrelation coefficient. On top periodicity is shown in seconds on the horizontal axis with relative amplitude on the vertical axis with major peak at 30 s. See text for other details for calculating the periodicity index.

Figure III.3 shows (bottom) the autocorrelation of the envelope transfer seen in Fig. III.2 and confirms by its clear rhythmical feature a prominent periodicity (2.3 cycles in 69 s). The same figure (top) shows the FFT of the autocorrelation, smoothing out the nonperiodic rhythms and again showing the periodicity at 30 s. The figure also demonstrates the way to determine the score for the degree of periodicity. The ratio of the height of the peak of 100 at 30 s to the next peak of 17 at 17.5 s ($\times 10$) = score of 58.8($100/17 \times 10$).

Table III.2 gives the periodicity scores for the different composers, showing that J.S. Bach most often had the *highest* scores of >30, J.C. Bach most often (14%) with scores of 25–29.9, and Mozart (11%) at 20–24.9. Note the significant difference between the scores over 25 for the latter three composers versus Chopin and 43 other composers. The lowest scores (10–14.9) with minimal periodicity were more often seen with Chopin and the other

Table III.2. Long-lasting periodicity. Different composers. Percent with given degree of periodicity.

		Scores—Degree of Periodicity				
Composer	No.	10–14.9	15–19.9	20–24.9	25–29.9	>30
Mozart	(45)	44*	29	11	9†	7‡
J.C. Bach	(37)	54*	27	3	14†	3‡
J.S. Bach	(67)	47*	24	6	13†	10‡
Chopin	(39)	59*	28	10	3†	0‡
Others	(43)	61*	28	9	2†	0‡

$^*p = 0.11$; $^{\dagger}p = 0.008$; $^{\ddagger}p = 0.01$.

composers, and least often with Mozart. The latter difference was not quite statistically significant.

Table III.3 shows the highest periodicity scores for the various composers. The highest were selections by J.C. Bach (71.4) and Mendelssohn (66.7) but generally the two Bachs and Mozart demonstrated high scores, with Chopin scores usually lower (21–32). Also seen are the periodicities in seconds varying between 10 and 60 s but with a mean of 30.6 s (median 30 s) for those particular selections.

One of the controls used in the study on epileptiform activity[5] was music by the modern composer Philip Glass. Figure III.4 (bottom) shows the autocorrelation function of this music, failing to demonstrate any clear long-term periodicity. The same figure (top) confirms the absence of any prominent peak of periodicity. The score using the ratio of the peak at 100 to the next-highest at 90 would be $100/90 = 1.1(\times 10) = 11$. In Table III.4 the musical selections with the lowest values are found (<17). Note that the other control piece used in the epilepsy study,[5] Old Time Piano Tunes, which failed to produce any effect, scored the low value of 16.

Short-lasting periodicities

Figure III.5 shows an example of the *short*-term periodicity in a Mozart sonata (K. 570—2nd movement) demonstrating 15 waves over a time shift of 10 s (bottom), equivalent to a periodicity of 1.5 Hz (top). However, Figure III.6 shows a similar periodicity in the control piece, Old Time Piano Tunes (#3), indicating 21 waves over a 10 s time shift (bottom), equivalent to a periodicity of 2.1 Hz (top).

Table III.3. Highest values for long-lasting periodicities.

		Index (×10)	Period (s)
I.	J.S. Bach		
	1. Suite for Orchestra #3 in D "Air"	50.0	13.5
	2. Concerto in E #3 allegro assai	45.5	35.0
	3. Goldberg Variations CD2, #1, Variation 16, Overture	45.5	12.0
	4. St. Matthew Passion Chorus	40.0	10.3
	5. Concert for Clavier & Orchestra BWV 1054, 3 allegro	40.0	10.0
II.	Mozart		
	1. Sonata in E Flat Major I Movement (K282)	50.0	24.0
	2. Sonata in C Major III Movement (K309)	43.5	17.0
	3. Sonata in A Minor II Movement (K310)	35.7	60.0
	4. Sonata in D for Keyboard III Movement (K576)	31.3	27.0
	5. Sonata in D Major III Movement (K448)	31.3	40.0
III.	J.C. Bach		
	1. Sonata in B Flat Major, Op. 5, No. 1. #2 Tempo di Menueto	71.4	10.2
	2. Sonata in C Minor, Op. 5, No. 6. #3 allegretto	50.0	30.0
	3. Sonata in G Major, Op. 5, No. 3. #1 allegro	33.3	32.0
	4. Sonata in E Major, Op. 5, No. 5. #1 allegro assai	31.3	40.0
	5. Sonata in E Major, Op. 5, No. 5. #2 adagio	30.3	17.5
IV.	F. Chopin		
	1. Waltz in D Flat Major, Op. 64, No. 1, Minute Waltz	32.3	10.3
	2. Funeral March from Sonata B Flat Minor, Op. 35/2	25.0	35.0
	3. Mazurka in C Sharp Minor, Op. 63, No. 3	23.8	50.0
	4. Prelude in D Flat Major, Op. 28/15, "Raindrops"	22.7	50.0
	5. Fantasie Impromptu in C Sharp Minor, Op. 66	21.3	40.0
V.	Others		
	1. Mendelsohn: Venetian Barcarole Song from "Song Without Words"	66.7	60.0
	2. Mendelsohn: Venetian Gondolier's Song	58.8	30.0
	3. Franck: Fugue	50.0	60.0
	4. CPE Bach Symphony No. 2 in E Flat Major, 1. allegro de molte	50.0	30.0
	5. Schumann: Dreaming from Scenes from Childhood, Op. 15/7	47.6	22.0

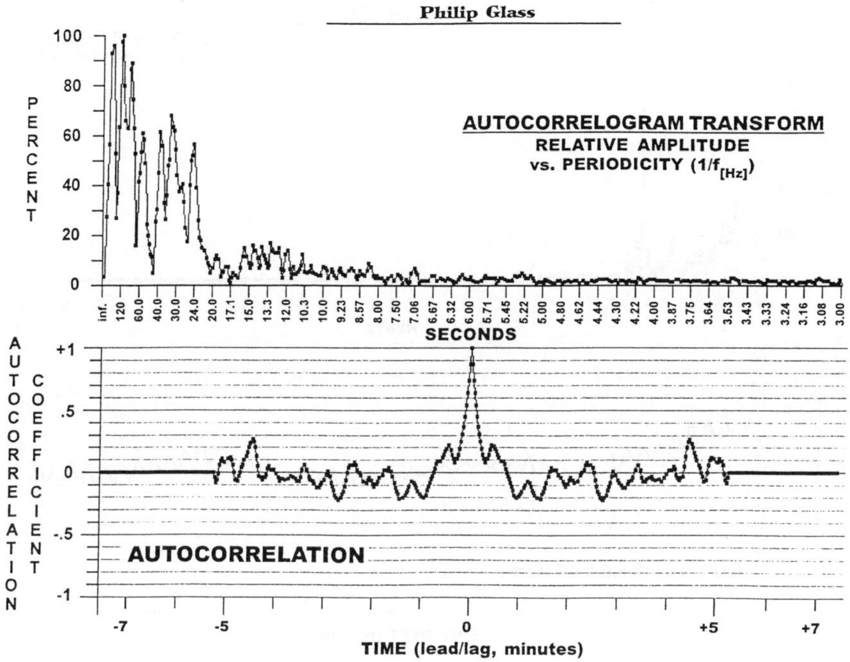

Fig. III.4. Autocorrelation (bottom) and Autocorrelation Transform (top) of Philip Glass selection. See legend of Figure III.3 for details of the axes. Note that no clear rhythmicity appears in the autocorrelation (bottom) or in the transform (top).

Table III.4. Lowest values for long lasting-periodicities.

1. W. Kilar: Orawa
2. Schubert-Tausig: Marcia militare
3. Klenner-Lewis: Just Friends
4. A. Skrjabin: Vers la flume
5. Rachmaninov: Prima danza sinfonica
6. J.S. Bach: Concerto for clavier and orchestra, BWV 1054, allegro
7. Mozart: Fantasia for piano in C minor – K 475 – I
8. Chopin: Etude in E major, Op. 10 #3
9. Chopin: Berceuse in D flat major, Op. 57
10. Brahms: Piano concerto No. 2 in B flat major Op. 83 Andante
11. Old Time Pop Tunes (Control) = Index = 16.2
12. Philip Glass (Control) = Index = 11.9

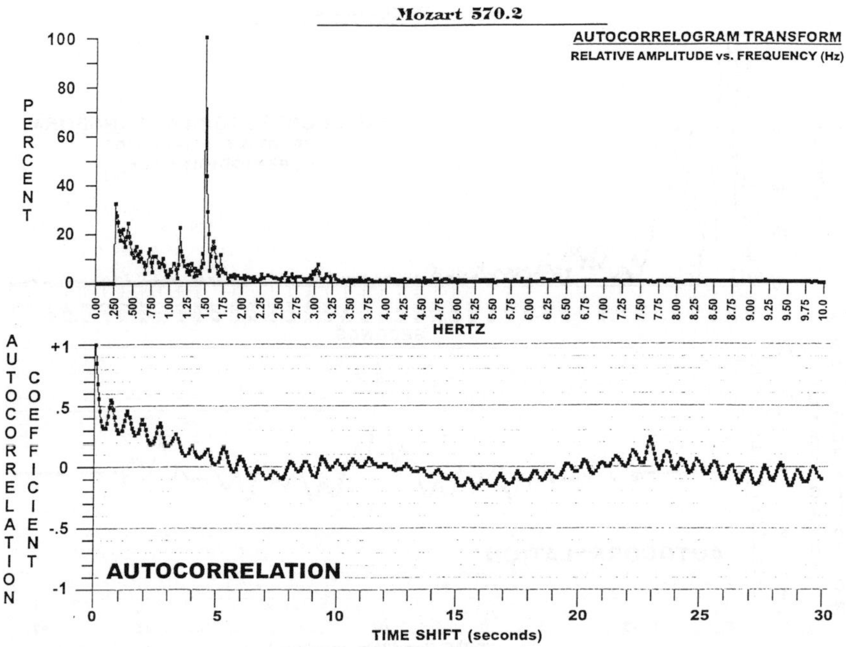

Fig. III.5. Autocorrelation (bottom) and Autocorrelation Transform (top) of Mozart (K.570—2nd movement). The horizontal axis shows time shift in only one direction to show longer shifts. See text for details for the periodicity at 1.5 Hz.

Table III.5 shows a summary of the short-lasting periodicities found in 290 pieces composed by Mozart, three different Bachs and Chopin and also 177 selections from 51 other composers. Although the number (%) that showed significant periodicity tended to be higher for Mozart and the Bachs, compared to the other composers, the number (%) at 100% (highest) was not significantly different. Also, the number of subharmonics or harmonics tended to be higher for the Mozart and the Bachs, but the second (×2) harmonics were not different. Finally, no clear differences were seen for the highest peaks over or under 1.0/s. In summary, no clear differences in short-term periodicity were generally noted between the musical selections of Mozart and the Bachs, compared to those of the other composers.

All of these results have shown that the music of Mozart and of the two Bachs are distinctive in that they demonstrate a *long-term* periodicity significantly more often than other composers, but no clear differences were seen

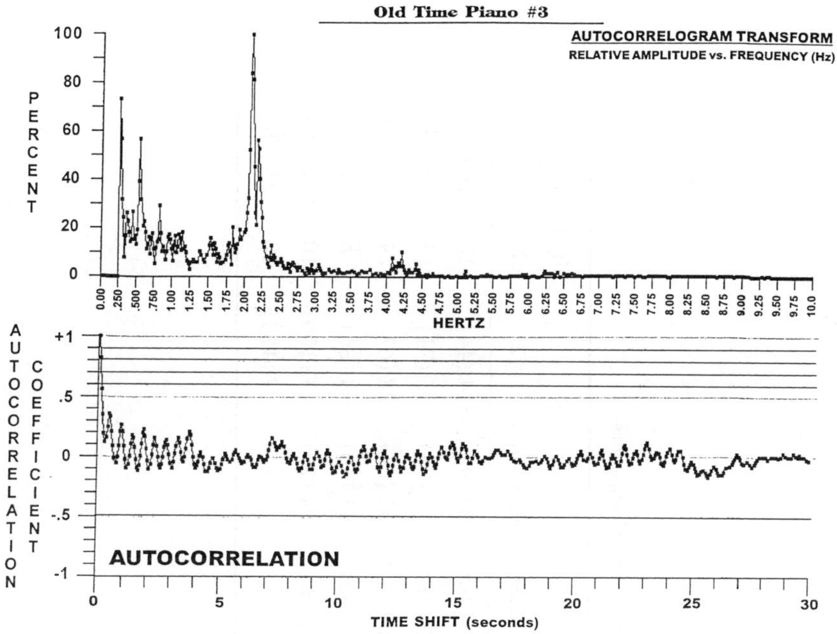

Fig. III.6. Autocorrelation (bottom) and Autocorrelation Transform (top) of Old Time Piano Tunes (#3). See text for details for the periodicity at 2.1 Hz.

between Mozart and the two Bachs and other composers with *short-term* periodic changes.

Discussion

The major point of this study is that the music of Mozart, J.S. and J.C. Bach was distinctive by the long-term periodicities found in our computer analyses (see Table III.2). These periodicities are consistent with a general theme, characteristic of Mozart music, that it is highly organized, presumably resonating with the superorganized cerebral cortex.[5] Johann Sebastian Bach, the father, and son Johann Christian Bach, Mozart's friend, also showed high periodicity scores (Table III.2) and with some expectation since they had influences on each other. If these periodic changes do represent a distinctive feature contributing to the Mozart effect as seen in our previous studies on epilepsy,[5,6] this long-term periodicity should not be evident in our two control musical selections that had no effect on our epilepsy patients. These controls did

Table III.5. Short-lasting periodicity. Composers.

Composer	No.	Not Sig.	Sig. (%)	# at 100%	Subharm.	Harmon.	×2	Highest Peak	
								<1.0	>1.0
Mozart	60	26	34 (57)	24 (71)	9 (26)	32 (94)	14 (44)	18	16 (47)
C.P.E. Bach	15	7	8 (53)	4 (50)	2 (25)	7 (88)	5 (71)	3	5 (63)
J.S. Bach	126	60	66 (52)	49 (74)	10 (15)	42 (64)	28 (67)	24	42 (64)
J.C. Bach	48	26	22 (46)	14 (64)	7 (32)	11 (50)	4 (36)	8	14 (64)
Chopin	41	27	14 (34)	11 (79)	1 (6)	4 (29)	4 (100)	10	4 (29)
Others (51)	177	144	33 (19)	22 (67)	1 (3)	7 (21)	7 (100)	10	23 (70)

not show such periodicity (see Table III.4, Figure III.4). From Table III.3, showing music with high degrees of periodicity, the prediction would be that many selections from the two Bachs and also certain selections from other composers, like *Gondolier's Song* of Mendelssohn (Figure III.3, Table III.3), should also be effective in reducing epileptic activity, as was previously reported with Mozart's *Sonata in D Major* (K.448).[5]

In the Introduction it was mentioned that a stimulus with some beneficial cognitive effect on the individual may have some relationship with the normal coding within the brain. The facts in evidence are that Mozart music (K.448) was shown in our past studies[5,6] to decrease abnormal epileptiform activity, thus tending to normalize these abnormal patterns, and that one main feature of such a musical stimulus in the present study is its long-term periodicity. Therefore, it seems possible that normal coding within the brain also may involve such periodic changes. Other known phenomena intrinsic within the brain with similar long-term periodicities include the "cyclic alternating pattern" (CAP), which appears mainly within sleep stages, repeating itself every 20–40 s.[9] Delamont *et al.*[10] mentioned that the CAP is now regarded as an *integrating mechanism* for the different parts of the central nervous system, including the autonomic system. These investigators showed that cardiac parasympathetic activity is related to the CAP with a maximal peak of 40 s. Parrino *et al.*[11] reported that the longest periods were 31 s in older subjects. The CAP is now considered to be related to bruxism,[12] nocturnal paroxysmal dystonia,[13] myoclonic seizures,[14] and periodic leg movements.[15] Thus, the CAP, as an integrating mechanism for the central nervous system, represents an intrinsic periodic change every 20–40 s and stimuli that vary at that same frequency or period may resonate with this intrinsic patterning to produce beneficial effects within the brain.

One other intrinsic phenomenon within the brain that may have some relationship to these periodicities found in the music, is the periodic change in normal sleep spindles. Steriade[16] has shown that one rhythm in the reticular thalamic nuclei responsible for the spindles is around 0.1 Hz (every 10 s) and Hughes[17] has reported that spindles, especially in the first year of life, tend to recur every 8–9 s. Such periodic changes may represent the fastest rates of 8–10 s of the long-term periodicities under present discussion.

The short-term periodicities, especially around 1–2 Hz (see Figures III.4–III.6), were not distinctive to the Mozart or Bach music and were found to be equally prominent in the control music used in the epilepsy studies,[5,6] Philip Glass music and Old Time Piano Tunes. Thus, one of our conclusions is that such short-term periodicity does not represent a distinctive characteristic of

Mozart music, to explain the beneficial effects of that music. It is not surprising that the short-term periodicities were not distinctive to Mozart music, since music like hard rock or "heavy metal," with the very prominent beat at around 1–2 Hz, has not been associated with any known beneficial behavior.

Other than the many studies showing the Mozart effect,[1–4] in part mentioned in the Introduction, there are many other studies on various types of music showing different beneficial effects. These include behavioral improvements in sleeping,[18] anxiety,[19] mood,[19] planning and monitoring capabilities,[20] time-keeping ability,[21] antiemesis,[22] accuracy and speed in answering questions.[23] In addition, quantitative changes have been reported and these include a *decrease* in (1) exercise lactate,[24] (2) norepinephrine,[24] (3) beta endorphins,[25] f(4) cortisol levels,[26](5) right frontal activation,[26] and (6) muscle rigidity,[19] and an *increase* in (1) normalized cardiovascular responses,[19] (2) blood flow in the right middle cerebral artery,[27] (3) Ig A,[28] (4) P600-event-related potential from the right anterior temporal area,[29] and (5) alpha power.[19]

The major conclusion of the present study is that one of the distinctive aspects of Mozart music (and likely of J.S. and J.C. Bach) is long-term periodicity that may well play a beneficial role in decreasing epileptic seizure activity and also may have some relationship to coding within the brain.

Summary

The goal of this study as to determine distinctive aspects of Mozart music that may explain the Mozart effect, specifically the decrease in seizure activity. As many as 81 musical selections of Mozart, but also 67 of J.C. Bach, 67 of J.S. Bach, 39 of Chopin and 148 from 55 other composers, were computer-analyzed to quantify the music in search of any distinctive aspect and later to determine the degree to which a dominant periodicity could be found. Long-term periodicity (especially 10–60 s, mean and median of 30 s) was found often in Mozart music but also that of the two Bachs, significantly more often than for the other composers, and was especially absent in the control music that had no effect on epileptic activity in previous studies. Short-term periodicities were not significantly different between Mozart and the Bachs versus the other composers. The conclusion is that one distinctive aspect of Mozart music is long-term periodicity that may well resonate within the cerebral cortex and also may be related to coding within the brain.

References

1. F.H. Rauscher, G.L. Shaw and K.N. Ky, Listening to Mozart enhances spatial-temporal reasoning: towards a neurophysiological basis, *Neuroscience Lett.* **185**, 44–7 (1995).
2. J. Sarnthein, A. von Stein, P. Rappelsberg, H. Petsche, F.H. Rauscher and G.L. Shaw, Persistent patterns of brain activity: an EEG coherence study of the positive effect of music on spatial-temporal reasoning, *Neurol. Res.* **19**, 107–16 (1997).
3. B.E. Rideout and C.M. Laubach, EEG correlates of enhanced spatial performance following exposure to music, *Percept. Motor Skills* **82**, 427–32 (1996).
4. F.H. Rauscher, G.L. Shaw, L.J. Levine, E.L. Wright, W.R. Dennis and R.I. Newcomb, Music training causes long-term enhancement of preschool children's spatial-temporal reasoning, *Neurol. Res.* **19**, 2–8 (1997).
5. J.R. Hughes, Y. Daaboul, J.J. Fino and G.L. Shaw, The "Mozart effect" on epileptiform activity, *Clinical Electroencephalogr.* **29**(3), 109–19.
6. J.R. Hughes, J.J. Fino and M. Melyn, Is there a chronic change of the "Mozart Effect" on epileptiform activity? *Clin Electroencephalogr.* **30**, 44–5 (1998).
7. G.L. Shaw, *Keeping Mozart in Mind* (Academic, San Diego, 1999).
8. R. Miller, *The Structure of Singing* (Schirmer, Macmillan., New York, 1986).
9. M.G. Terzano, D. Mancia, M.R. Salati, G. Constani, A. Decembrino and L. Parrino, The cyclic alternating pattern as a physiological component of normal NREM sleep, *Sleep* **8**, 137–45 (1985).
10. R.S. Delamont, P.O. Julu and G.A. Jamal, Periodicity of a noninvasive measure of cardiac vagal tone during non-rapid eye movement sleep in non-sleep deprived and sleep-deprived normal subjects, *J. Clin. Neurophysiol.* **16**(2): 146–53 (1999).
11. L. Parrino, M. Roselli, M.C. Spaggari, A. Smerieri and M.G. Terzano, Cyclic alternating pattern (CAP) in normal sleep: polysomnographic parameters in different age groups, *Electroencephalogr. Clin. Neurophysiol.* **107**(6), 439–50 (1998).
12. G.M. Macaluso, P. Guerra, P. Di Giovanni, M. Boselli, L. Parrino and M.G. Terzano, Bruxism is a disorder related to periodic arousals from sleep, *J. Dent. Res.* 77(4), 565–73 (1998).
13. M.G. Terzano, M.F. Monge-Strauss, F. Mikol, M.G. Spagyiari and L. Parrino, Cyclic alternating pattern as a provocative factor in nocturnal paroxysmal dystonia, *Epilepsia* **38**(9): 1015–25 (1997).
14. A. Palomino, M. Carballo, E. Rodriguez *et al.*, Analysis of the changes in sleep EEG recording of patients with juvenile myoclonic epilepsy, *Revue Neurol.* **27**(159), 801–4 (1998).
15. D.W. Droste, J.K. Krauss, G. Hagedorn and M. Raps, Periodic leg movements are part of the B-wave rhythm and the cyclic alternating pattern, *Acta Neurol. Scand.* **94**(5), 347–52 (1996).

16. M. Steriade, Cellular substrates of brain rhythms. In: E. Niedermeyer, F. Lopes da Silva, *Electroencephalography*, 3rd ed. (Williams and Wilkins, Baltimore, 1993), pp. 27–62.
17. J.R. Hughes, Development of sleep spindles in the first year of life, *Clin. Electroencephalogr.* **27**(3), 107–15 (1996).
18. I. Levin, "Music of the Brain" in the treatment of insomnia patients, *Zh. Nevropatol. Psikhiatr. Im. S. S. Korsakoff* **97**(4), 39–43 (1997).
19. V.A. Gumeniuk, N.I. Batova, T.S. Mel'nikova, *et al.*, Systems analysis of colour music corrective effect, *Vestn. Ross. Akad. Med. Nauk.* **2**, 18–25 (1998).
20. C. Palmer and C. Drake, Monitoring and planning capacities in the acquisition of music performance skills, *Can J. Exp. Psychol.* **51**(4), 369–84 (1997).
21. B.H. Repp, Variations on a theme by Chopin: relations between perception and production of timing in music, *J. Exp. Psychol. Hum. Percep. Perform.* **24**(3), 291–311 (1998).
22. S. Ezzone, C. Baker, R. Rosselet and E. Terepka, Music as an adjunct to antiemetic therapy, *Oncol. Nurse Forum* **25**(9), 1551–6 (1998).
23. T. Cockerton, S. Moore and D. Norman, Cognitive test performance and background music, *Percept Motor Skills* **85**(3 Pt 2), 1435–8 (1997).
24. L. Szmedra and D.W. Bacharach, Effect of music on perceived exertion, plasma lactate, norepinephrine and cardiovascular hemodynamics during treadmill running, *Inter. J. Sports Med.* **19**(1), 32–7 (1998).
25. C.H. McKinney, F.C. Tims, A.M. Kumar and M. Kumar, The effect of selected classical music and spontaneous imagery on plasma beta-endorphin, *J. Behav. Med.* **20**(1), 85–99 (1997).
26. T. Field, A. Martinez, T. Nawrocki, J. Pickens, N.A. Fox and S. Schanberg, Music shifts frontal EEG in depressed adolescents, *Adolescence* **33**(129), 109–16 (1998).
27. J. Vollmer-Haase, K. Finke, W. Hartje and M. Bulla-Hellwig, Hemispheric dominance in the processing of J.S. Bach fugues: a transcranial Doppler sonography (TCD) study with musicians, *Neuropsychologia* **36**(9), 857–67 (1998).
28. C.J. Charnetski, F.X. Brennan Jr and J.F. Harrison, Effect of music and auditory stimuli on secretory immunoglobulin A (IgA), *Percept. Motor Skills* **87**, 1163–70 (1998).
29. A.D. Patel, E. Gibson, J. Ratner, M. Besson and P.J. Holcomb, Processing syntactic relations in language and music: an event-related potential study, *J. Cogn. Neurosci.* **10**(6), 717–33 (1998).

IV. Characteristics of the Melodic Line in Mozart Music

Introduction

The previous section (III) showed that Mozart music was distinctive by the long-term periodic changes of the acoustic *power* of this music. However, the positioning of a note with reference to other notes to create a melody is one of the most important aspects of music. The goal of this study was to investigate the incidence of periodic changes in the *melodic line* of Mozart music, compared to other well-known composers. Thus, the repetition of a given melody throughout a musical selection was studied as another example of periodic change.

Method

MIDI (Musical Industry Digital Interface) files were used in this study, and these files are a mathematical representation of the actual sheet music for a given musical selection and this type of file can be downloaded from the Internet. The file stores each note, frequency, its duration, timing, attack or rise time, and decay time, and therefore the entire score is stored sequentially as electronic data. A program (150 ft. in length) was written to count the gross number of notes, their incidence, the scaled degrees or steps referring to the position of a given note within the musical key. Also counted were the number of naturals, flats, or sharps, the incidence of note duration, and acoustic harmonic intervals between notes played at the same time. In the case of dual pianos with four tracks from the four hands, the harmonic data were analyzed in two ways. First, the data were viewed as all four tracks playing at the same time as the ear would hear it and then converted into a single track; in addition, each track was analyzed separately, and later the data were combined. The melodic data, viewing the sequence of notes as a melody, were analyzed in a similar way, both into a single track and separated as four tracks. When more than one note could have been part of a melody, the highest note was accepted as part of the melodic line, as traditionally is the case. The computer could then determine the number of times that a given note sequence appeared within the entire musical score and the sequences were counted from a minimum of four notes to the maximal number that was repeated.

A repeating sequence of *notes*, as part of a melodic line, was printed out by the computer, according to the track involved, the measure, and the beat within the measure, and all repeating melodic note sequences were so listed.

The same analysis was performed for melodic *intervals*, referring to the same tonal distance between notes, rather than the exact same notes. An example is that the interval between notes A and C is the same as between B and D, but both pairs may be used in a melodic line. Finally, the same analysis was used for melodic contours, referring to the direction of a note sequence—whether it was the same, above or below the previous note. The same analysis was applied to *reversals* of sequences, referring to a forward sequence of notes that would also be played in the reverse or backward direction. Reversal analysis applied to notes, intervals, and contours. All of the data are summarized into the note, interval, and contour sequences occurring at each sequence length, and once a note was counted in a given sequence, it was not counted again in any other sequence. Sequence length was counted from longest to shortest and the cumulative value was plotted as a function of sequence length. The final value to represent these data was called the *repetitive melodic index*, the percentage of all notes, intervals, or contours involved in repeating sequences of four or more notes and three or more intervals, or contours. The computer then plotted out these data and the curves were plotted to include not only four notes but all sequence lengths.

The computer also designated the absolute *duration* of each note in a given sequence, the *cadence*, referring to the same relative magnitude of change in duration from one note to the next and the *swing*, referring not to any given magnitude, but only if a note was longer or shorter that the previous one. Examples of a duration would be alternating 8th and 16th notes, cadence as alternating notes with half the duration of the previous note and swing as an alternating long note, followed by a shorter note. Reversal analysis also applied to these three variables and the computer then plotted all of these data for each sequence length of four or more repeating durations and three or more cadences or swings.

The number of musical selections was 330 for Mozart, 155 for J.S. Bach, 61 Beethoven, 58 Chopin, and 23 for Chopin, accounting for over 1 918 000 analyzed notes. The musical selections were chosen at random, usually depending on the availability of MIDI files, which included more piano sonatas than other forms, especially because they constituted 30% of the Mozart music. An analysis was done of the various kinds of music from Mozart, which included (for this particular analysis) 76 piano sonatas, 33 symphonies, 28 minuets, 26 piano concertos, 12 overtures, 6 nocturnes, and 3 rondos. The average deviation of the melodic index from the mean for those 10 different forms was only 5.8% for notes and 3.6% for intervals. Also for J.S. Bach 41 piano sonatas, 29 suites, 17 concertos, 15 preludes, 14 fugues, 6 partitas, and 3 toccatas were analyzed and the average deviation from the mean for the melodic index of notes was only 3.0%. Thus, the selection of a given form of music made no significant difference in our analysis for a given composer.

In summary, for each musical selection the computer plotted in 12 curves, representing all sequence lengths, the incidence of repeating (1) notes, (2) intervals, (3) contours, (4) durations, (5) cadences, (6) swings, and (7–12) reversals of (1–6).

Results

Figure IV.1 shows 12 different indices that characterize the melodic line and the results of the sequence length of four *notes.* The major finding was the

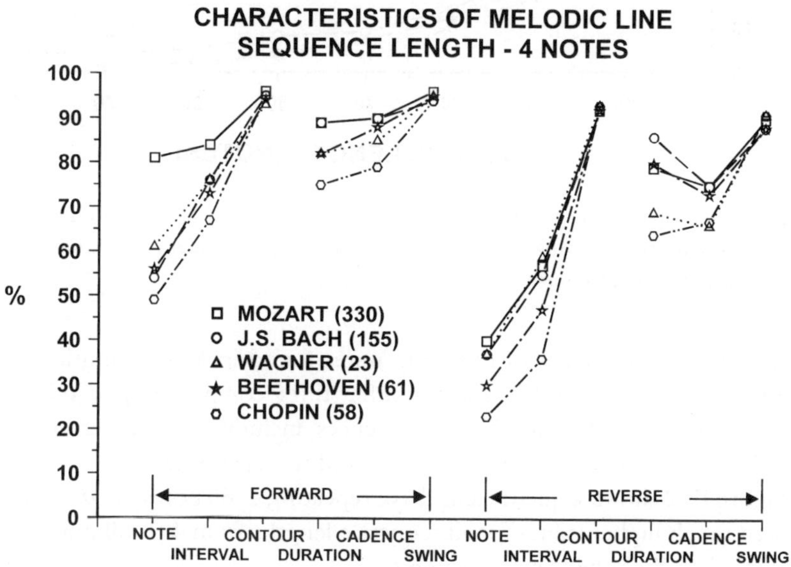

Fig. IV.1. Characteristics of the melodic line. Sequence length of four notes. On the horizontal axis are indicated (1) notes, (2) intervals, (3) contours, (4) durations, (5) cadences, and (6) swings, followed by the reversal of (1)–(6). On the vertical axis is percent (%) that the given characteristic was found. Mozart showed significantly higher values for notes, compared to Wagner ($p = 0.03$) and the other three composers ($p < 0.0001$). Also, for intervals Mozart showed higher values than Wagner ($p = 0.02$), Beethoven and Bach ($p =< 0.01$), and Chopin ($p < 0.0001$). For durations a difference was seen between Mozart sand Chopin ($p = 0.002$), and for reversed notes, intervals, and durations also with Chopin ($p < 0.005$).

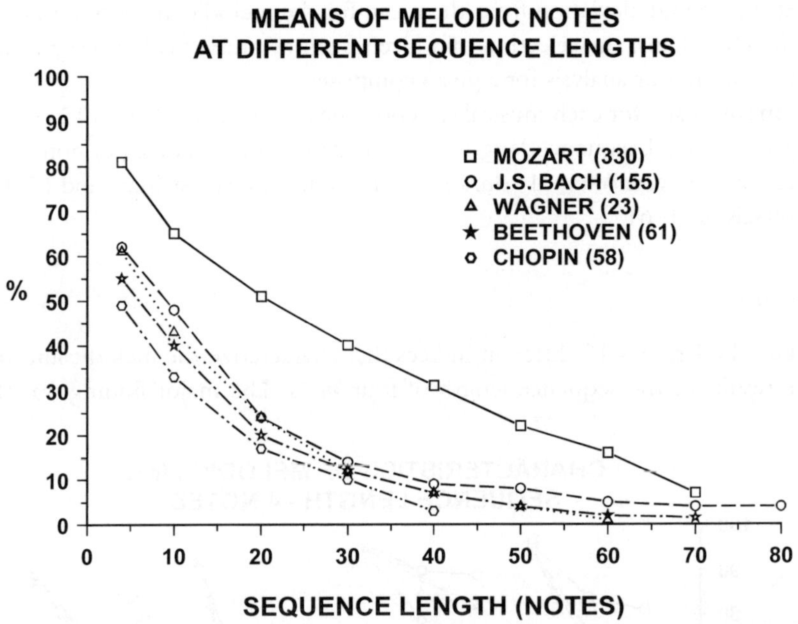

Fig. IV.2. Characteristics of the melodic line. Sequence lengths of 4–80 notes. For all sequences from 4–60 Mozart showed significantly higher values ($p < 0.0001$) than for the other four composers.

significantly higher values of repeating notes found in Mozart music, compared to Wagner ($p = 0.03$) and the other three composers ($p < 0.0001$). See the legend for other significant differences, including the higher values of Mozart for repeating intervals, durations, and reversed notes.

Figure IV.2 shows sequence lengths of repeating 4–80 notes. Mozart music showed much higher values for all sequence lengths from 4 to 60 notes ($p < 0.0001$) than the other four composers.

Discussion

The major finding in this section is that Mozart music includes a repeating melodic line much more often than music from the four other prominent composers, J.S. Bach, Beethoven, Wagner, and Chopin. These latter findings are consistent with the general theme of this chapter, that Mozart in his genius featured repetition in his music, not only melodies at various sequence lengths but also periodic changes in the amplitude or power of the music (see Section III). Part of his genius is to repeat themes in a way that is not boring, but instead engaging to the listener. Thus, a theme would be repeated, not necessarily with the same notes but with different notes and the same interval (see results, Figure IV.1). In addition he may reverse the melodic line, and Figure IV.1 shows that the value of *reversed* notes was highest in Mozart music. Finally, the theme may be repeated with different notes and different intervals but with the same duration; Figure IV.1 shows that the highest values were from the music of Mozart and J.S. Bach for this variable.

On a broader scope, repetition and periodic changes are found in all aspects of our brain function and also of our bodily functions. The periodic changes of Mozart music, therefore, resonate well with all of the other periodic changes that characterize brain and bodily functions.

On still a broader scope, Gray *et al.*[1] have made the point that singing birds have the same rhythm and pitch permutations and combinations of notes and retention of melodies as man. Whales have similar phrases, sing over seven octaves with the same intervals, elaboration of themes, and *repetition of refrains* as man. The similarity of the music of birds and whales to that of man may lead to the speculation of a universal music. Our chapter provides evidence that Mozart is the leading proponent of this universal music.

Reference

1. P.M. Gray, B. Krause, J. Atema, R. Payne, C. Krumhansl and L. Baptista, The music of nature and the nature of music, *Science* **291**, 52–6 (2001).

Chapter 14

The Amusias

Jason Warren

Music is the pleasure the human soul experiences in counting without being aware that it is counting.

—Leibniz

Introduction

"Amusia" refers to a neurological deficit in music perception, recognition or production, attributable to a central cause. Music, like civilisation itself, is easy to recognise but difficult to define; Leibniz's attempt reminds us that it has a physical character, which must be apprehended before the brain can invest it with meaning. Alongside language, music can be considered a highly evolved species of patterned sound, imbued by the brain with semantic and affective significance. While comparisons between music and language are commonplace, clinical analogies such as "expressive" and "receptive" amusia, "musical alexia", "agraphia" and "apraxia" are potentially misleading, and do not indicate the intricate perceptual analysis which must occur for music, as for all complex acoustic phenomena.[1] The acoustic and cognitive properties of music, while they are comparable in formal complexity, are quite different from those of speech and other environmental sounds.[1–9] It would be remarkable were these properties not extracted and represented by distinct neural mechanisms, which are of considerable interest in their own right.

The clinical study of the amusias is subject to a number of caveats. Although all normal individuals can recognise music, musicality (unlike language) is subject to wide individual variation, heavily influenced by exposure and training. Musical functions are difficult to assess reproducibly, even in trained musicians, and batteries such as those of Botez and Wertheim[10] and Peretz[11] are time-consuming to administer. Elements of music such as "pitch", "melody" and "timbre" are problematic to define and isolate. These difficulties may be compounded by the presence of aphasia or attentional deficits, while a more general disorder of complex sound processing, not specific for music, may be overlooked.[1] Functional recovery and neural plasticity[12] may account for apparent discrepancies between patients assessed at different stages following a brain lesion, with different types of lesion or with pre-existing brain damage (especially chronic epilepsy). The clinical literature on the amusias therefore poses substantial problems of interpretation. Detailed case studies of musical deficits are nonetheless very valuable, since they provide circumstantial evidence that particular brain regions are necessary (though not necessarily sufficient) to support musical functions, an inference which cannot be drawn from the study of the intact brain.[13]

Development of the Concept of Amusia

Interest in the neurology of music is, of course, not new: Thomas Willis, for example, localised musical functions in the cerebellum.[14] The term "amusia" was coined by Steinhals in 1871.[14] Dissociations between aspects of musical function (reading, writing, playing and singing) were described by Fischer in 1867 and by Proust in 1872;[15] the sparing of musical abilities in aphasic patients had already been recognised for over a century, and the reverse dissociation was described by Mann.[16] Edgren in 1895 and Brodmann in 1914 concluded that "musical agnosia" was produced by lesions of one or both anterior temporal lobes.[14] In the 1920s, Henschen distinguished motor amusia (vocal and instrumental apraxia, musical agraphia) from sensory amusia (musical deafness, amnestic amusia, musical alexia), and postulated discrete "centres" for musical functions (such as reading music, singing and specific instruments) in the dominant hemisphere.[3] Kleist[17] also espoused a localisationist approach to the amusias: he identified discrete impairments of tonal and interval sense and melodic pattern following temporal lobe lesions, and proposed a detailed classification of motor and sensory amusias.[15] A symbolic analogy between music and language was drawn by Feuchtwanger,[18] who postulated corresponding bilateral representations in the superior temporal gyri.[3,14] Ustvedt[19] regarded attempts to localise musical functions as misguided, emphasising the diversity of clinical deficits and concluding that "amusia is simply a shorthand term for a heterogeneous collection of rather complicated symptom groups".[15] Interestingly, Ustvedt also proposed that a subcortical network of structures subserves emotional aspects of the musical experience.[14] Hécaen[20] linked disordered sound recognition and musical understanding with non-dominant and dominant hemisphere lesions, respectively. Barbizet[21] asserted that the right hemisphere mediates perceptual and executive musical functions, while the left hemisphere is responsible for musical recognition and memory, symbolic manipulation and integration. Wertheim[14] associated receptive amusia with dominant anterior temporal lesions and expressive amusia with non-dominant frontal lesions, while Benton[15] concluded that expressive amusia generally follows anterior lesions, and receptive amusia temporal lobe lesions, in either hemisphere.

More recently, the concepts of distributed networks, hierarchical and parallel processing have largely replaced older, localisationist notions in the literature of the amusias. Brust[3] asserted that neither the presence nor absence of aphasia, nor hemispheric lateralisation, predicts the presence, type or severity of amusia. The importance of inter-hemispheric cooperation in normal musical functioning was stressed by Peretz,[11] who maintained that the right hemisphere represents melody as a global contour, while the left fills in the fine structure of pitch intervals between notes.

A variety of specific auditory processing deficits producing amusia have been described,[1,7,22–26] leading Griffiths *et al.*[1,7] to emphasise that amusia may represent a disorder of complex sound processing. This step in the perceptual analysis of the sound patterns embodied in music, speech and environmental sounds is interposed between the initial encoding of the acoustic signal, and high-level semantic processes, which link sound patterns with stored symbolic representations and memories.[1]

Milner[27] described deficits of musical judgement, especially involving timbre and tonal memory, in a series of patients who had undergone right temporal lobectomies for epilepsy. This line of enquiry has been advanced with great sophistication by Zatorre and others[9,28–36] in patients with a variety of more or less selective temporal and other focal cerebral resections. Liégeois-Chauvel[36] partitioned the temporal lobes for different aspects of musical processing, based on the study of patients with anterior and posterior temporal lobectomies. These case series illustrate an important distinction in the clinical literature between amusia as a cardinal symptom of a brain lesion (frequently the subject of individual case reports), and musical deficits uncovered as a result of systematic study of patients with brain lesions, usually temporal lobe resections or strokes. The two methods of case ascertainment define symptom-led and lesion-led approaches, respectively. They represent quite different patient populations, and should be regarded as complementary.[1]

Analysis of Published Cases: A Classification of the Amusias

Overview

The symptom-led literature on the amusias is summarised in Tables 1–3, and the lesion-led literature in Tables 4–5, drawing on representative cases for which anatomical correlation is available. Figure 1 depicts key brain areas involved in music processing. Sites of lesions which result in disturbed processing of various aspects of music, derived from both the symptom-led and the lesion-led literature, have been superimposed in Figure 2; it should be emphasised that Figure 2 does not represent a functional map of music processing. Despite the heterogeneity of clinical findings, certain general principles emerge.

Musicality is a highly fractionated neuropsychological function, with many perceptual and cognitive subcomponents. This is illustrated by the numerous dissociations which have been described: between music and other examples of patterned sound;[7,23,26,28,37,38] between music and language;[6] between global and local,[11,39] frequency-based and time-based,[38,40] structural and affective[41] properties of music; between music perception and recognition;[42,43] and between musical processing and expression.[10,44]

Amusias of greater or lesser selectivity have been described with lesions involving the temporal, frontal and parietal lobes and subcortical structures, and may follow damage to either or both hemispheres, suggesting that widely distributed anatomical networks subserve music processing and expression. An uncertain proportion of these cases represent disconnection syndromes, in which interruption of fibre pathways exerts remote effects on areas critical for musical processing.[22] The most severe deficits follow bilateral or right-sided lesions (Table 1), generally involving primary auditory cortex in medial Heschl's gyrus or secondary auditory areas including lateral Heschl's gyrus, superior temporal gyrus and planum temporale (Figure 1).

Initially, patients may have cortical deafness, or loss of perception of sound.[6,45] If perception of sounds is disordered despite preserved hearing, the condition can be characterised as an auditory (apperceptive) agnosia.[1] To the extent that music shares acoustic properties with speech and environmental noises, derangements of musical processing are predicted in conjunction with deficits involving these other classes of patterned sound. Such patients have a disorder of complex sound processing,[1,7,22] which interferes with perceptual analysis rather than semantic representation; thus, patients may be unable to understand speech, although language as assessed by reading and

Table 1. Representative cases of amusia: patients with associated deficits of complex sound processing.

Author	Complex sound deficits	Language deficit?	Lesion
Spreen *et al.*, 1965	65 y.o. RH male, "unable to understand the meaning of common sounds", discriminate musical instruments or pitch intervals; speech sounds normal	No	R sup temporal, insula, inf parietal, inf and middle frontal infarction (post-mortem)
Oppenheimer & Newcombe, 1978	64 y.o. RH male, unable to understand speech, impaired perception of environmental sounds and music	Transient; expressive aprosody	Bilat sup temporal (incl L Heschl's), L inf frontal and insula, R inf parietal infarcts (post-mortem)
Mazzucchi *et al.*, 1982	58 y.o. RH male guitarist, difficulty identifying voices, environmental sounds, instruments and "grasping" music, distortions of melodies, loss of pleasure in music; able to identify pitch, melodies, rhythm, sing and play guitar	No	R temporal infarct (CT)
Miceli, 1982	56 y.o. RH female pianist, unable to understand any sounds, recognise or sing melodies, notes, chords, rhythms, instruments; spectral analysis defect	Yes	R > L sup temporal infarcts (CT)
Auerbach *et al.*, 1982	58 y.o. RH male, speech and music "like noise", unable to recognise tunes or musical instruments or sing; difficulty in perceiving consonants; able to discriminate ascending vs descending tonal sequences, many environmental sounds, voices (though not languages); temporal resolution disorder	No	Bilat sup temporal (sparing L Heschl's) and auditory radiation, R frontal and parietal infarcts (CT)

Table 1. Continued.

Author	Complex sound deficits	Language deficit?	Lesion
Coslett *et al.*, 1984	48 y.o. RH male, unable to understand speech, impaired identification of familiar songs, unable to reproduce rhythms; able to recognise environmental sounds	Mild; affective prosody normal	Bilat sup temporal (incl L Heschl's), R supramarginal and inf frontal infarcts (CT)
Lechevalier *et al.*, 1984	33 y.o. RH female, unable to identify rhythm, pitches, melodies, different types of music, speech or non-verbal noises; preserved affective response to music	Yes	L > R temporal damage 2° meningitis (CT)
Motomura *et al.*, 1986	69 y.o. RH male, unable to distinguish speech, music, other sounds, detect melodies or rhythms; raised pure tone thresholds; temporal resolution/summation disorder	No	R post hemisphere haemorrhage involving internal capsule, old L post thalamic infarct (CT/MRI)
Tanaka *et al.*, 1987	26 y.o. RH female pianist, unable to understand speech or sing, difficulty identifying musical instruments, impaired discrimination of auditory, tactile, visual rhythms, tonal patterns; able to recognise some environmental sounds, nursery rhymes; supramodal temporal resolution defect	Mild; expressive aprosody	R>L mid and sup temporal (incl Heschl's), auditory radiation, parietal infarcts (MRI)
Mendez & Geehan, 1988; Tramo *et al.*, 1990	Case 1: 60 y.o. RH male, all sounds disagreeable ("hum"), unable to recognise environmental sounds, speech	Mild; expressive aprosody	Bilat sup temporal, temporal pole, parietal infarcts (CT)

	Case 2: 23 y.o. ambidextrous male, all sounds "like a buzzing noise", unable to recognise melodies; able to recognise most environmental sounds; temporal pattern analysis defect	Yes; expressive aprosody	Bilat Heschl's, L parieto-temporal, R fronto-parieto-temporal, auditory radiation and basal ganglia infarcts (CT/MRI)
Lambert *et al.*, 1989	28 y.o. RH female, initially unable to discriminate speech, music, other sounds; later impaired naming of environmental sounds and instruments, unable to recognise familiar musical phrases or categories; able to reproduce rhythm	No	Intraventricular haemorrhage (CT/MRI)
Eustache *et al.*, 1990	Case 2: 64 y.o RH male bugler, impaired discrimination (despite identification) of phonemes and tunes, impaired reproduction of rhythm, melodies, naming of environmental sounds and instruments; able to sing when words supplied	No	R lentiform nucleus, external capsule, inf frontal infarction (CT)
Fujii *et al.*, 1990	55 y.o. RH male, impaired recognition of environmental sounds, tonal memory, discrimination of rhythm, timbre (relatively sparing pitch); able to sing from memory	No; prosody normal	R post temporal haemorrhage (CT)

Table 1. Continued.

Author	Complex sound deficits	Language deficit?	Lesion
Praamstra *et al.*, 1991	57 y.o. RH male, sounds and music "strange", unable to understand speech, difficulty identifying non-verbal sounds	Pre-existing	Bilat sup temporal (incl L Heschl's), R angular gyrus, L frontal and parietal infarcts (CT)
Takahashi *et al.*, 1992	55 y.o. RH male, unable to understand speech, difficulty discriminating pitch, melody, rhythm; able to recognise melodies, musical mood, instruments, non-verbal sounds	No; receptive aprosody	L thalamic haematoma involving auditory radiations, sparing Heschl's gyrus (CT/MRI)
Godefroy *et al.*, 1995	58 y.o. RH female, unable to understand speech, environmental sounds or music	No	Bilat external capsule and auditory radiation haemorrhages (MRI); hypometabolism of temporal and parietal cortices on ^{15}O PET
Habib *et al.*, 1995	44 y.o. RH female, "totally unable to recognise famous tunes", severe pitch discrimination deficit, impaired emotional response to music, poor identification of voices and non-verbal sounds, difficulty singing, unable to play piano	No; expressive and receptive aprosody	Bilat insula, partial R Heschl's infarcts (CT/MRI)
Johkura *et al.*, 1998	46 y.o. RH male, "unable to recognise any sounds", unable to identify songs, impaired discrimination of pitch intervals; able to discriminate rhythms and sing	No	Inferior colliculi haemorrhage (MRI)

Abbreviations: ant, anterior; AVM, arteriovenous malformation; bilat, bilateral; CT, computerised tomography; esp, especially; incl, including; inf, inferior; L, left; LH, left-handed; MCA, middle cerebral artery; MRI, magnetic resonance imaging; PET, positron emission tomography; post, posterior; R, right; RH, right-handed; sup, superior.

Table 2. Representative cases of amusia: musical without other complex sound deficits. Abbreviations as in Table 1.

Author	Musical deficits	Language deficit?	Lesion
Roeser & Daly, 1974	49 y.o. RH female, music "fuzzy and blurred" in L ear	No	R thalamic tumour (angiography)
Mavlov, 1980	61 y.o. RH male violinist, unable to identify familiar tunes, sing, reproduce or compare rhythms in auditory, visual or tactile domains; able to reproduce tone sequences	Yes	L MCA territory infarct (angiography)
Mackworth-Young, 1983	35 y.o. RH male trumpeter, sequential impairments of pitch, timbre, rhythm perception, impaired production of pitch, rhythm; musical palinacusis	No	R temporo-parietal damage 2° encephalitis (CT)
Eustache *et al.*, 1990	Case 1: 31 y.o. RH male, unable to identify (but able to discriminate) musical phrases, unable to sing	Mild	L ant temporal and parietal infarction (CT)
Sidtis & Feldmann, 1990	52 y.o. RH male, voices and music "flat and monotonous"; rhythm perception normal	No; receptive aprosody	R MCA infarct (CT)
Mazzoni *et al.*, 1993	24 y.o. ambidextrous male guitarist, difficulty understanding musical structure, loss of aesthetic response to music	No; receptive aprosody	R temporo-parietal haemorrhage 2° AVM (CT/MRI)
Peretz *et al.*, 1994; Peretz, 1996	Case CN: 35 y.o. RH female, unable to recognise or sing familiar tunes, no sense of familiarity, initially impaired perception of pitch variations (sparing rhythm), persistent inability to memorise music; able to recognise emotional tone of music	No; expressive aprosody (receptive normal)	Bilat sup temporal (sparing Heschl's), R insula and inf frontal infarcts (CT)
	Case GL: 61 y.o. RH male, unable to recognise familiar music, loss of enjoyment in music, unable to discriminate scale (pitch contour, rhythm spared); able to sing spontaneously	Yes; receptive aprosody	Bilat sup temporal (incl L Heschl's), temporal pole, insula, inf frontal infarcts (CT)

Table 2. Continued.

Author	Musical deficits	Language deficit?	Lesion
Griffiths *et al.*, 1997	75 y.o. RH male, impaired recognition of tunes, unpleasant quality of music; able to sing from memory; impaired discrimination of transitions in rapid tone sequences	No; receptive prosody normal	R post sup temporal, insula, inf parietal, antero-lateral occipital infarction (MRI)
Peretz & Gagnon, 1999	40 y.o. RH female, unable to recognise or discriminate musical phrases (metre relatively spared), or sing; able to judge emotional tone of melodies	No	Bilat sup temporal (incl L Heschl's) and insula, L mid, inf temporal, frontal operculum and inf parietal, R inf and mid frontal infarcts (CT)
Piccirilli *et al.*, 2000	20 y.o LH male guitarist, music monotonous, unpleasant in quality, unable to recognise tunes, unable to play guitar or sing; able to recognise scales and metres, recognise and reproduce rhythmic patterns	Transient; expressive aprosody	L sup temporal (incl Heschl's) infarction and atrophy 2° AVM (MRI)
Ayotte *et al.*, 2000	Case NR: 51 y.o. RH female, unable to recognise musical phrases, discriminate melodic and temporal sequences; able to supply song titles from spoken lyrics	No	R sup temporal (incl Heschl's), temporal pole, insula infarction (CT)
	Case RC: 44 y.o. RH male, unable to recognise musical phrases, discriminate melodic and temporal sequences; able to supply song titles from spoken lyrics	No	R sup temporal gyrus (incl Heschl's gyrus), temporal pole, insula infarction (CT); also clipping of L MCA aneurysm

Table 3. Representative cases of amusia: disorders of musical reading, writing, or praxis. Abbreviations as in Table 1.

Author	Musical deficits	Language deficit?	Lesion
Botez & Wertheim, 1959	26 y.o. RH male, unable to sing or play accordion (pitch transposition, intonational and rhythm errors), impaired reproduced and spontaneous melody and rhythm (esp playing); able to recognise familiar melodies, discriminate pitch, analyse chords, recognise own errors	Mild; expressive aprosody	R post frontal tumour (operation)
Levin & Rose, 1979	58 y.o. RH drummer, inability to read musical notes (able to read other musical symbols), impaired discrimination of tonal sequences, initially also pitch and timbre; able to discriminate rhythmic patterns, play drums	Alexia without agraphia	L trigonal intraventricular meningioma (CT) with surgical division of splenium
Brust, 1980	Case 1: 22 y.o. RH female music student, impaired writing and reading of music (esp pitch); musical comprehension and non-graphic expression intact	Yes; normal prosody	L inf temporal meningioma, temporo-parietal infarct (CT)
	Case 2: 42 y.o. RH male double-bassist, music sounding "not right", unable to imitate (though able to identify) notes or melodies, unable to recognise metre or rhythm, unable to sing, play, read or write music	Yes; normal prosody	L parieto-temporal infarct (CT)
McFarland & Fortin, 1982	78 y.o. RH male organist, unable to play, difficulty reproducing rhythmic patterns, identifying familiar pieces; able to sing	No	R sup temporal, supramarginal gyrus infarction (CT)

Table 3. Continued.

Author	Musical deficits	Language deficit?	Lesion
Judd *et al.*, 1983	77 y.o. RH male composer, impaired reading and writing of music (esp pitch), impaired naming of notes, musical and visual memory; able to detect pitch and tempo errors, compose and conduct	Initially; later alexia without agraphia	L occipito-temporal haemorrhage (CT)
Basso & Capitani, 1985	67 y.o. male conductor, impaired writing of music; able to read music, play piano and conduct	Yes; normal prosody	L temporo-parieto-occipital infarction (CT)
Takeda *et al.*, 1990	65 y.o. RH female saimsen player, pitch errors on singing or playing, mild disturbance of tonal memory; rhythm spared	No; normal prosody	R temporal haemorrhage (CT/MRI)
Confavreux *et al.*, 1992	63 y.o. RH female singer, progressive loss of ability to sing, unable to recognise well-known pieces, discriminate rhythms; able to discriminate, read and write notes	No; expressive aprosody, speech apraxia	R > L temporo-insular atrophy (CT/MRI)
Polk & Kertesz, 1993	Case 1: 58 y.o. RH male guitarist, progressive inability to read and write music, reproduce rhythms; able to discriminate pitch, recognise tunes	Yes	L > R diffuse cerebral atrophy (CT/MRI)
	Case 2: 53 y.o. ambidextrous female pianist, progressive apraxia (incl piano playing), unable to write music, impaired reading of music, disorganised production of pitch and metre; able to reproduce simple rhythms, discriminate pitch, recognise tunes	Agraphia; normal prosody	R > L parieto-occipital atrophy (CT/MRI)

Horikoshi *et al.*, 1997	26 y.o. RH female pianist, impaired ability to read music (esp pitch); able to play from memory, write music to dictation	Yes	L occipito-temporal / parasplenial AVM (MRI)
Beversdorf & Heilman, 1998	65 y.o. RH female musician, loss of ability to read music	Alexia without agraphia	L > R post cortical degeneration (PET)
Cappelletti *et al.*, 2000	51 y.o. RH female musician, unable to read or write notes; able to read other musical symbols, play familiar and novel pieces	No aphasia, agraphia, alexia	L postero-lateral temporal, R occipito-temporal damage 2° encephalitis (MRI)
Midorikawa & Kawamura, 2000	53 y.o. RH female pianist, difficulty writing music (errors of rhythm rather than pitch), reproducing complex rhythms; able to write single notes, read music, recognise tunes, sing, play	Transient agraphia	L sup parietal lobule gliosis (MRI)

Table 4. Representative case series examining effects of temporal lobectomy and other selective surgical resections on music processing, in patients with intractable epilepsy. All patients were left-hemisphere-dominant for language, and most had no formal musical training.

Author	Resection	Side (no.)	Musical deficits
Zatorre, 1985	Anterior* temporal	L (28)	Melody recognition
		R (30)	Scale and contour discrimination, melody recognition
Zatorre, 1988	Anterior temporal	L (15), R (15)	R*: Extraction of fundamental pitch from a complex tone
	Anterior* temporal	L (16), R (18)	
Kester *et al.* 1991	Anterior temporal	L (9), R (12)	R: Metre and tempo perception
Zatorre & Samson, 1991	Anterior* temporal	L (26), R (26)	R: Short-term tonal pitch retention
	Frontal (variable)	R (13)	
Samson & Zatorre, 1991	Anterior* temporal	L (22)	Lyric and song recognition
		R (21)	Melody recognition
Samson & Zatorre, 1992	Anterior* temporal	L (20), R (20)	Learning and delayed recognition of melodies and nonsense words (especially melodies after R, words after L)
Zatorre & Halpern, 1993	Anterior temporal	L (14), R*(14)	R: Musical imagery and pitch retention for songs
Samson & Zatorre, 1994	Anterior* temporal	L (15), R (15)	R: Timbre discrimination (spectral and temporal information)
Liégeois-Chauvel *et al.*, 1998	Temporal, sparing STG	L (14)	Pitch interval discrimination
		R (19)	Pitch interval discrimination
	Anterior STG	L (5)	Metre discrimination
		R (8)	Metre discrimination
	Including posterior STG*	L (3)	Pitch interval discrimination
		R (5)	Pitch interval and contour discrimination
Penhune *et al.*, 1999	Anterior* temporal	L (7), R (9)	R*: Auditory rhythm retention
	Anterior temporal	L (18), R (15)	

Key: L, left; R, right; STG, superior temporal gyrus; *partial resection of Heschl's gyrus in some patients.

Table 5. Representative case series examining effects of other forms of brain damage on music processing. All patients were left-hemisphere-dominant for language unless otherwise indicated, and most had no formal musical training.

Author	Lesion	Side (no.)	Musical deficits
Shapiro *et al.*, 1981	Anterior (pre-Rolandic)[†]	L (5)	None identified
	Anterior	R (7)	Pitch, rhythm, phrasing
	Central (pre-, post-Rolandic)	L (6), R (5)	Rhythm, phrasing
	Posterior (temporo-parietal)	L (5)	None identified
Kinsella *et al.*, 1988	Hemispheric stroke (anterior, central, posterior, subcortical)	L (15), R (15)	Generalised impairment of singing quality, no lateralised pitch or rhythm impairment
Peretz, 1990	Hemispheric stroke (no further details)	L (8)	Pitch interval, rhythm discrimination, melody recognition
		R (8)	Pitch interval, contour, rhythm discrimination, melody recognition
Prior *et al.*, 1990	MCA territory stroke	L (13)	Rhythm perception and reproduction, singing familiar and novel tunes
		R (13)	Rhythm reproduction, singing familiar tunes

Table 5. Continued.

Author	Lesion	Side (no.)	Musical deficits
Ayotte *et al.*, 2000	MCA territory stroke	L‡ (7)	Memory recognition
		R (10)	Scale, contour, interval discrimination, memory recognition
		B (3)	Scale, contour, interval, metre discrimination, memory recognition
Schuppert *et al.*, 2000	Cortical stroke (anterior or posterior)	L‡ (12)	Pitch value, interval, contour, rhythm, metre discrimination; dissociated (local vs global) deficits within pitch and temporal domains
		R (8)	Pitch value, interval, contour, rhythm, metre, "affective appreciation"; no dissociated (local vs global) deficits within pitch or temporal domains
Ehrlé *et al.*, 2001	Mesial temporal sclerosis	L (8), R (10)	L: Rapid anisochrony discrimination

Key: B, bilateral; L, left; MCA, middle cerebral artery; R, right; †nature of lesion not specified; ‡language lateralisation not clear in all cases.

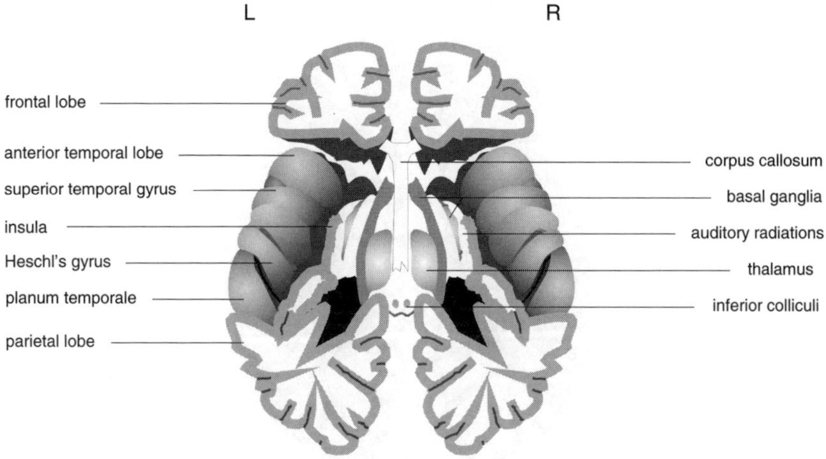

Fig. 1. Schematic axial slice of the brain at the level of the superior temporal gyri, showing structures involved in music processing.

writing is intact (see Table 1). Various patterns of auditory agnosia are possible (Tables 1 and 2): music may be involved together with both speech and environmental sounds;[22,25,42,45–49] with speech, sparing environmental sounds,[23,42,50,51] with environmental sounds, sparing speech;[37,52,53] or in relative isolation.[7,38,39,41,54] Rarely if ever is music selectively spared, though it may recover before other types of sounds.[1,6]

Although aphasia not infrequently accompanies amusia (Tables 1 and 2), there are obvious limitations to sophisticated musical assessment in this situation, as well as ascertainment bias,[4] which make interpretation difficult. Excluded from the tables are reports of intact musical faculties in aphasic musicians and composers.[4,55,56] This "mirror image" of amusia without aphasia completes a double dissociation, and must be taken into account in formulating models of music processing. The relationship of musicality to prosody (the stress, pitch and intonational variations which convey the "melody" of speech) has unfortunately not been studied systematically (Tables 1–3); nevertheless it is evident that perception of musical melody can be affected without receptive aprosody.[7]

A hierarchy of music processing deficits can be identified,[4,47] ranging from impaired extraction of acoustic properties[7] to musical associative agnosias, in which access to music-specific memories appears to be lost.[43] Although frameworks for music processing based on local and global feature extraction[11] and two-stage recognition[39] have been proposed, the place of musical

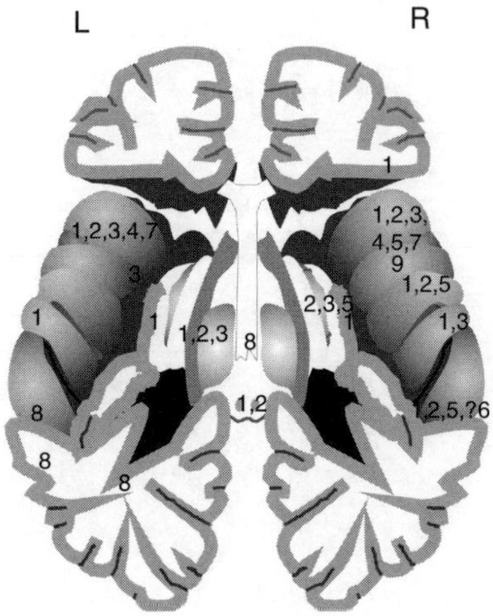

Fig. 2. Sites of lesions which disturb music processing (based on Tables 1–5). Anatomical landmarks as shown in Figure 1. Numerals indicate musical subcomponent(s) affected by damage at that site. Both lesion-led and symptom-led studies are represented (see text for explanation). Key: 1, pitch (scale, chord and interval); 2, melody; 3, rhythm; 4, metre; 5, timbre; 6, emotional tone; 7, musical long-term memory; 8, musical reading and writing; 9, musical praxis.

subcomponents within the hierarchy is still open to question (Figure 3). This reflects both the difficulty of providing operational definitions for concepts such as "pitch" and "timbre", and the frequent perceptual and representational interactions between musical subcomponents at different levels of abstraction.[57] "Melody", for example, has been used in the literature to refer specifically to pitch sequence contour, but also in the sense of entire musical pieces, with complex temporal (rhythmic and metrical) as well as semantic properties.

The following is a tentative taxonomy of the amusias.

Pitch, harmony and pitch interval

Musical tones (like vowels) are composed of sets of harmonically related sinusoids, with pitch corresponding to the fundamental frequency of the harmonic series.[58] However, the perception of pitch in music is far more dependent on the intervals between successive notes and their harmonic context (chords, scales and keys) than on absolute frequency values,[57] as illustrated

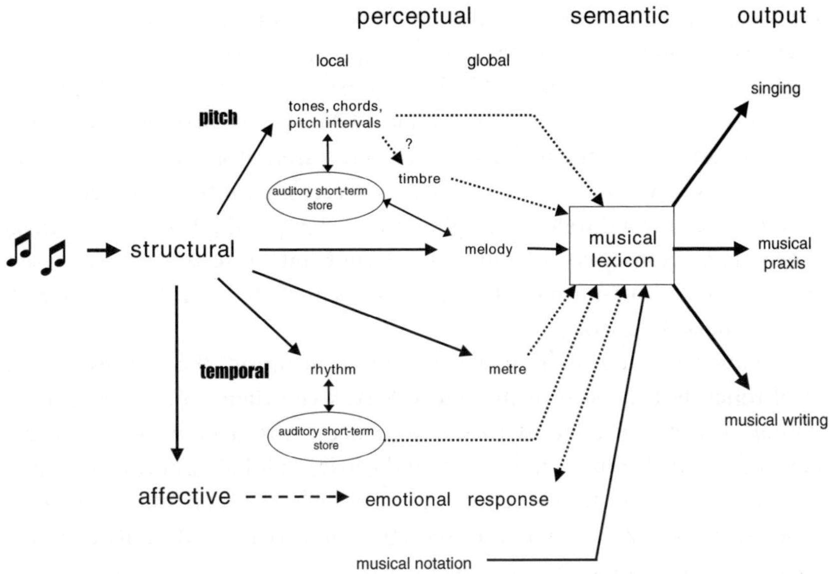

Fig. 3. Hierarchical model of music processing, based on clinical data. Arrows indicate the postulated direction of information flow, and the extensive interaction between musical subcomponents. Links for which limited evidence is available are represented with dashed arrows (see text for details).

by preservation of simple pitch perception by lesions which impair musical discrimination.[59] The brain is able to perceive virtual pitch, in which a pitch corresponding to a missing fundamental is heard.[57] While the "rules" governing tonal hierarchies (scales) and harmonic relationships may be learned, the tendency for tones separated by octave intervals to be perceived as similar or "equivalent" is observed even in the musically untrained, and tonal hierarchies can be abstracted cross-culturally.[57]

Pure tone perception is variably affected by bilateral lesions involving Heschl's gyri, secondary auditory cortical and subcortical areas in humans, and considerable functional recovery may occur.[24,26,45,50,53] Tonal consonance perception may be permanently damaged by complete bilateral lesions of Heschl's gyri and partial lesions of secondary auditory cortex, however limited perception of harmonic relationships is still possible in this situation, suggesting that "broad tuning" may occur in auditory association or subcortical structures.[26] Removal of the right Heschl's gyrus impairs perception of the missing fundamental in complex tones.[29] Tonal interval discrimination (for example, deciding whether a two-tone sequence is ascending or descending) may be disrupted by right[60] or bilateral[25] temporo-parietal lesions, and may depend on frequency of presentation.[23] Impairment may also follow bilateral insula[53] or subcortical lesions.[24,51] Discrimination of pitch intervals requires auditory short term memory: the patient of Mackworth-Young[60] with right temporo-parietal damage had disordered perception of sequential pitch intervals and scales, despite retained ability to perceive chords. Short-term pitch retention is disturbed following right anterior temporal lobectomy restricted to secondary auditory cortex and also by right frontal resections,[31] which suggests that tonal short-term working memory is mediated by a distributed right fronto-temporal network.

In sequential pitch patterns such as those in music, the pitches of individual tones and the size of the intervals between them can be regarded as a "local" feature, in contrast to the sequence contour or melody, which is independent of absolute pitch values and carries "global" information about the sequence as a whole. This contrast forms the basis for an influential model proposed by Peretz,[11] based on observations in patients with unilateral brain damage, and corroborated by Liégeois-Chauvel *et al.*,[36] Ayotte *et al.*[39] and Schuppert *et al.*[12] According to this model, the right hemisphere encodes a global melody representation, which provides a reference for the extraction of local information about pitch intervals by the left hemisphere. Damage to either hemisphere can therefore interfere with the extraction of pitch interval information. However, there is evidence that either hemisphere can use both scale and contour information when the other is damaged,[28] and that pitch discrimination can be spared relative to other musical functions.[27,52]

Pitch perception is traditionally held to depend on extraction of spectral information (analysis of the component frequencies of the auditory signal). However, pitch can be extracted using temporal (time interval) information alone, as illustrated by the musical tone created when noise is periodically reflected from a surface.[58] The distinction between local and global properties of a musical sequence may reflect short-term versus longer-term time structure. Fine time structure analysis of local pitch information in short tone sequences may be deranged following a right supero-posterior temporal lobe lesion,[7] and impaired temporal resolution of auditory events may underlie the deficits of both speech and music perception observed with bilateral posterior temporal lobe lesions.[23–25]

Melody (pitch contour)

Evidence that melodic pattern analysis is mediated by subsystems located in secondary auditory cortex, which integrate information over longer time scales (hundreds of milliseconds) than those responsible for pitch interval processing (typically tens of milliseconds) in primary auditory cortex, has emerged both from functional imaging observations in normal subjects[58,61] and from psychophysical studies in patients with discrete lesions.[7,35] Melodic deficits are typically prominent in the setting of right or bi-temporal damage (Table 2). Processing of pitch contour is specifically disrupted by resections involving secondary auditory cortex in the right posterior superior temporal gyrus.[36] Although right temporal resections disturb melodic discrimination and retention, resections of either anterior temporal lobe may interfere with recognition.[28,33,35] and yet recognition of melodies may still be possible despite bilateral temporal lobe damage which affects tonal pattern analysis.[25] Temporal lobectomy studies implicate both Heschl's gyri in melody processing, perhaps in maintaining the short-term "auditory trace".[28]

Under normal circumstances, the two hemispheres cooperate in processing melodies. Melody storage in the right temporal lobe is modulated by information processed in the left, including verbal cues, such as song lyrics.[32] Schuppert *et al.*[12] found defects in pitch contour perception following unilateral left as well as right hemisphere lesions, and suggested that bilateral temporoparietal pathways are used to communicate between subsystems mediating local and global properties of the musical stimulus. The patient described by Levin and Rose[62] had difficulty discriminating tonal sequences following callosal section.

Rhythm and metre

Rhythm is conveyed by the durations of notes, rests and their grouping, whereas metre refers to a regular pattern of accents (strong versus weak beats) in a periodic pattern, corresponding to the bar in Western music, which is independent of the absolute durations of notes and rests.[36,57] Both describe the temporal (time interval) architecture of a piece of music, and can be viewed (analogously to pitch and melody) as conveying information about local and global structure, respectively. Rhythm and metre deficits frequently dissociate from the corresponding pitch processing deficits.[11,12,38,40,44,48,54,62] Impaired perception of rhythmic pattern disrupts musical recognition[40] and expression.[10] Rhythm, however, is not specific to music or even the auditory domain. Rhythmicity can be perceived in periodic visual and tactile stimuli,[57] and disorders of rhythm processing are often "supramodal", in the sense that they involve the perception of rhythm via different sensory channels.[25,40]

Left, right and bilateral temporo-parietal lesions disturb rhythm perception and production.[3,12,25,40,50,60,63,64] Right anterior temporal resections which include secondary auditory cortex in the antero-lateral part of Heschl's gyrus impair auditory rhythm reproduction selectively.[9] However, rapid anisochrony discrimination (perception of irregularity of inter-tone interval length at rapid rates of presentation, of the order of 80 msec) is specifically impaired in patients with left mesial temporal damage.[65] This observation may be specific for fast sequential auditory processing, or alternatively, reflect a short-term auditory memory deficit. It may also indicate that processing of rhythm, like pitch, has regional specificity depending on critical time windows. Subcortical lesions may also affect rhythm discrimination: the patient of Takahashi *et al.*[51] had a left thalamic haemorrhage which involved the auditory radiations but spared primary auditory cortex.

Metre has been studied less systematically than other musical subcomponents. Discrimination of metre is impaired following right anterior temporal lobectomy,[30] and the anterior superior temporal gyrus may be critical;[36] however (as for rhythm), a consistent lateralisation has not emerged. These findings may reflect defective semantic categorisation of metrical patterns (for example, "march" or "waltz"), which normally engages the anterior temporal lobe.[36]

Preserved metre judgements despite impaired rhythm discrimination have been observed in patients with unilateral damage to either hemisphere,[11] and the reverse dissociation following anterior temporal lobectomies.[36] Schuppert *et al.*[12] identified patients with both dissociations following unilateral left anterior (though not right-sided) strokes. Rhythm processing was largely spared in the study of Ayotte *et al.*,[39] and results for metre were highly variable.

Timbre

Timbre, sometimes loosely equated with "tone colour", is difficult to define precisely, but undoubtedly crucial to musical appreciation, as the uniquely recognisable voices of human singers and musical instruments attest. The spectral composition of a tone, its initial segment or "attack" and temporal envelope, are all integral to its timbre.[34] This implies that a deficit in discriminating the precise order of acoustic signals would affect timbre perception, and thus (like other musical subcomponents) it might depend on temporal processing mechanisms. Disturbed timbre (tone quality, musical instrument) discrimination has been described following right temporal,[52,60,66] right basal ganglia and postero-inferior frontal,[42] bilateral superior temporal,[23,38] bilateral temporoparietal[25] and left trigonal[62] lesions. With the exception of the patient of Mazzucchi *et al.*,[66] additional musical deficits were identified; this patient also had difficulty discriminating environmental sounds and voices based on timbral features. Samson and Zatorre[34] found that processing of both spectral and time cues in synthetic timbral stimuli was impaired following right anterior temporal lobectomy.

Emotional tone

Neural correlates of musical emotion are poorly understood, however they are likely to be at least partly distinct from the areas which process musical structure, as illustrated by patients who selectively retain[38,41,43,47,51] or lose[67] emotional discriminations and response to music. Mazzoni *et al.*[67] identified no discrete perceptual deficits in their patient, a guitarist, who lost aesthetic pleasure in music and had difficulty grasping the structure of musical pieces; the lesion in this case was a right temporo-parietal haemorrhage. Schuppert *et al.*[12] observed reduced affective musical appreciation chiefly following right hemisphere damage. Clearly, processing of structural and affective features is normally integrated: many patients with amusia complain that music has acquired an unpleasant dissonant, "flat", "dull" or "fuzzy" quality.[7,38,53,54,66] In cases where musical discrimination is damaged, emotional judgments may be based on a limited number of perceptual (for example, metre and tempo) cues.[41]

Musical associative agnosia and musical long-term memory

By analogy with other neuropsychological functions, music recognition can be conceptualised as a two-stage process:[39] auditory analysis, followed by activation of a "musical lexicon" which encodes, stores and retrieves music-specific long-term memories.[43] Access to the lexicon appears to be determined mainly by melody or local pitch information,[11,38] however, rhythmic cues are probably also used.[40] Many patients with amusia have derangements of perceptual analysis, which can be classified as "apperceptive" agnosias.[7,38,39]

In contrast, Eustache *et al.*[42] and Peretz[43] described patients who were unable to identify musical pieces, to sing tunes from memory or to memorise novel music although they could still discriminate various properties of a musical piece. They were able to use verbal cues (lyrics or titles) to achieve normal identification. This pattern is consistent with damage to the musical lexicon itself, or disconnection of the lexicon from the channels of auditory analysis.[22] Association of musical percepts with corresponding musical long-term memories would no longer be possible, producing music-specific "associative" agnosia.

There is evidence that musical apperceptive agnosia results from damage to the right hemisphere, associative agnosia from left-sided or bilateral damage,[28,39,42] implying that the right hemisphere mediates perceptual access to musical memories, "while the neural correlates of the memory component of the recognition system are more elusive".[39] It is clear that perceptual processing, encoding and retrieval of items from musical long-term memory are generally interdependent and have a neural substrate which is at least partly shared;[11,22,23,32,33,35,41,54] however, recognition may still be possible when discrimination is impaired.[25,42] Our understanding of how the musical lexicon is organised and accessed remains limited: patients M.H. and C.N., for example, exhibited some evidence of familiarity with well-known pieces under restricted conditions, indicating that engagement of the lexicon is not all-or-none.[42,43]

Musical (singing and instrumental) apraxia

Isolated deficits of musical expression appear to be rare.[10,68,69] Although this pattern may follow lesions of the central or anterior right hemisphere, musical praxis[3,70] and musical subcomponents of singing[71] do not show clear hemispheric lateralisation. Representative cases of musical apraxia are summarised in Table 3. The celebrated, progressive amusia of Maurice Ravel, which affected chiefly musical expression and was accompanied by disturbances of language and limb praxis,[72] may have been a musical apraxia; though not confirmed pathologically, Pick's disease or another frontotemporal dementia would be plausible diagnoses.[73] Deficits of musical praxis may accompany orofacial apraxia.[74] Alternatively, musical praxis may be spared despite non-musical orofacial and limb apraxia.[44,75]

It is likely that music processing and production both normally engage the lexicon of stored musical representations,[38] and, indeed, perceptual deficits frequently degrade musical expression.[23,25,40,41,53,54,60] Classifications of amusia as "expressive" or "receptive" are therefore difficult to defend. However, over-learned, musical "tactile-motor loops"[4] may come to operate largely autonomously of higher cognitive controls, allowing some patients to continue to sing or play their instrument even as musical perceptual processing disintegrates.[44]

Musical alexia and agraphia

Although they both use symbolic lexicons which require semantic processing, verbal and musical notational systems are likely to demand quite different perceptual strategies for their decipherment. Music is written using a much smaller number of lexical items which are visually more ambiguous and visuospatially more complex than most scripts.[4,5] While musical and verbal alexia generally occur together,[3,15,62,70,76] observed dissociations imply that their neuroanatomical substrates overlap only in part.[5,56,75,77] Representative cases of musical alexia and agraphia are summarised in Table 3. Musical alexia often follows damage to the posterior left hemisphere; right hemisphere lesions usually produce a more general disorder of music processing.[5] Similar observations apply to musical agraphia.[78] The patient of Midorikawa and Kawamura,[78] with predominantly musical agraphia, had a lesion involving the left superior parietal lobule; that of Assal and Buttet,[79] with preserved musical writing but verbal agraphia, involvement of the left inferior parietal lobule. The patient of Cappelletti *et al.*,[77] with alexia and agraphia selective for music, had sustained damage to right occipito-temporal and left postero-lateral temporal areas which spared the left supramarginal gyrus, implicated in verbal reading. The authors suggested that access to stored, abstract representations of musical notes via their written symbols was lost in this case, although the representations themselves were intact, since the patient retained the ability to play notes to spoken command. The deficit was specific for musical notes, not extending to numerals and other non-verbal symbols.

Examples of selective derangements in reading and writing pitch[3,5,70] and rhythm[78] symbols have been described, which may indicate defects of visuospatial feedback and short-term rehearsal, respectively. Identification of musical symbols appears to be influenced by their context.[5] Reading of notes may be affected selectively, relative to other musical symbols.[3,62,77] These notational subclasses may differ in several ways: along the pitch versus rhythm dimensions,[3] in the extent to which they undergo verbal processing,[70] or to which they engage dorsal ("where") versus ventral ("what") visual streams.[76]

Conclusions

The rich clinical phenomenology of the amusias makes simple classification schemes, based on hemispheric lateralisation or an expressive–receptive dichotomy, untenable. The hierarchical framework for musical processing presented in Figure 3 attempts a synthesis of the clinical data, but must remain at best provisional. This model treats music as an example of complex, patterned sound, with structural (pitch and temporal) and affective properties, which are interdependent, but processed partly in parallel. Local and global properties are analysed over distinct time windows. Disordered processing specific to different levels of acoustic temporal structure may constitute a unifying mechanism underlying many of the amusias. It appears that some properties of the musical stimulus (for example, tonal characteristics) are processed by both hemispheres; hemispheric lateralisation may only emerge in the extraction of higher order temporal structure (for example, pitch contour—or melody—by the right hemisphere). Once processed, the various subcomponents of the musical stimulus may access a common lexicon of stored musical representations or long-term memories. The lexicon in turn has several possible forms of output, including the motor subroutines engaged in singing or playing an instrument.

As is the case for all complex neuropsychological functions, no lesion-based description of musicality can be complete in itself. The clinical study of the amusias will continue to suggest and inform fresh lines of enquiry, which must be pursued using complementary approaches, such as functional brain imaging. The neurologist will continue to have a legitimate role in the elucidation of these fascinating maladies, which after all touch one of the ornaments of our humanity.

Acknowledgement

I am indebted to Dr T.D. Griffiths for discussions pertaining to this topic.

References

1. T.D. Griffiths, A. Rees and G.G.R. Green, Disorders of human complex sound processing, *Neurocase* **5**, 365–78 (1999).
2. R.F. Voss and J. Clarke, "1/f noise" in music and speech, *Nature* **258**, 317–8 (1975).
3. J.C.M. Brust, Music and language: musical alexia and agraphia, *Brain* **103**, 367–92 (1980).
4. O.S.M. Marin, Neurological aspects of music perception and performance. In: D. Deutsch (ed.), *The Psychology of Music* (Harcourt Brace, 1982), pp. 453–77.
5. J. Judd, H. Gardner and N. Geshwind, Alexia without agraphia in a composer, *Brain* **106**, 435–57 (1983).

6. O. Godefroy, D. Leys, A. Furby *et al.*, Psychoacoustical deficits related to bilateral subcortical hemorrhages: a case with apperceptive auditory agnosia, *Cortex* **31**, 149–59 (1995).
7. T.D. Griffiths, A. Rees, C. Witton, P.M. Cross, R.A. Shakir and G.G.R. Green, Spatial and temporal auditory processing deficits following right hemisphere infarction: a psychophysical study, *Brain* **120**, 785–94 (1997).
8. A. Cutler and C. Clifton, Comprehending spoken language: a blueprint of the listener. In: C.M. Brown and P. Hagoort (eds.), *The Neurocognition of Language* (OUP, 1999), pp. 123–55.
9. V.B. Penhune, R.J. Zatorre and W.H. Feindel, The role of auditory cortex in retention of rhythmic patterns as studied in patients with temporal lobe removals including Heschl's gyrus, *Neuropsychologia* **37**, 315–31 (1999).
10. M.I. Botez and N. Wertheim, Expressive aphasia and amusia following right frontal lesion in a right handed man, *Brain* **82**, 186–202 (1959).
11. I. Peretz, Processing of local and global musical information by unilateral brain-damaged patients, *Brain* **113**, 1185–1205 (1990).
12. M. Schuppert, T.F. Munte, B.M. Wieringa and E. Altenmuller, Receptive amusia: evidence for cross-hemispheric neural networks underlying music processing startegies, *Brain* **123**, 546–59 (2000).
13. M. D'Esposito, Functional neuroimaging of cognition, *Sem. Neurol.* **20**, 487–98 (2000).
14. N. Wertheim, The amusias. In: P.J. Vinken and G.W. Bruyn (eds.), *Handbook of Clinical Neurology*, Vol. 4 (New Holland, Amsterdam, 1969), pp. 195–206.
15. A.L. Benton, The amusias. In: R.A. Henson and M. Critchley (eds.), *Music and the Brain* (Heinemann, London, 1977), pp. 378–97.
16. L. Mann, *Casuistische Beiträge zur Hirnchirurgie und Hirnlocalization Monatschr. Psychiat. Neurol.* **4**, 369–78 (1898).
17. K. Kleist, *Gehirnpathologische und lokalisatorische Ergebnisse über Hörstörungen, Gerauschtaubheiten und Amusien*, *Mschr. Psychiat. Neurol.* **68**, 853–71 (1928).
18. E. Feuchtwanger, *Amusie. Studien zur Psychologie der akustischen Wahrnehmung und Vorstellung und ihrer Strukturgebiete besonders in Musik und Sprache* (Springer, Berlin, 1930).
19. H.I. Ustvedt, *Über die Untersuchung der musikalischen Funktionen bei Patienten mit Gehirnleiden, besonders bei Patienten mit Aphasie*, *Acta. Med. Scand.* Suppl 86, 1–186 (1937).
20. H. Hécaen, Clinical symptomatology in right and left hemispheric lesions. In: V.B. Mountcastle (ed.), *Interhemispheric Relations and Cerebral Dominance* (Johns Hopkins, Baltimore, 1962), pp. 215–43.
21. J. Barbizet, *Role de l'hémisphère droit dans les perceptions auditives.* In: J. Barbizet, M. Ben Hamida and P. Duizabo (eds.), *Le Monde de L'Hemiplegie Gauche* (Masson, Paris, 1972).

22. G. Miceli, The processing of speech sounds in a patient with cortical auditory disorder, *Neuropsychologia* **20**, 5–20 (1982).
23. S.H. Auerbach, T. Allard, M. Naeser, M.P. Alexander and M.L. Albert, Pure word deafness: analysis of a case with bilateral lesions and a defect at the prephonemic level, *Brain* **105**, 271–300 (1982).
24. N. Motomura, A. Yamadori, E. Mori and F. Tamaru, Auditory agnosia: analysis of a case with bilateral subcortical lesions, *Brain* **109**, 379–91 (1986).
25. Y. Tanaka, A. Yamadori and E. Mori, Pure word deafness following bilateral lesions: a psychophysical analysis, *Brain* **110**, 381–403 (1987).
26. M.J. Tramo, J.J. Bharucha and F.E. Musiek, Music perception and cognition following bilateral lesions of auditory cortex, *J. Cogn. Neurosci.* **2**, 195–212 (1990).
27. B. Milner, Laterality effects in audition. In: V.B. Mountcastle (ed.), *Interhemispheric Relations and Cerebral Dominance* (Johns Hopkins, Baltimore, 1962), pp. 177–95.
28. R.J. Zatorre, Discrimination and recognition of tonal melodies after unilateral cerebral excisions, *Neuropsychologia* **23**, 31–41 (1985).
29. R.J. Zatorre, Pitch perception of complex tones and human temporal lobe function, *J. Acoust. Soc. Am.* **84**, 566–72 (1988).
30. D.B. Kester, A.J. Saykin, M.R. Sperling, M.J. O'Connor, L.J. Robinson and R.C. Gur, Acute effect of anterior temporal lobectomy on musical processing, *Neuropsychologia* **29**, 703–8 (1991).
31. R.J. Zatorre and S. Samson, Role of the right temporal neocortex in retention of pitch in auditory short term memory, *Brain* **114**, 2403–17 (1991).
32. S. Samson and R.J. Zatorre, Recognition memory for text and melody of songs after unilateral temporal lobe lesion: evidence for dual encoding, *J. Exp. Psychol. [Learn Mem. Cogn.]* **17**, 793–804 (1991).
33. S. Samson and R.J. Zatorre, Learning and retention of melodic and verbal information after unilateral temporal lobectomy, *Neuropsychologia* **30**, 815–26 (1992).
34. S. Samson and R.J. Zatorre, Contribution of the right temporal lobe to musical timbre discrimination, *Neuropsychologia* **32**, 231–40 (1994).
35. R.J. Zatorre and A.R. Halpern, Effect of unilateral temporal-lobe excision on perception and imagery of songs, *Neuropsychologia* **31**, 221–32 (1993).
36. C. Liégeois-Chauvel, I. Peretz, M. Babai *et al.*, Contribution of different cortical areas in the temporal lobes to music processing, *Brain* **121**, 1853–67 (1998).
37. O. Spreen, A.L. Benton and R.W. Fincham, Auditory agnosia without aphasia, *Arch. Neurol.* **13**, 84–92 (1965).
38. I. Peretz, R. Kolinsky, M. Tramo *et al.*, Functional dissociations following bilateral lesions of auditory cortex, *Brain* **117**, 1283–1301 (1994).

39. J. Ayotte, I. Peretz, I. Rousseau, C. Bard and M. Bojanowski, Patterns of music agnosia associated with middle cerebral artery infarcts, *Brain* **123**, 1926–38 (2000).
40. L. Mavlov, Amusia due to rhythm agnosia in a musician with left hemisphere damage: a non-auditory supramodal defect, *Cortex* **16**, 331–8 (1980).
41. I. Peretz and L. Gagnon, Dissociation between recognition and emotional judgements for melodies, *Neurocase* **5**, 21–30 (1999).
42. F. Eustache, B. Lechevalier, F. Viader and J. Lambert, Identification and discrimination disorders in auditory perception: a report on two cases, *Neuropsychologia* **28**, 257–70 (1990).
43. I. Peretz, Can we lose memory for music? A case of music agnosia in a nonmusician, *J. Cogn. Neurosci.* **8**, 481–96 (1996).
44. M. Polk and A. Kertesz, Music and language in degenerative disease of the brain, *Brain Cogn.* **22**, 98–117 (1993).
45. M.F. Mendez and G.R. Geehan, Cortical auditory disorders: clinical and psychoacoustic features, *J. Neurol. Neurosurg. Psychiatry* **51**, 1–9 (1988).
46. D.R. Oppenheimer and F. Newcombe, Clinical and anatomic findings in a case of auditory agnosia, *Arch. Neurol.* **35**, 712–9 (1978).
47. B. Lechevalier, Y. Rossa, F. Eustache, C. Schupp, L. Boner and C. Bazin, Un cas de surdité corticale épargnant en partie la musique, *Rev. Neurol.* **140**, 190–201 (1984).
48. J. Lambert, F. Eustache, B. Lechevalier, Y. Rossa and F. Viader, Auditory agnosia with relative sparing of speech perception, *Cortex* **25**, 71–82 (1989).
49. P. Praamstra, P. Hagoort, B. Maassen and T. Crul, Word deafness and auditory cortical function: a case history and hypothesis, *Brain* **114**, 1197–1225 (1991).
50. H.B. Coslett, H.R. Brashear and K.M. Heilman, Pure word deafness after bilateral primary auditory cortex infarcts, *Neurology* **34**, 347–52 (1984).
51. N. Takahashi, M. Kawamura, H. Shinotou, K. Hirayama, K. Kaga and M. Shindo, Pure word deafness due to left hemisphere damage, *Cortex* **28**, 295–303 (1992).
52. T. Fujii, R. Fukatsu, S. Watabe *et al.*, Auditory sound agnosia without aphasia following a right temporal lobe lesion, *Cortex* **26**, 263–8 (1990).
53. M. Habib, G. Daquin, L. Milandre *et al.*, Mutism and auditory agnosia due to bilateral insular damage—role of the insula in human communication, *Neuropsychologia* **33**, 327–39 (1995).
54. M. Piccirilli, T. Sciarma and S. Luzzi, Modularity of music: evidence from a case of pure amusia, *J. Neurol. Neurosurg. Psychiatry* **69**, 541–5 (2000).
55. A.R. Luria, L.S. Tsvetkova and D.S. Futer, Aphasia in a composer, *J. Neurol. Sci.* **2**, 288–92 (1965).
56. G. Assal, *Aphasie de Wernicke sans amusie chez un pianiste*, *Rev. Neurol.* **129**, 251–5 (1973).

57. C. Krumhansl, Rhythm and pitch in music cognition, *Psychol. Bull.* **126**, 159–79 (2000).
58. T.D. Griffiths, C. Büchel, R.S.J. Frackowiak and R.D. Patterson, Analysis of temporal structure in sound by the human brain, *Nat. Neurosci.* **1**, 422–7 (1998).
59. K. Johkura, S. Matsumoto, O. Hasegawa and Y. Kuroiwa, Defective auditory recognition after small hemorrhage in the inferior colliculi, *J. Neurol. Sci.* **161**, 91–6 (1998).
60. C.G. Mackworth-Young, Sequential musical symptoms in a professional musician with presumed encephalitis, *Cortex* **19**, 413–9 (1983).
61. R.J. Zatorre, A.C. Evans and E. Meyer, Neural mechanisms underlying melodic perception and memory for pitch, *J. Neurosci.* **14**, 1908–19 (1994).
62. H.S. Levin and J.E. Rose, Alexia without agraphia in a musician after transcallosal removal of a left intraventricular meningioma, *Neurosurgery* **4**, 168–74 (1979).
63. B.E. Shapiro, M. Grossman and H. Gardner, Selective musical processing deficits in brain damaged populations, *Neuropsychologia* **19**, 161–9 (1981).
64. M. Prior, G. Kinsella and J. Giese, Assessment of musical processing in brain-damaged patients: implications for laterality of music, *J. Clin. Exp. Neuropsychol.* **12**, 301–12 (1990).
65. N. Ehrlé, S. Samson and M. Baulac, Processing of rapid auditory information in epileptic patients with left temporal lobe damage, *Neuropsychologia* **39**, 525–31 (2001).
66. A. Mazzucchi, C. Marchini, R. Budai and M. Parma, A case of receptive amusia with prominent timbre perception defect, *J. Neurol. Neurosurg. Psychiatry* **45**, 644–7 (1982).
67. M. Mazzoni, P. Moretti, L. Pardossi, M. Vista, A. Muratorio and M. Puglioli, A case of music imperception, *J. Neurol. Neurosurg. Psychiatry* **56**, 322–4 (1993).
68. H.R. McFarland and D. Fortin, Amusia due to right temporoparietal infarct, *Arch. Neurol.* **39**, 725–7 (1982).
69. K. Takeda, M. Bandou and Y. Nishimura, Motor amusia following a right temporal lobe hemorrhage—a case report, *Rinsho Shink* **30**, 78–83 (1990).
70. T. Horikoshi, Y. Asari, A. Watanabe *et al.*, Music alexia in a patient with mild pure alexia: disturbed visual perception of nonverbal meaningful figures, *Cortex* **33**, 187–94 (1997).
71. G. Kinsella, M.R. Prior and G. Murray, Singing ability after right and left sided brain damage: a research note, *Cortex* **24**, 165–9 (1988).
72. T. Alajouanine, Aphasia and artistic realization, *Brain* **71**, 229–41 (1948).
73. R.J. Alonso and R.M. Pascuzzi, Ravel's neurological illness, *Sem. Neurol.* **19**, 53–7 (1999).
74. C. Confavreux, B. Croisile, P. Garassus, G. Aimard and M. Trillet, Progressive amusia and aprosody, *Arch. Neurol.* **49**, 971–6 (1992).

75. A. Basso and E. Capitani, Spared musical abilities in a conductor with global aphasia and ideomotor apraxia, *J. Neurol. Neurosurg. Psychiatry* **48**, 407–12 (1985).
76. D.Q. Beversdorf and K.M. Heilman, Progressive ventral posterior cortical degeneration presenting as alexia for music and words, *Neurology* **50**, 657–9 (1998).
77. M. Cappelletti, H. Waley-Cohen, B. Butterworth and M. Kopelman, A selective loss of the ability to read and to write music, *Neurocase* **6**, 321–32 (2000).
78. A. Midorikawa and M. Kawamura, A case of musical agraphia, *NeuroReport* **11**, 3053–7 (2000).
79. G. Assal and J. Buttet, *Agraphie et conservation de l'écriture musicale chez un professeur de piano bilingue*, *Rev. Neurol.* **139**(10), 569–74 (1983).
80. R.J. Roeser and D.D. Daly, Auditory cortex disconnection associated with thalamic tumor, *Neurology* **24**, 555–9 (1974).
81. J.J. Sidtis and E. Feldmann, Transient ischemic attacks presenting with a loss of pitch perception, *Cortex* **26**, 469–71 (1990).

Chapter 15

Music and the Brain: A Musicologist's Viewpoint

Paul Robertson

Our culture needs to know why we are musical. It may even be that our survival requires that we understand ourselves better musically. Increasingly interconnected through the technology of information, we need more and more complex, subtle and beautiful models of thought and experience with which to cope with this process of change and relate to it. Music, I believe, may be our richest language for expressing this complexity, subtlety and emotional insight.

Study of how sound energy creates patterns in form has been going on for centuries, probably millennia. The system most familiar to us in the West is cymatics. As I speak, my voice creates molecular energy. That energy is cross-sectioned by the membranes of the hearer's ear and the energy patterns are then translated in the brain and recreated into the rich and multidimensional sound world we all inhabit. It is possible to cross-section the sound and make a visual pattern. If you stretch a membrane across a drum skin and put sand on it, then sing or make some other sound near the drum, the molecular energy makes the particles dance on the surface. This is more than a metaphor; it is a different perception of our earliest auditory neural development, the symmetries of energy that play a fundamental role in our perceptual system and our life.

Mapping the Musical Brain

About 18 years ago I attended a lecture on what was then the brave new world of neurology. The lecturer spoke particularly about the hemispheres of the brain and our extraordinary dual perception system. At the end of the evening I asked him what, with regard to the functioning of the hemispheres of the brain, could be said about the development of music. His answer created a whole new life for me: "I think that's one of the most important questions that could be asked at this time, so much so that I recommend you go and find the answers for yourself."

He put me in touch with Dr Peter Fenwick, an eminent neuropsychiatrist. For two years Peter and I attempted to have a conversation, but our domains and our language of skills were so different that we couldn't communicate. Gradually, however, we began to build up a model of what might be happening in terms of brain function, brain response, and the evolution of musical language and musical response.

Before Peter and I started work it had been discovered that the two halves of the brain preferentially process different combinations of sounds. Concordant sounds, which have low frequency ratios and are preferred by all mammals, are preferentially processed in the right side of the brain. Discords are preferentially processed in the left side. We know that the right side of the brain is emotional, spatial and non-verbal whereas the left side is verbal, sequential, and highly involved with the development of language. Peter and I were therefore able to postulate that a composer who, for whatever reason, was drawn to a propensity for left-brain musical language would inevitably use discordant, arrhythmic musical language. Schoenberg was driven by an internal intellectual imperative to an increasingly discordant left-brain musical language. I think he was also driven by verbal language. Much of his music is created around language structures, after which the words are thrown away, leaving discordant prosodic shapes.

A composer or indeed a music world that seeks the language of emotion and enhanced meaning without words will tend towards concordance. It is no accident that Western religious music strongly favours such sound because it is associated with the right brain and actually has the effect of enhancing our sense of emotional well-being and coherence.

Where Music Is More Powerful Than Words

There is a chilling illustration of what happens if the right side of the brain is missing. The doctor of a patient who had had a large part of his right hemisphere removed asked him how he felt. The answer, delivered in a robotic tone, was "With my hands." The literal meaning of language was there but not the emotional depth and connotation. Equally significantly, the prosody, the musicality of the voice had gone.

What happens when the left side of the brain is damaged is illustrated powerfully and sadly by my friend Stephen Wade. He suffered a massive stroke of the left hemisphere and now, while his personality is intact, he cannot speak, read or write. To make the situation even more poignant, he previously earned his living as a multilingual telephonist, so words were his world and his life. He has lost the use of the right side of his body and has also lost short-term memory. You can no longer ask him "Would you like a cup of tea or a cup of coffee?" because while he is processing the world "tea" he loses the world "coffee". So what can he do?

Stephen had always been an amateur composer and somehow, miraculously, his musical self remains intact. The hand that can no longer write words can still write music. He can also improvise at the piano. With his voice he can make only unintelligible sounds but he can express his feelings through music. He is obviously an intact musician and he comes across as an intact person. He knows exactly what he wants to try to achieve but he cannot communicate anything in words, only in music.

For me it is increasingly self-evident that what is true for the individual is true for groups and for society itself. Just as someone who has suffered a stroke can no longer speak but can communicate through music, groups which are prevented from speaking by political repression will carry on their tradition in music, song an dance. I believe that metaphor offers a great deal to us.

There is an extraordinarily subtle and yet-to-be-explored relationship between music and language. Our understanding so far leads us to believe that musical expression, like verbal language, is based on the communication between mother and child. This tends to be prosodic, billing and cooing, and it requires extraordinary and beautiful brain structures. There is no point in crying to express distress if your parent does not have the brain system to connect the sound with an emotion. The structures that allow this connection are absolutely fundamental, built into each of us as part of our birthright, our evolution. I believe that those structures of sound and emotion go on to create a musical language, what might be called the development of prosody, the exquisite exploration of communication of emotion through sound. They also underlie spoken language, which is another form of communication through sound.

We get glimpses of the syntax of such communications. The notorious tritone, the musical interval consisting of three whole tones, was outlawed in medieval music because it was believed to be the Devil's interval. We now know that we inevitably hear tritone connection according to where we learned our mother tongue. An English-speaking American will come up with a subjective interpretation, which is distinctly and predictably different from that of someone brought up in the southern counties of England. The researcher who discovered this, Diana Deutsch, was disturbed because there was one aberrant individual in the study which otherwise confirmed the finding. Eventually he admitted that he was an illegal immigrant and had lied about his place of origin. For us the important thing about this finding is that subtle musical codes, musical recognitions and responses, are built into us as part of our ability to communicate before we have language skills. They are the syntax of emotional communication and that is why we need to understand music better.

The Universal "Mummy"

Another example, observed across cultures, is the little falling phrase known as the mummy interval. It is familiar to all parents, usually in the middle of the night: "Mummy", and famously, "I want a drink of Wa-ter." It appears to be universal, another glimpse of why and perhaps how music speaks to us even when we don't know it's happening.

Haydn was a deeply religious man and when he came to set *Christ's Seven Last Words from the Cross* he delved as deeply as he could into his personal emotional experience. In Christ's words to Mary and St John, "Mother, behold thy son. Son, behold they mother", we hear the mummy interval. Another example of music expressing deep feeling is found in Brahms, who was brought up—more or less dragged up—in a brothel. In the bars and brothels of Hamburg there was always a gypsy orchestra, and in Brahms' last work, the *Clarinet Quintet*, he makes an allusion to that music, a single glimpse of his childhood.

This touches on the whole gamut of the immense therapeutic and emotional potential of music. One of its great gifts is that it allows us a complete experience of ourselves, often without words. Sometimes words are too painful or too clumsy to carry the completeness of who and what we are. This aspect of music is too large for me to explore here.

For most of us, our auditory and musical development took place before birth and in the early months of life. We have a remarkable gift. Let me give a personal example.

The telephone rings, I answer it, and the voice at the other end says, in a certain tone, "Hello." I reply, "Hello, mum. What's wrong?" That is an impressive transaction. I have recognized the meaning of the word "hello", in itself no mean feat; as far as I know, no other animal can do it. I have recognized the individual voice, and this on an instrument that gives only a limited cross-section of sound frequency. Most significantly of all, I have recognized in an instant the emotional tonality of the person speaking to me.

The Musical World of Autistics

The development that allowed me to do all that is often halted in people who have suffered specific brain damage. They may have great gifts but, through no fault of their own, they are incapable of either generating or recognizing emotional signals, or at least limited in their ability to do so. None the less, music can give these autistic individuals an opportunity to build up a greater gamut of emotional connection and inner coherence.

Tony de Blois suffered significant brain damage during his birth and was born blind. At the age of two he still wasn't sitting up. His mother, a piano teacher, almost in desperation gave him a little electronic keyboard and guided his hands towards it—in itself a long-winded business. Little Tony discovered that if he moved his arms up and down, sound was elicited. Already that is significant. The great gift of human intelligence is that we can recognise events in the outside world and create change by will and design and anticipation. Such a gift is not easily found by a blind, autistic child, unable to sit up, but Tony discovered the keyboard. For three weeks all he did was bang it. Then, to her amazement, his mother heard the first few notes of *Twinkle, Twinkle, Little Star*. Tony is now grown up and, whilst still unable to tie his own shoelaces, has repertoire of more than 8000 pieces.

One theory of brain development is that within broad bands of biologically dictated opportunities for growth, stages of development within the brain, the neurons themselves are relatively random. According to this hypothesis there is a kind of Darwinian evolution within the neurons and in the connections between them. That is why a newborn baby moves randomly, and gradually, by self-observation and trial and error, refines its movements until it has precise control. It could be that Tony de Blois' development is just such a refining process of the memory.

Tony's mother believes that music has helped him to express himself in ordinary language, "When he was little," she said, "we used to sing *Autumn Leaves* and we'd go out there and we'd play in the leaves and we'd talk about autumn leaves. When I taught him how to swim I'd have him put his head on my shoulder and we'd sing *Put Your Head on My Shoulder*.... I was trying to give him meaning from the words that were in the songs because I felt that the music was the key to Tony and how to work with him."

Tony himself can describe how, after hearing a tune once, he can pick it out on the piano. He can play the classics and improvise jazz. He can imitate birdsong, trains, and the sirens of emergency vehicles on the piano. He can use it to express his own feelings at any particular time and maintains there is nothing he couldn't say in music. When asked to express what he felt about his mother he played a lyrical, ornamented version of *Twinkle, Twinkle, Little Star*.

The Greatest Human Gift

One aspect of the arts—for me, of music in particular—is that they offer an opportunity to discover and refine particular emotions. This ability to recognise, express, and then, in high art perhaps, synthesise emotions is one of the highest if not the single highest medium we have. Virtually all the great musical repertoire consists of paradoxical emotions, emotions that almost cannot exist in ordinary life, drawn together. It happens in Mozart and in Schoenberg. In *Opus 131*, Beethoven takes four notes etched in pain and creates a mighty fugue with them. What greater gift could there be for a human being?

When we explore sound in terms of frequency, we can play tricks with it. When white light is passed through a prism a spectrum of colour comes out at the other side. Each colour has a frequency, which can be translated into sound. By translating the frequencies of red, white and blue one can play the French flag. That is the playful end of the process but such relationships are extremely powerful. The ancient Greeks formalized frequencies of sound into patterns and mathematical aesthetics. A harmonic series of notes can be mathematically analysed into something that formalizes into musical scales and these scales become the seven ages of man or the seven days of the week or the seven deadly sins. If you continue mathematically applying divisions into a 12-step you end up with the 12 hours on the clock or the 12 months of the year.

We are informed by musical patterns more than we know and such information carries on into immensely subtle structures. Throughout history it has been understood, as part of our human gift, that music is closely connected with our sense of being and of well-being. The healing bow "Goma" is a single structure with the string down the side and it makes one great complex package of sound. Prof. Nigel Osborne took one second of the sound of the healing bow and expanded it into a three-minute piece, which can be played by a string quartet. When we hear it we are climbing inside the music, just as a microscope climbs inside the structure of a piece of matter. That is the musical mind beginning to move towards a scientific, objective exploration of itself and of emotion.

Measuring Emotion

As musicians move towards scientific explanation, we find scientists moving towards a music experience. Manfred Clynes is probably the most exceptional of them. He was a top-class professional pianist who moved into psychology and neurology and then into artificial intelligence. He has found a way of measuring the physiology of affect—in other words, how we are physically when we are feeling something specific. We know that anger, joy and love have their own language, both body language and tone of voice. They are interconnected. If we measure them in terms of brain chemistry or muscle tonality or tone of voice, we will find conformity. You can't have the emotion of anger without the whole of its expression, and if that is a predictable change it can be measured.

Clynes chose to measure muscle changes in the most passive finger of the passive left hand. He invited people to emote—something we can do easily by visualizing or even evoking words—and this caused muscle tonality to change predictably in everyone. A little button measured pressure up and down, away and towards. For example, thinking of love involves a gesture that both releases pressure and draws towards, while anger presses down and away. That gives two pieces of information that can be put into two algorithms. Clynes made measurements in different cultures all over the world and found that human beings tend to emote the same way. If we did not, we would not be human. It's almost a tautology. Then the brilliance came in. Klein took a computer, which played music—which tends not to be pleasing, computers being a little literal in their reading—and created an interactive program, which allowed cursors to make subtle rhythmic pulse changes in the computer playing. He was looking at what happened between different affective languages. He discovered not only that emotions have their own contours but that specific individuals have their own contours too. Klein has created what might be called archetypal forms for each major composer, and even non-musicians will tend to find the right form for the appropriate composer. There is a rightness, a justness about it. I believe that these things are recognizable in the way we walk, perhaps in our handwriting. They are certainly implicated in music.

As human beings we are driven, controlled, affected by pulse and rhythm. That is certain from our earliest days, even before we have a pulse of our own, when our mother's pulse is informing us. Changes in pulse are deeply significant to us and communicate emotion. In *Opus 50, No. 2* Beethoven uses a pulse identical to a foetal heartbeat. There is also a breathing melody. That is part of how we respond; it is what creates musical language. Breathing, walking, even the natural span of our arms, our movements, are all rhythmically defined and the connection between motion and emotion is no accident. We emote through movement and we change our emotion by changing our movements.

Music to Control Pain

Ralf Spintge, a German anaesthetist, uses music to control pain. "The first thing we see," he reported, "is that we can save sedative drugs for premedication. In anaesthesia and even in my pain clinic I can work without any sedative drugs nowadays. A group of patients who are going to get central nerve blocks, which is an unpleasant procedure, don't get a sedative drug for this procedure because they get music. This is an important thing for a doctor, but there's something more. You can obviously enhance the motivation of the patients for post-operative rehabilitation exercises. The co-operation, the compliance between patient and therapist is much improved."

Dr Spintge described how the music therapist designs programmes, which control the level of patients' activity. "We start with a simple melody done by a single instrument. Then we add voices, thus increasing the dynamic range of the piece of music, and this helps the patient to get up, to be more active. We keep it on a certain level and then we go back. We take away one voice after the other until we have again the single instrument with the simple melody, and it runs out. We have even designed it so that it follows exactly the time schedule of that procedure. It's 12 minutes and that's it. And it works nicely."

The obvious question is whether the music is merely distracting the patient or whether it is tying in to a more fundamental system. Dr Spintge believes that two factors are involved. "One is that it's a distraction. When you ask, especially young people, 'What do you feel when you, listen to that music?' they say 'I'm going away from this situation to my discotheque' or something like that. At the same time we have seen that we can significantly reduce the amount of pain experienced by the patient and we can significantly decrease the level of stress hormones in the blood. And not only with our European patients. I did the same research with Japanese, which is completely different cultural background, but it worked the same way."

But what is it in music that works the magic? "This is the decisive question," said Dr Spintge. "My feeling is, from all my experience, that it might be rhythm which is the main stimulus or the most important parameter. We are running a research programme where we are trying to combine the knowledge in neuro-physiology about the rhythmic control of all vital functions with music and rhythm."

Persistence of the Musical Response

That level of change is only because there are universal templates of response that are shared cross-culturally by all of us. We are designed to be musically responsive and when we lose the music we lose a great part of ourselves. It is almost certain that one in four of us will suffer Alzheimer's disease in our later years. As people lose themselves, along with the ability to recognise their nearest and dearest, finally not knowing who are where they are, it is common that the musical response remains. I met a lady who was deeply demented and could not even speak. She had been a piano teacher, and if she was in a room with a piano and someone began to sing, she would shamble across to the piano and begin playing, always in the right key. Suddenly a fully intact person was there, a laughing and happy person. Sadly, as soon as the music went, that person was lost.

Such things occur all the time. When my father was on his deathbed he was not demented but his body had given up long before the rest of him. It was Christmastime and all we could think of doing was to go in with the kids and play Christmas carols. My father was fiercely anti-religious and hadn't been to church for 70 years or more but he sat up in bed, despite the fact that he was in a desperate state, and for half an hour he sang carols, all the words of every verse from memory. They were deeply embedded in him with emotion connections.

This can happen with musical hallucinations, which we know are associated with precise areas of the brain. There was a man who got in his car to drive to see his family and found, to his delight, that in the car there was an uninterrupted medley of brass band music, which he loved . However, he was a bit disturbed when he got to the end of his journey, because the brass band music followed him into the house and continued day and night. It turned out that he had a fairly discrete lesion in the area of the brain that evokes specific musical memory. Interestingly, it would appear that those complete musical memories always belong to the ages between 8 and 12. We are locked into these extraordinarily precise musical developments. We need to know that individually and we need to known it culturally.

If we are losing our integrity as a person, for whatever reason, and music offers a way of reintegrating ourselves, that must be equally true of cultures. A culture can be cancerous, autistic or in a condition of terrible self-destruction, an act of madness. We know the human race is highly gifted to do this. Ordinary people with ordinary lives and ordinary aspirations can be caught up in it. Friends of mine went to Sarajevo during the siege and followed two young girls through streets where snipers were firing into an underground car park they called "Our Place". All those who went there risked their lives. Why did they go? Because the Sarajevo Philharmonic Orchestra was playing there.

It is now culturally possible to share the information I have been describing and for people to listen. It is also possible to explore much of this work in the language and the terms that our culture recognizes; at present this means scientific language. A number of groups want to go forwards and make a musical brain map. There are groups working with music therapy and music healing in war-torn areas. Nigel Osborne and I hope to set running the notion of a pan-European collaborative research project to map the musical brain. There is collaborative research on the use of music with dementia and Parkinson's disease. I am involved with groups which wish to further work on chronic pan.

Making Things Happen

All this needs to happen but unless there is active change at every level, personal, political, financial, these things cannot happen. The time is clearly right for these things to occur within the medical domain and the world of teaching. We live in a world which is beginning to focus not on morbid processes but on well-being. You cannot have well-being unless you are exploring yourself fully, and that includes an aesthetic experience of yourself, an emotional fulfilment.

I will end with a description of what is likely to remain the single most beautiful expression of anything I would seek to express about music, about how music is deeply implicated in what we are, how we become what we are as human beings, and our potential. We do not exist in isolation but know ourselves by means of a greater communication and a greater community. We can have a full exploration of ourselves not only through our minds and bodies but through our emotions too. Anything less and we are less than human.

My closing illustration concerns the inspired music therapist Paul Nordoff working with a child who was inhabiting his own personal Sarajevo. They had meetings of 10–15 minutes and on the first occasion the child could respond to human contact only by fighting, screaming and kicking. The music therapist simply played a simple tune repeatedly. At the third meeting the therapist was playing a simple melody followed by repeated chords. The child screamed less frequently and the therapist sang with the music. The ninth time they met, the child and the therapist repeated sounds and sang words made by each other. There was no screaming, only laughter.

Chapter 16

The Convulsionary Samuel Johnson and the Miaowing of Mozart

Milo Keynes

Introduction

The case for "the great convulsionary", Samuel Johnson, having the Gilles de la Tourette syndrome is necessarily circumstantial but entirely convincing. He was observed to have innumerable strange rituals and compulsions, tics, gesticulations, and a great range of involuntary ejaculations and mimicries. Sacks[1] has written that "one cannot avoid thinking that his enormous spontaneity, antics, and lightning quick wit had an organic connection with his accelerated motor impulsive state".

In 1985, Fog and Regeur[2] suggested at a congress of psychiatry in Vienna the possibility that Mozart's "tics and vocalisations" might be explained by the Tourette syndrome. It will be argued, however, that with Mozart the hyperactivity, tics, sudden impulses and odd motor behaviours, echolalia, palilalia (rapid repetition of words and phrases) and driven inner rhythms that so often accompany the syndrome were not manifest.[3,4]

In mediaeval times the syndrome of involuntary movements and bizarre vocalisations often employing foul language was taken as evidence of diabolical possession, and could be treated by burning. In 1884, Georges Gilles de la Tourette (1855–1909) joined the great neurologist J.M. Charcot (1825–1893) at the Salpêtrière in Paris, and, as he had already shown interest in convulsive movement disorders, Charcot directed him to make further study of these. Gilles de la Tourette published his classic description[5] of the syndrome that bears his name the next year when he described nine cases and insisted it was a neurological disorder and not a form of insanity or psychiatric illness. His career after this was brief, as in 1893 he was shot in the head by a paranoid young woman who believed herself to be under his hypnotic influence, though he did not die until 1909 from a different sort of brain damage, that of neurosyphilis.

Gilles de la Tourette Syndrome

Tourette's syndrome, which is inherited as an autosomal dominant with variable penetrance, is an uncommon disorder that has its onset in childhood, and in most cases the initial symptom is of involuntary tic-like movements, which are irregular and brisk.[6] The face is most commonly affected with eye-blinking and grimacing, followed with diminishing frequency by more caudal parts of the body. About 50% of patients develop more complicated movements, such as stamping or uncontrollable touching of people or objects.[7]

Abnormal vocalisations are eventually produced by all patients, though this is rare as an initial symptom. They can be meaningless grunts, barks, hisses or whistles, the production of formed words, sudden cursing and swearing, or coprolalia. The symptom of coprolalia (literally "babbling about faeces") is seen in about 50% of cases, and usually consists of forced utterance of single obscenities, but rarely can take the form of elaborate phrases or sentences; it spontaneously disappears in about one-third of patients in later life.[6] Echolalia (the forced repetition of heard words or phrases) is only observed in 20% of cases.

Tourette's syndrome is not truly progressive, but has a fluctuating course. Complete remission is rare, but the symptoms change over a period of months, both in severity and in the groups of muscles affected. Patients can usually suppress their symptoms for short periods, though this may be terminated by an explosive outburst. Symptoms disappear during sleep, lessen with rest or on concentration, but are made worse by anxiety and stress.[6]

There are different forms of the disease. At one extreme is the stereotypic form with simple motor tics, iterations, perseverations, and brief, explosive vocalisations. At the other extreme is an elaborate, innovatory, phantasmagoric form which is remarkable for its mimicry, antics, playfulness, extravagance, inventions and dramatisations.[1] Stereotypic Tourette's syndrome is usually distressing, though perhaps little more than an annoyance, but phantasmagoric Tourette's syndrome, while it may cause distress and disability, interacts with a person's character, stimulating perception and imagination, though whether creativity is truly enhanced is uncertain.

The Convulsionary Samuel Johnson

Samuel Johnson (1709–1784) had miserable health all his life, with extreme myopia, deafness, the scrofula, dyspepsia, emphysema, chronic bronchitis, gout, a stroke, dropsy and "morbid melancholy", besides his convulsive movements and vocalisations.[4] Writing about Johnson was long an interest of the great neurologist Russell Brain, FRS (1895–1966), later Lord Brain. In his collection of essays, *Some Reflections on Genius*,[8] the chapter entitled "The Great Convulsionary" furnishes much of the evidence for making the diagnosis of Tourette's syndrome. Brain firmly believed that Johnson's movements—mainly because the movements were not involuntary, but also because of the compulsive element in the elaborate rituals, with Johnson's inner need to perform the ceremonials correctly, and to repeat the performance if any detail was omitted—showed a psychic pattern, and were due to a purely psychological disorder and not due to organic brain disease. In this he was followed by L.C. McHenry,[9] and both, in effect, disagreed with the diagnosis of Tourette syndrome championed by T.J. Murray[10] in 1979. Other diagnoses have included Sydenham's chorea, epilepsy and athetoid cerebral palsy.

It is unclear at what age Johnson's abnormal movements began, but there are descriptions of his awkwardness as a child, and at the age of seven his appearance was described "as little better than that of an idiot". A teacher said of him while he was at Lichfield Grammar School that he was "a great overgrown boy, rolling clumsily about on his form as his body in some peculiar way responded to his mental efforts".[11] The first clear accounts of his convulsive starts and odd gesticulations appear in the diaries of his friends when he was a young man, though Johnson himself hardly ever referred to them, either in conversation or in writing. Many found it difficult to reconcile his superb intellect, eloquence and wit with his slovenly appearance, and on first meeting him were often surprised and shocked by his tics and gesticulations.

Johnson's movements included grimacing, mouth opening, eye blinks, lip twitching and shoulder, arm and leg jerks. He was refused several jobs as a teacher because of what was called a haughty, ill-natured manner and facial grimacing, and because his bizarre movements might have become the subject of ridicule with the schoolchildren. When Johnson began his own school at Edial in his mid-twenties, David Garrick (1717–1779), who was one of his three pupils, used to find his oddities and mannerisms amusing, and would imitate them, even in later life, much to Johnson's annoyance.[11] Frances Reynolds (1729–1807),[12] Sir Joshua's painter sister, remembered how men, women and children gathered round him, laughing and jeering at his extraordinary gestures.

Fanny Burney (1752–1840), who became Mme d'Arblay on marriage in 1793, gave a vivid portrait[13] of Johnson:

> "He is, indeed, very ill-favoured! Yet he has naturally a noble figure; tall, stout, grand and authorative: but he stoops horribly; his back is quite round: his mouth is continually opening and shutting, as if he were chewing something; he has a singular method of twirling his fingers, and twisting his hands: his vast body is in constant agitation, see-sawing backwards and forwards: his feet are never a moment quiet; and his whole great person looked often as if it were going to roll itself, quite voluntarily, from his chair to the floor."

The most detailed account[12] of his movements is that given by Frances Reynolds when she describes:

> "... his extraordinary gestures or anticks with his hands and feet, particularly when passing over the threshold of a Door, or rather before he would venture to pass through any door-way.... But the strange positions in which he would place his feet (generally I think before he began his straddles, as if necessarily preparatory) are scarcely credible. Sometimes he would make the back part of his heels to touch, sometimes the extremity of his toes, as if endeavouring to form a triangle, or some geometrical figure, and as for his gestures with his hands, they were equally strange: sometimes he would hold them up with some of his fingers bent, as if he had been seized with the cramp, and sometimes at his Breast in motion like those of a jockey on full speed; and often would he lift them up as high as he could stretch over his head for some minutes. But the manoeuvre that used the most particularly to engage the attention of the company was his stretching out his arm with a full cup of tea in his hand, in every direction, often to the great annoyance of the person who sat next to him, indeed to the imminent danger of their cloaths, perhaps of a Lady's Court dress; sometimes he would twist himself round with his face close to the back of his chair, and finish his cup of tea, breathing very hard, as if making a laborious effort to accomplish it.
>
> "What could have induced him to practise such extraordinary gestures who can divine: his head, his hands and his feet often in motion at the same time. Many people have supposed that they were natural effects of a nervous disorder, but had that been the case he could not have sat still when he chose, which he did, and so still when sitting for his picture.... It was not only at the entrance of a Door that he exhibited his gigantick straddles, but often in the middle of a Room, as if trying to make the floor to shake."

James Boswell (1740–1795)[14] in his biography describes how Johnson, "while talking or even musing as he sat in his chair, he commonly held his head to one side towards his right shoulder, and shook it in a tremulous manner, moving his body backwards and forwards, and rubbing his left knee in the same direction, with the palm of his hand." Lord Chesterfield (1694–1773) wrote in a letter to his son on 28 February 1751[15]:

> "His figure (without being deformed) seems made to disgrace or ridicule the common structure of the human body. His legs and arms are never in the position which according to the situation of his body they ought to be in. They are constantly employed in committing acts of hostility on the graces."

Johnson's eccentricities were not limited to "convulsions" but included involuntary vocalisations. While sitting in a tavern or a private drawing room, or when walking in the street, Johnson was often noted to talk to himself, when, according to Boswell, he might utter "pious ejaculations, for sometimes his voice grows stronger, and parts of the Lord's Prayer have been distinctly overheard", and sometimes he could be heard repeating snippets of Shakespeare or lines from an ode of Horace. Other mouthings were the blurting out of grunts, hummings and whistles, besides other meaningless and unintelligible moans, clucking sounds, sighs and heavy breathing, as well as the echolalia, or repetitions of phrases and poems or expressions just heard.

The best account of his involuntary vocalisation comes from Boswell[14]:

> "In the intervals of articulating he made various sounds with his mouth, sometimes as if ruminating, or what is called chewing the cud, sometimes giving a half whistle, sometimes making his tongue play backwards from the roof of his mouth, as if clucking like a hen, and sometimes protruding it against his upper gums in front, as if pronouncing quickly under his breath, *too, too, too*: all this accompanied sometimes with a thoughtful look, but more frequently with a smile. Generally when he had concluded a period, in the course of a dispute, by which time he was a good deal exhausted by violence and vociferation, he used to blow out his breath like a Whale. This I supposed was a relief to his lungs; and seemed in him to be a contemptuous mode of expression, as if he had made the arguments of his opponent fly like chaff before the wind."

We cannot be sure that Johnson's vocalisations were not scatological, as this may have been covered up by his friends in their writings. For instance, Mrs Piozzi, in whose house, when she was Mrs Thrale, Johnson had resided from 1765 to 1781, remarked: "... hearing a man [*Johnson*] so wildly proclaim what he could at least persuade no one to believe; and what, if true, would only have been so very unfit to reveal."[16] He was never known to swear, and had a low opinion of those who did. He once asked a man to desist from using profanities and left the room when he refused to do so. But, if his vocalisations had been scatological, it would have been something that his religiosity could hardly have endured.

In this discussion, Johnson's complex obsessional compulsive behaviour, as further described by Frances Reynolds,[12] has been little mentioned, with its elaborate rituals and his inner need to perform the ceremonials correctly and to repeat the performance if any detail had been omitted. Boswell[14] described Johnson's odd habit of always measuring his way out of a room with his feet. He would start off step by step until he reached the doorway. If he arrived there on the wrong foot he would go back and do it again until he came to the door with the correct foot. Boswell also made references to Johnson's tendency to mild self-destructive or damaging behaviour, such as continually hitting his legs, as well as rubbing them, and also cutting his fingernails deeply. Boswell said: "Not only did he pare his nails to the quick, but scraped the joints of his fingers with a pen-knife till they seemed quite red and raw." Some of Johnson's other compulsive habits included never walking on the cracks between paving stones and touching every post along the street or road as he walked. If he missed a post he would keep his friends waiting while he went back to touch it.

Jadresic[17] has discussed obsessionality, and Murray[10] compulsivity and the tendency to carry out self-destructive acts, in patients with Gilles de la Tourette syndrome. Samuel Johnson's symptoms fit best into the group of patients in whom the presentation is dominated by obsessional compulsive behavioural rituals and mannerisms, with relatively few tics and vocalisations.[18]

The Miaowing of Mozart

Karoline Pichler (1769–1843), a poet and diarist, mentioned in her memoirs[19] Mozart's scatty behaviour and joker mentality, his character shown up by silly jokes and an irresponsible way of life, with his inability, she thought, to show any great intellectual capacity beyond his music. She recalled an incident where, when making an improvisation on *Non più andrai* (from Act I of *Figaro*),

> ". . . he suddenly tired of it, jumped up, and in the mad mood which so often came over him, he began to leap over tables and chairs, miaow like a cat, and turn somersaults like an unruly boy."

In subsequent literature this single miaowing incident has been recounted as if it occurred many times, and has become a major reason for diagnosing Tourette's syndrome in Mozart.

Eleven out of 25 people who recorded their personal memories of Wolfgang Mozart (1756–1791) later told of his perpetual movements and mannerisms, which have been called facial and bodily tics by some.[20] Schlichtegroll wrote of Mozart in *Nekrolog*[21]:

> "He was thin and pale; and although the actual shape of his face was extraordinary, his expression was memorable in nothing save in its extreme variability. His features would alter from one instant to another, yet never revealing anything save the pleasure or distress that he happened to feel in that immediate instant. He had one inveterate habit or idiosyncrasy which, as a general rule, is a symptom of stupidity: his body was perpetually in motion; he would play incessantly with his hands, or tap restlessly on the floor with his feet."

In 1828, Sophie Haibel (1763–1864), youngest sister of Mozart's wife, Constanze (1762–1842), wrote in her memoir[22] of Mozart's continual movement, which here sounds to have been more like mannerism than classical tic:

> "Even when he was washing his hands in the morning, he paced up and down. . . . never standing still, tapping one heel against the other. . . and always deep in thought. At table, he would often twist up and tightly crumple a corner of a napkin and rub it to and fro across his upper lip, while appearing to be unaware of what he was doing, and often making extraordinary grimaces with his mouth at the same time. In his leisure he was always passionately attached to the latest fad, whether it was riding or billiards. To keep him from company of an unworthy kind, his wife patiently shared everything with him. Otherwise his hands and feet were always in motion, he was forever playing with something, for instance his hat, pockets, watch-fob, tables, chairs—as if they were the keyboard of a clavier."

And Constanze's eldest sister, Josepha Hofer (1758–1819), reiterated "the restless movements of his hands" and the "movements of his lips" at the opera, while Constanze herself told of his impatient stamping with his feet and his *Sapperlotte* exclamations when things did not go smoothly at orchestral rehearsals. She also mentioned his ability to do something else at the same time as composing, that he composed walking about the apartment, quite abstracted, and how he would then sit down by her, ask for ink and paper, and notate the music as she recounted the day's events at his request.[23] She added that "he could never entirely abstract himself from his musical thoughts, and composed while playing billiards, or conversing with friends". Otto Jahn wrote in his biography[24] of Mozart:

> "We have already observed that musical ideas occupied him during all bodily exercises, such as riding, bowls and billiard playing. General conversation, as Frau Haibel says, did not disturb his mental labours."

What is known about Mozart's "movements" has now been described, but, before considering his "vocalisations", what of his behaviour that has been described as "flamboyant, frivolous and hypomanic"[25]? Mozart's prickly social sensitivity, with his concern for proper behaviour, was likely in part to have derived from the feeling of social disadvantage that his short stature of 4 feet 11 inches (1.5 m) would have given him, as there was then such a large height difference between the nobility and upper classes and the working classes.[26]

He was not helped by his physical appearance, and could be found unattractive with his strangely shaped head, pale and pockmarked face, large nose, receding chin and deformed left ear, though with, according to the Irish tenor Michael Kelly (1762–1826), a "profusion of fine fair hair, of which he was rather vain", which most of the time he kept tidy and elegantly powdered. Mozart tended to dress in keeping with the fashion of the day, and favoured expensive clothes in vivid colours, particularly red, regarded as extravagant by some, but more likely was all too necessary for the maintenance of his social position and in moving comfortably in aristocratic circles.

With his undistinguished appearance, and lacking in charisma and the elementary graces and skills necessary for easy communication with others, Mozart appears to have had an arrogant, frustrated, childish and irresponsible character, though not one with obsessional features. He had an extremely optimistic nature, as well as high self-esteem: the possibility of failure was inconceivable. He delighted in creativity, exulted in showing brilliance and innovation in his musical composition and performance, and enjoyed astonishing his audiences. He needed public acclaim, but with his exuberant self-confidence and, seeming correctly to sense that he was more important than other musicians, his obvious awareness of his supreme musical talent could be irritating to others. To his contemporaries he was capricious, hurtful, tactless and spiteful in a world dominated by birth, patronage and privilege, where natural ability counted for little.

From childhood Mozart showed a lifelong penchant for nonsense words and odd-sounding names and nicknames—he wrote nonsense letters or quasi-nonsense passages in his correspondence with his family, and relished puns, "spoonerisms", anagrams, repetitions and word alliterations and assonances.[25,27] There is, besides, the scatology—use of "filthy" words particularly relating to excrement and defecation, though not pornography—found in his letters.[28]

There are, however, only three instances of Mozart speaking such filthy words—twice when he told of it in letters to his father in October and

November 1777, and once when it was mentioned in the autobiography[23] of his brother-in-law, Joseph Lange (1751–1831), written in 1808:

> "Never was Mozart less recognisably a great man in his conversation and actions than when he was busied with an important work. At such times he not only spoke confusedly and disconnectedly, but occasionally made jests of a nature which one did not expect of him, indeed he even deliberately forgot himself in his behaviour.... Either he intentionally concealed his inner tensions behind superficial frivolity...or he took delight in throwing into sharp contrast the divine ideas of his music and these sudden outbursts of commonplace banalities, and in giving himself pleasure by seeming to make fun of himself."

Here there is just a suggestion that the obscenities were spoken illogically and inappropriately, but in the two letters the obscene words were placed appropriately to the context, such as:

> "I did frequently, without any difficulty, but quite easily, perpetrate... rhymes, the same being, moreover, sheer garbage, that is, on such subjects as muck, shitting and arse-licking."[27]

The scatology in the letters was first exposed in English in 1938 when Emily Anderson published her edition of the letters of the Mozart family.[27] Examination of the 374 letters written by Wolfgang Mozart shows scatological writing (coprographia) in 39, or 10.5%, which mention shit (29 times), arse and arse hole (27), muck (17), fart (6), piddling or pissing (6),[28] but without the words being placed illogically, if not inappropriately. Twenty-three of all Mozart's letters (6.2%) contain obvious word games and word scrambling, repetitions of words just heard or written by someone else, and repetitions of his own words—the last two called, respectively, "echographia" and "paligraphia" by Simkin.[28] Simkin found that the coprographia–echographia–paligraphia in 63, or 17%, of the letters occurred at periods of stress in 1770, 1777–81, 1783, 1789 and 1791, and that the recipients of the "unusual" letters were principally—as for the vast majority of the correspondence that remains—five close relatives, with only one each to four friends.

Mozart's behaviour has already been considered, and in considering the question of hypomania (or of him showing the hyperactivity of Gilles de la Tourette syndrome), it is likely that some of the possible episodes of it were associated with his musical self-confidence, such as the exhilaration of sustained creativity, or the euphoria that follows public performance. But can the times when he apparently showed sudden impulses, great productivity, reduced need for sleep, gregariousness, love of nonsense words, punning and inappropriate joking, and frivolous and odd behaviour be accepted as periods of hypomania? I do not think there is nearly enough certainty to answer in the affirmative.

From the foregoing, I do not think that Mozart suffered from Gilles de la Tourette syndrome: to do so presupposes that his movement mannerisms were true tics, and that the hyperactivity shown by the sudden impulses, odd behaviour and love of nonsense words was part of the disease. Bearing out the experience of clinical neurologists, there is no mention in the medical literature of coprographia as a symptom of the syndrome. If there were, the filthy words might be expected to occur, at least at times, in an inappropriate and uncontrolled manner, as they do in coprolalia, and this was a symptom that Mozart does not appear to have had. It is not known whether or not the symptoms, if they were those of Tourette's syndrome, started in childhood or adolescence, or whether there was a family history of this genetic disorder. The absence of a description of compulsive involuntary movements in the symptomatology, with only the controlled presence of obscenities in the letters in way of scatology, rules out the diagnosis of Tourette's syndrome in Mozart.

References

1. O. Sacks, Tourette's syndrome and creativity, *B.M.J.* **305**, 1515–6 (1992).
2. R. Fog and L. Regeur, Did Mozart suffer from Tourette's syndrome? *Proceedings of World Congress of Psychiatry* (Vienna, 1985).
3. M. Keynes, The personality and illnesses of Wolfgang Amadeus Mozart, *J. Med. Biography* **2**, 217–32 (1994).
4. M. Keynes, The miserable health of Dr Samuel Johnson, *J. Med. Biography* **3**, 161–9 (1995).
5. G. Gilles de la Tourette, *Étude sur une affection nerveuse, caraterisée par de l'incoordination motrice, accompagnée d'écholalie et de coprolalie*, *Arch. Neurol. (Paris)* **9**, 19–42, 158–200 (1885).
6. M. Lawden, Gilles de la Tourette syndrome: a review, *J.R.S.M.* **79**, 282–8 (1986).
7. A.J. Lees, M. Robertson, M.R. Trimble and N.M.F. Murray, A clinical study of Gilles de la Tourette syndrome in the United Kingdom, *J. Neurol. Neurosurg. Psychiatry* **47**, 1–8 (1984).
8. R. Brain, The Great Convulsionary. In *Some Reflections on Genius* (Pitman, London, 1960).
9. L.C. McHenry, Neurological disorders of Dr Samuel Johnson, *J.R.S.M.* **78**, 485–91 (1985).
10. T.J. Murray, Dr Samuel Johnson's movement disorder, *B.M.J.* **i**, 1610–4 (1979).
11. G.B. Hill (ed.), *Johnsonian Miscellanies* (Oxford, 1897), 2 vols.

12. F. Reynolds, in *Johnsonian Miscellanies*, G.B. Hill (ed.) (Oxford, 1897), 2 vols.
13. Mme. d'Arblay [Frances (Fanny) Burney], *Diary and Letters of Mme. d'Arblay, 1842–6*, A. Dobson (ed.) (London, 1904–5), 6 vols.
14. J. Boswell, *The Life of Samuel Johnson LL.D.* (C. Dilly, London, 1787), 2 vols.
15. Earl of Chesterfield, *Letters Written by the Late Right Honourable Philip Dormer Stanhope, Earl of Chesterfield, to His Son, Philip Stanhope* (J. Dodsley, London, 1774), 2 vols.
16. H.L. Piozzi (formerly Mrs Thrale), *Anecdotes of the Late Samuel Johnson, LL.D., During the Last Twenty Years of His Life* (T. Payne, London, 1786).
17. D. Jadresic, Obsessionality in Tourette syndrome, *Lancet* **341**, 1063 (1993).
18. A.J. Lees, Gilles de la Tourette syndrome & some celebrated ticqueurs. In: *Tics and Related Disorders* (Churchill Livingstone, Edinburgh, 1985).
19. K. Pichler, *Denkwürdigkeiten aus meinem Leben,* E.K. Blümml (ed.) (Munich, 1915).
20. B. Simkin, The case for Mozart's affliction with Tourette syndrome, *J. Conductor's Guild* **12**, 50–64 (1991).
21. F. Schlichtegroll, Nekrolog (1793). In: H.B. Stendahl, *Haydn, Mozart and Metastasio* (1814), R.N. Coe (ed.) (Calder & Boyars, London, 1972).
22. S. Haibel, Memoir of W.A. Mozart, 1828. In: O.E. Deutsch, *Mozart: A Documentary Biography*, transl. E. Blom, P. Branscombe and J. Noble (Adam & Charles Black, London, 1965).
23. O.E. Deutsch, *Mozart: A Documentary Biography*, transl. E. Blom, P. Branscombe and J. Noble (Adam & Charles Black, London, 1965).
24. O. Jahn, *W. A. Mozart*, 4 vols. (Leipzig, 1856–9); *Life of Mozart*, transl. P.D. Townsend, 3 vols. (Novello, Ewer & Co, London, 1891).
25. P.J. Davies, Mozart's manic-depressive tendencies, *J.R.S.M.* **128**, 123–6, 191–6 (1987).
26. A. Steptoe, *The Mozart–Da Ponte Operas* (Clarendon, Oxford, 1988).
27. E. Anderson (ed.), *The Letters of Mozart and His Family* (Macmillan, London, 1938).
28. B. Simkin, Mozart's scatological disorder, *B.M.J.* **305**, 1563–7 (1992).

Chapter 17

The Influence of Shakespeare on Charcot's Neurological Teaching

Christopher G. Goetz

Introduction

J.-M. Charcot was the first Clinical Professor of Diseases of the Nervous System at the Salpêtrière Hospital in Paris (Figure 1). He conducted dramatic teaching sessions in the hospital amphitheater twice weekly, a carefully rehearsed lecture on Fridays, and an impromptu case discussion on Tuesdays.[1] Whereas the Friday lectures presented Charcot's scientific ideas in their clearest form, the Tuesday lessons focused on Charcot's diagnostic methods in a relaxed and natural manner.[2,3] In the Tuesday presentations, he drew on references from many cultural and historical backgrounds. Knowing that his audience was composed of nonmedical as well as medical observers, and foreign as well as French-speaking participants, Charcot drew on examples from art, history, and literature to illustrate his diagnostic points and complement the patient material he discussed.

Although not an admirer of most poetry, Charcot showed a special respect for Shakespeare and cited the Englishman's quotations on frequent occasions (Figure 2). Charcot's incorporation of Shakespearean citations into his neurological teaching served several purposes. Occasionally, he drew on Shakespeare's words to illustrate a specific neurological observation. More often, he lauded Shakespeare as an exemplary observer of human behavior and emphasized the clinical importance of careful and dispassionate documentation. In these broader references, he used Shakespeare's words to communicate philosophical principles related to the field of medicine and the role the physician. Outside these professional contexts, Charcot's personal anglophilia brought Shakespeare into his family life and social circles. In using quotations from

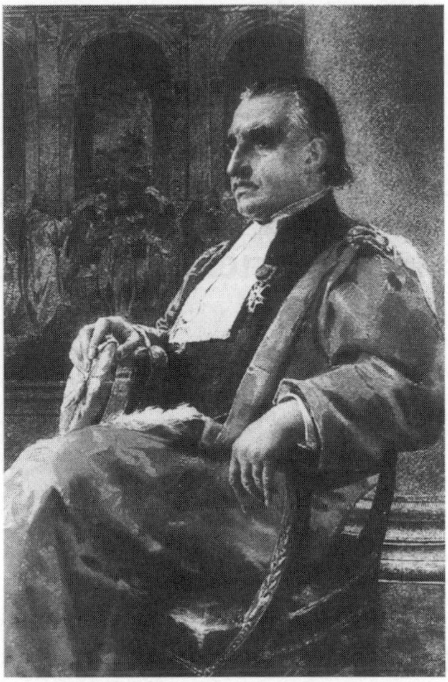

Fig. 1. Portrait of Jean-Martin Charcot (1825–1893) in his academic robes.[1]

Shakespeare on a frequent basis, Charcot effectively presented himself as a worldly man of culture before his international audience, his students, friends, and family, creating an appropriate image of sophistication that belied his very humble working class origins.

Shakespeare's Neurological Observations

Modern analysts have documented the neurological richness of Shakespeare's writing, especially in the depiction of epilepsy (*Julius Caesar*, *The Tempest*, *King Lear*, *Henry IV* [Part 2], *Othello*).[4] In a case of a seizure patient whose epileptic attacks (probably absence status) included ambulations through Paris in an unconscious daze, Charcot discussed references to Shakespeare in his consideration of the possible diagnosis of somnambulism. He stated to his students: "I would not profess to be an expert on somnambulism, and in fact, there are no experts on this subject."[3] Afterwards, Charcot's students were assigned night watch duty to observe somnambulic episodes, and thereby witnessed his patients' spells firsthand. The resultant observations were some of the earliest medical descriptions of such nocturnal behaviors.

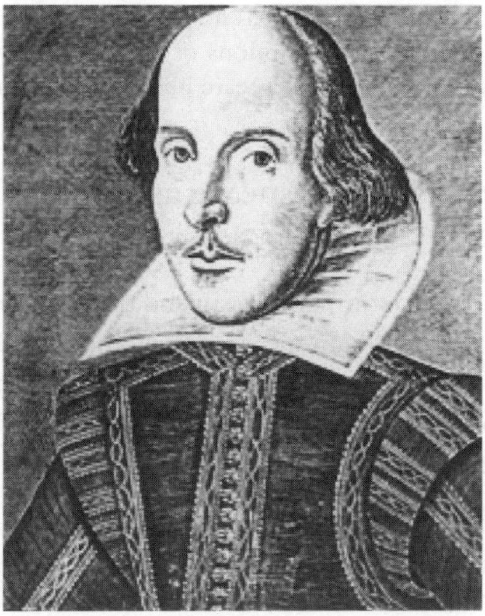

Fig. 2. Portrait of William Shakespeare.

For addedinformation, however, Charcot suggested that his audience refer to Shakespeare:

> "His eyes were open. In *Macbeth* there is a very significant observation on somnambulism. The doctor sees Lady Macbeth get up and begin her somnambulic activity, turns to the other characters on stage, and, supposing them better informed than they are, exclaims: 'Look, her eyes are open!' Indeed, in somnambulism, whether the eyes are open or closed is the most important question. . . . Shakespeare . . . was a remarkable medical observer. Shakespeare and Joseph Franck give in fact the same definition of somnambulism; such an agreement between poet and physician is singularly remarkable."[3]

Charcot also used Shakespeare as a neurological reference source in the context of the disputed diagnosis of "senile tremor". As an outgrowth of his studies of Parkinson's disease and multiple sclerosis, Charcot developed an extensive classification of tremor types, based on their frequency and the activities that provoked them. Taking an adamant stand against the concept that tremor was a natural accompaniment of normal aging, he rejected "senile tremor" as a separate nosographic entity. After reviewing his data from the Salpêtrière service where 2000 elderly inpatients lived, he turned to Shakespeare's renditions of elderly figures:

> "Do not commit the error that many others do and misrepresent tremor as a natural accompaniment of old age. Remember that our venerated Dean,

> Dr. Chevreul, today 102 years old, has no tremor whatsoever. And you must remember in his marvelous descriptions of old age (*Henry IV* and *As You Like It*), the master observer Shakespeare never speaks of tremor."[3]

Broader References: Shakespeare as Observer and Philosopher

Although the references to somnambulism and tremor were directly applicable to a medical diagnosis in a Shakespearean play, most Shakespearean citations in Charcot's teaching were used for more general emphasis. Henry Meige, Charcot's student and colleague, wrote on the professor's special respect for Shakespeare's skills:

> "With a well-known reverence, he honored Shakespeare, whom he had read and reread and whose writing he annotated by hand. He particularly prized the English playwright's philosophy as it was based on an attentive study of nature. In Shakespeare's work, Charcot saw a model for analyzing human sentiments and passions. He found in Shakespeare the same rigorous observational technique of the human race that he himself applied in clinical medicine."[5]

Charcot turned to Shakespeare's keen philosophical views when he analyzed neurological disease and the role of the physician. Speaking on the diagnosis of repetitive movements that he termed "rhythmic chorea" but that today would likely be diagnosed as psychogenic mannerisms, Charcot stated:

> "Rhythm and cadence, these are the characteristic features that I have stressed as the hallmarks of so many hysterical phenomena. In rhythmic chorea, specifically, the rhythm is so regular that a ballet master could record and reproduce the strange and often complex movements executed by these patients in the midst of their spells. 'There is a method in their madness,' as Shakespeare wrote in *Hamlet*."[3]

The "method" in Charcot's allusion referred to the methodical reproducibility of the movements, and not to a psychological motive. Charcot prided himself on his observational impartiality, stating: "In fact all I am is a photographer."[3] He left the analysis of his patients' psychological "methods" entirely to his later students, including Freud.

In another broader reference, Charcot used Shakespeare to explain the benefit of sleep to his audience. Although Charcot's interest in sleep focused primarily on abnormal and induced states, specifically somnambulism, hysterical sleep, and hypnotic trances, he also appreciated the important restorative function of normal sleep, especially in a patient recovering from neurological injury. In discussing such a case, he said:

> "He walks better, suggesting that his arachnoid pain has abated. His sleep is no longer disrupted by terrifying nightmares; one can even say that it has become for him 'the balm of hurt minds,' as Shakespeare says."[3]

Charcot's main neurological contribution was his application of the *méthode anatomoclinique*, whereby he correlated specific clinical signs with discreet neuroanatomical lesions.[1] This discipline involved the careful examination and clinical documentation of patients throughout the evolution of their neurological disease and painstaking autopsy analysis after death. The two-arm process was feasible only at a large institution like the Salpêtrière, where patients lived chronically and died as wards of the state. Although Charcot was an active practicing neurologist with a large private clientele, his investment in treatments and interventions was always modest in comparison to his scientific studies of natural disease progression.[6] In teaching his students about the variety of diseases and the gamut of neurological manifestations, he emphasized that nature outstripped man's imagination. He closed his final work, *Faith Healing* (*La foi qui guérit*), with the following Shakespearean quotation:

> There are more things in heaven and earth than are dreamt of in your philosophy.[7]

Against the vast array of degenerative and progressive illnesses surrounding him, Charcot became a somber and fatalistic scientist. In his dark, monastic study, he painted Shakespearean quotations, evoking the vanity of life and the futility of medicine:

> As flies to wanton boys, are we to the gods,
> They kill us for their sport.

Shakespeare in Charcot's Personal Life

Charcot's interest in Shakespeare extended to his private life, and his reverence for the English poet was longstanding and common knowledge to his family and friends.[8,9] On St Martin's Day, November 11th, Charcot's children and pupils regularly prepared a revue or theatrical program based on Shakespeare. In his biography of Charcot, Guillain recounts how these productions were staged in the professor's private study, and how, as the party date approached, Charcot always conveniently allowed himself to be chased from his otherwise private sanctum (Figure 3).[8]

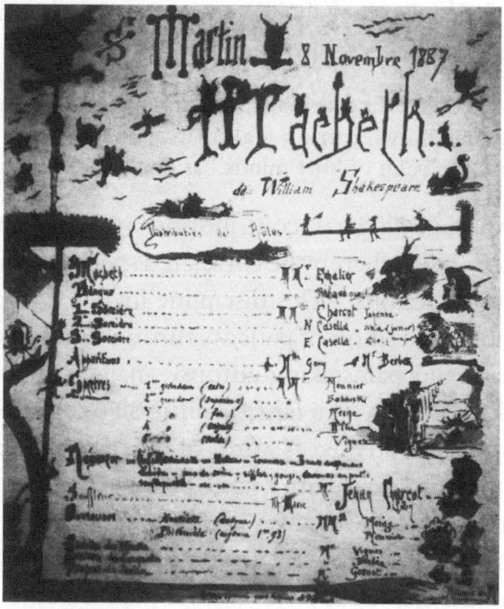

Fig. 3. Program from 1887 St Martin's Day celebration (Charcot's saint day) in the Charcot home, with Charcot's students and children in the cast.[1]

Charcot's intimate and eccentric friend, Duchenne de Boulogne, also had an interest in Shakespeare. For his classic photographic essay on the muscles of facial expression, G.B.A. Duchenne selected an actress dressed as Lady Macbeth and photographed her assuming a wide variety of facial poses to capture the nuances of cruelty and suffering (Figure 4).[10]

One aspect of Shakespeare's dramas especially appreciated by Charcot as a clinician was the particular mixture of the real and the unreal. Ghosts and spirits haunt the stage of many of Shakespeare's masterpieces, and Charcot was known to marvel at these characters, especially the sorceresses in *Macbeth*.[9] Charcot similarly marveled at the spectacular behaviors of the hysterics who crowded his wards, and whose symptoms were often mixtures of real and elaborated disease. He spent much of his research effort analyzing the bizarre behaviors of his hysterical patients who often unwittingly mimicked the witches and spirits of the Shakespearean stage. He coauthored the text *Les démoniaques dans l'art*, in which he found examples from paintings, etchings, and sculpture of subjects who would have fit his diagnosis of hysteria but could easily have played the supernatural scenes of Shakespearean drama.[11]

Where and when Charcot would have been originally exposed to Shakespeare remains unclear. He grew up as the son of a carriage builder

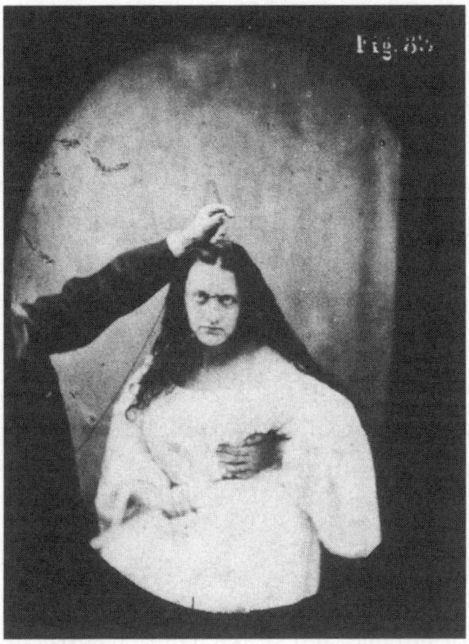

Fig. 4. Duchenne de Boulogne, Charcot's close friend and colleague, conducting electrical stimulation of selected facial muscles. In this photograph, the experimental subject is an actress in the role of Lady Macbeth. Duchenne uses the electrical stimulator to induce selected forehead muscle contraction to reveal the expression of cruelty "under the impression of her horrible invocation."[10]

and decorator in the working class environment of central Paris, and it is unlikely that exposure to Shakespeare came from his younger years at home or school. After medical school, Charcot had the fortune to be employed by a wealthy financier, Fould, and thereby began his European travels as a private physician.[9] He traveled to Italy, but there is no mention of England in his early medical years. After his marriage, his economic security was assured, and he traveled more widely. His son's childhood letters document that the family evacuated Paris in 1870 at the time of the anticipated Prussian invasion. Although Charcot stayed behind to continue his hospital responsibilities during the crisis, the family relocated to London, where Charcot visited them at least once.[12] The Charcot family had a number of English friends, and during his years as a professor, Charcot was known to have grandly entertained political, medical, and cultural personages of all nationalities in his palatial mansion on the Boulevard St Germain.[1] As evidenced by his private library and the extensive correspondence that still exists, he read and corresponded in English with ease. From the available evidence, however, it is most logical to estimate that he developed these skills primarily during his middle years.

Clearly, Charcot's references to Shakespeare did not occur in isolation. During his classroom presentations, citations from *Tristram Shandy*, other English works, and numerous British authors revealed his anglophilia. Such literary allusions were balanced by references to other cultures, leaving the modern reader of his classroom notes with the impression of a well-read, multifaceted, and highly cultured gentleman. A great advocate of visual art, Charcot himself was a painter and ceramist as well as a modest art collector, priding himself on paintings primarily from the Flemish and Dutch realism schools. He and his wife were both familiar faces within the art world of his epoch.[13] In this larger context, his familiarity with Shakespeare served Charcot in a social sense, conscious or unconscious, to create the image of a refined member of the *fin de siècle* bourgeoisie.

References

1. C.G. Goetz, M. Bonduelle and T. Gelfand, *Charcot: Constructing Neurology* (Oxford University Press, New York, 1995).
2. J.-M. Charcot, *Oeuvres Complètes*, 9 volumes (Bureaux du Progrès Médical, Paris, 1874–1892).
3. J.-M. Charcot, *Leçons du Mardi à la Salpêtrière* (Bureaux du Progrès Médical, Paris, 1887–1888). [Specific references cited by dates of classroom presentations: somnambulism, Jan. 31, 1888; tremor, July 24, 1888; rhythmical chorea, Oct. 23, 1888; Charcot as photographer, Feb. 7, 1888; sleep, Dec. 18, 1888.]
4. A.C. Kail, *The Medical Mind of Shakespeare* (Williams and Wilkins, Philadelphia, 1986).
5. H. Meige, Charcot artiste, *Nouv Icon Salpêtrière* **11**, 489–516 (1898) (citation, p. 504).
6. C.G. Goetz and M. Bonduelle, Charcot as therapeutic interventionist and treating neurologist, *Neurology* **45**, 2102–6 (1995).
7. J.M. Charcot, *La foi qui guérit, Revue Hebdomadaire* 7, 112–32 (1892) (citation, p. 132).
8. G. Guillain, *JM Charcot, His Life, His Work* (Hoeber, New York, 1959).
9. A. Souques and H. Meige, Charcot, *Biogr. Méd.* **13**, 321–52 (1939).
10. G.B.A. Duchenne, *Mécanisme de la physionomie humaine* (Renovard, Paris, 1862).
11. J.-M. Charcot and P. Richer, *Les Démoniaques dans l'art* (Delahaye et Lecrosnier, Paris, 1887).
12. J.-B. Charcot, Charcot in the Franco-Prussian war, *Military Surgeon* **37**, 153–4 (1926).
13. D. Silverman, *Art Nouveau in Fin-de-Siècle France* (University of California Press, Berkeley, 1989).

Chapter 18

Epilepsy in Literature: Writers' Experiences and Their Reflection in Literary Works

Peter Wolf

Epilepsy is a frequent subject in fiction, and one of the questions arising in this respect is how well-informed the authors are about epilepsy, and how they came by this information (Table 1). Many relied upon secondary literature, but we know that others have observed seizures. Thus, Muriel Spark[1] was inspired to write her novel *The Bachelors* (1960) when she observed a man in the street having a convulsive seizure (*personal communication*). *The Blindfold* (1992), by Siri Hustvedt, is a work which has one of the most breathtaking descriptions of an epileptic seizure including the reactions of the observers, and, for this author, the sight of a woman having a seizure in the street is one of the strongest memories of her first visit, as a girl of seven, to a big city, Chicago.[2]

Experiences of Epilepsy in Close Relatives

Impressive as the observation of a seizure in a foreigner may be, it belongs primarily to the realm of perceptions. Seizures seen in close relatives add emotional dimensions. Through the character Toby Withers in two of the novels by Janet Frame (b. 1924), *Owls Do Cry* (1957) and *The Edge of the Alphabet* (1962), the author's memories of her epileptic brother[3] have become part of a poetic cosmos where she relates Toby's seizure experiences in metaphors of great intensity:[4] "A dark cloak would be thrown over his head by Jesus or God, and he would struggle inside the cloak, pushing at the velvet folds, waving his arms and legs in the air till the sun took pity, descending in a dazzling crane

Table 1(a). Authors with epilepsy who write about it.

Tryggve Andersen (Norway)
Hubert Aquin (Canada)
Andreas Burnier (Netherlands)
Ernesto Dalgas (Denmark)
Fyodor M. Dostoyevsky (Russia)
Margiad Evans (England)
Margaret Gibson (Canada)
Susan Hawthorne (Australia)
Monika Maron (Germany, single seizure)
Richard Pollak (USA)
Rosita Steenbeek (Netherlands)
Herbjørg Wassmo (Norway)

Table 1(b). Writers with other first-hand experiences of epilepsy.

Majgull Axelsson (Sweden; sister with symptomatic epilepsy)
Laura Doermer (Germany; son with epilepsy)
Janet Frame (New Zealand; brother with epilepsy)
Siri Hustvedt (USA; observation of a seizure)
Klaus Merz (Switzerland; father had epilepsy)
Kenzaburo Oe (Japan; son with epilepsy)
Christoph Ransmayr (Austria; seizures in a classmate)
Muriel Spark (England; observation of a seizure)
Alfred Tennyson (England; father had epilepsy)

of light to haul, but, alas, preserve, where in all the sky, Toby wondered, this cloak of stifling recurring dream."

Swiss author Klaus Merz (b. 1945) keeps much closer to the reality of his father's epilepsy when he uses it in two of his stories, *Im Schläfengebiet* ("In the Temple's Realm", 1994) and *Jakob schläft* ("Jacob Sleeps", 1997). The latter work is the history of a family where "illness in general had precendence", and where there also is a paralyzed and hydrocephalic younger brother called Sonne ("Sun"): a sensation in the village where they live. In a series of utterly condensed episodes full of both grief and love, "the climax of the involuntary histrionics certainly was father's roadside Grand Mal. It was on a Sunday morning stroll that he fell in the middle of the village. Like on command the good Samaritans came out of their houses and formed a huge dome of curious bodies around us. Sonne stood within the sinister choir and gazed helplessly out of his cart, whereas I, pale, knelt besides the jerking father and, within the sourish chime of evaporations, ministered to him as well as possible. After an eternity which had transformed my brother and myself into two small old men, the sun was now in the zenith, and the smell of burnt meat was in the air, father woke and glanced around him. He gave me a nod, rose slowly and turned the tide. He brought his clothes in order, blew his nose in his Sunday handkerchief, pulled his dark blue beret down on his forehead and aligned sights to a point far on the horizon. He took hold of my brother's cabriolet and put his arm around my shoulders. Without vouchsafing the bewildered Sunday troops another glance, we stepped out of a black tunnel into the brightest afternoon I ever had experienced."

The villagers' attitude, a monstrous combination of curiosity and rejection, could not have been more clearly characterized with many words. The defiant sarcasm of the response to this attitude is refreshing.

However, highly intensive perceptions such as these are unusual, whereas works written by authors who themselves suffered from seizures will always be of particular interest. Not that all writers who are known to have had epilepsy wrote about it in their literary works. Gustave Flaubert (1821–1880), for example, did not although he seems to have planned a novel, *La spirale*, built on his experiences of vivid visual and psychic auras which included a sensation of his soul leaving him "as one feels blood gushing out of an open wound". He was quite hesitant about this project of a novel, and it was never written. In a letter to Louise Colet he said: "It is necessary to wait until I am far removed from these experiences in order to render a precise and factual account of them without any danger to myself or to my work." Only an allusion to his ictal experiences has been suggested to exist in *Madame Bovary*.[5]

Joaquím M. Machado de Assis (1839–1908)

A different case is the great classic of Brazilian literature Machado de Assis. Machado seems to have been scared by the social stigma connected with epilepsy. He went as far as to change the simile, in the first edition of one of his novels, from "She rolled on the floor, epileptic" into "she rolled on the floor, convulsive" in the later editions, to avoid any allusion to his own condition, which he tried to hide although it was well known to his contemporaries.[6]

Machado, however, was a writer who excelled in double understandings, subtle allusions and open endings, and there seems to be at least one camouflaged allusion to epilepsy in his novel *Quincas Borba* (1891). The book's anti-hero, Rubião, strolls through Rio de Janeiro and then follows a sinister procession which ends in the public hanging of a murderer: "The fatal moment fortunately was short; the criminal dangled his legs and jerked, with a dextrous swing the hangman let him ride through the air; confused voices ran through the crowd, Rubião uttered a cry and lost his perception." The chapter ends here, leaving it to the reader's imagination whether this was a simple faint or more. But the scene stands out, as it does not belong to the time stream of the tale. It occurs as a memory flashback of the protagonist, and this is the only flashback in the novel. Also, the description of a public execution is suggestive of literary associations. The book was written about 15 years after his fellow epileptic writer Dostoyevsky's novel *The Idiot* had appeared. Machado was an extremely well-read author, fully familiar with European literature, and the passage just quoted, apart from its ambiguity in itself and considering its unique formal position in the book, can be read as an allusion to Dostoyevsky's frequent scenes of violence, especially to Prince Myshkin's account, in *The Idiot*, of his witnessing an execution. Like Myshkin, Rubião has inherited a fortune, and the two stories end in similar decline and disaster. This very subtle, indirect and sophisticated allusion seems to have been the farthest Machado de Assis wanted to go by way of talking about epilepsy.

Fyodor Mikhailovich Dostoyevsky (1821–1881)

The reason why the name Dostoyevsky will always come first to mind when writers with epilepsy are mentioned, apart from his literary excellence, is certainly the prominent place he gives to epilepsy in his work. The stories and novels where epilepsy appears include the following:

Chozyayka ("A Young Woman", 1847)
Unishennye y oskorblennye ("The Insulted and the Injured", 1861)
Prestuplenye y Nakasanye ("Crime and Punishment", 1866)
Idiot (1868/69)
Vechnyj mush ("The Lifelong Husband", 1869)
Besy ("The Devils", 1871/72)
Bratya Karamazovy ("The Brothers Karamazov", 1879/80)

It is common knowledge that Dostoyevsky in *The Idiot* drew extensively on his own experiences when he described the prodromal stage leading up to Prince Myshkin's grand mal seizure,[7] and the Prince's seizure at an evening reception where he breaks a precious Chinese vase. The character Kyrillov's words in *The Devils* are famous where he describes the aura experience as a transformation of time into eternity: in these five or six seconds one feels "the presence of eternal harmony in its highest consummation".

However, a comparison of the various epilepsy motives in Dostoyevsky's writings[8] has rarely been made but is instructive. Thus, the motive of the hate–friendship relationship between two men which is prominent in *The Idiot* is varied in *The Lifelong Husband*, which was written at about the same time. In the latter, there is Lisa, an eight-year-old child who is seized by a fit when she witnesses a suicide. The fit is described by a naive observer but it is left open whether it was an epileptic attack or not, whereas *The Idiot* leaves no doubt about the diagnosis.

In many of Dostoyevsky's works, big emotions precipitate seizures. The famous scene in *The Idiot* where Myshkin falls with a seizure at the very moment when his friend–adversary Rogoshin moves to kill him (the seizure saving Myshkin's life) has its counterpart, in the early short story "A Young Woman", by the seizure which the character Murin has when he is about to shoot his adversary with a rifle—which saves *him* from committing a murder. The girl Nelly, in *The Insulted and the Injured*, has seizures in a series of emotionally upsetting situations, and Svidrigaylov, in *Crime and Punishment*, talking about his desperate love for Raskolnikov's sister Dunya, says: "I truly thought I was getting the falling sickness." The most astonishing example, however, is the epileptic character Smerdyakov in *The Brothers Karamazov*, who fakes seizures to get an alibi for the time when he killed his father, and then the malingering turns into truth, and he develops a severe, life-threatening status epilepticus.

Thus, talking about even great emotions is an understatement: whenever seizures appear in the work of Dostoyevsky, there is a question of life and death, of suicide or murder. This is perhaps most obvious in the deeply pessimistic *Devils*, where almost all major characters end violently, by murder or suicide. Kyrillov, who has isolated auras and is not aware that they mean epilepsy, commits suicide in consequence of the aura experience, which, according to him, man in his mundane shape cannot endure: "You have to physically transform yourself or die." This is closely related to his belief that man in his present physical shape cannot endure the awareness that there is no God. The physical transformation which the aura experience seems to call for would mean that man becomes God. If God exists, all will is His. Kyrillov commits suicide to demonstrate his independent will, and thus prove God's non-existence and become the man–god.

Dostoyevsky knew that epilepsy can manifest itself with isolated auras only, and knew even more about the aura, for example that it could be arrested[9]: in *The Idiot*, Prince Myshkin has an aura during an evening reception, but it is interrupted by a sudden shock when he, in his exalted state, overthrows and breaks a precious vase. As may happen in such cases, the aura reappears after an interval and evolves into a convulsive seizure.

Kyrillov is not aware that his ecstatic experiences mean that he has epilepsy, which is not uncommon in persons who for a long period of time get only isolated auras. One such case was the Norwegian writer Tryggve Andersen (1867–1920). As Aarli[10] discovered from the hospital files, Andersen drew extensively on his aura symptoms in his novel *Mot kvæld* ("Towards Evening"), when he described complex visual hallucinations in his leading character Erik Holk. At the time when he wrote the novel, the diagnosis of epilepsy had not yet been made, and he was unaware of its possibility.

Margiad Evans (Peggy Eileen Arabella Williams née Whistler, 1909–1958)

Of particular interest is the report of English writer Margiad Evans, who in her autobiographical book *A Ray of Darkness* (1952) describes in every possible detail the events which for more than one year preceded and led up to her first grand mal seizure on May 11, 1950.[a] She had known isolated auras since early childhood, but never seen them as anything pathological. On the contrary, they were precious to her because, in them, she would experience the co-appearance of opposite perceptions, and this particularly opened her creativity to the literary form of the oxymoron, which is the combination of two opposites in one expression. "To see, or to observe one thing, and at that same instant for the soul (it is too instantaneous for the mind) to give birth to its matching half, its sunny shadow. Such swift mental images I had constantly and they made me very happy. For that was why I was born, to be able to do just that and nothing else."

---

a. According to her biographer,[11] Evans later wrote another account of the progress of her disease, *The Nightingale Silenced*, but this was not published. The writer died from a brain tumour in 1958.

The very title of her book is an oxymoron, and a selection of oxymora from the book further includes:

- loud silence
- silent music
- sunny shadow
- voiceless call
- when is light so expressed as at midnight,
  or darkness so clear as at noonday?

They abound in the chapter where she describes her auras, and it is of course interesting whether she indeed uses oxymora often in her writings. Unfortunately, not all of her work is now available. In her first novel, *Country Dance*, which she wrote at the age of 23, there is nothing of the sort, but this book is written in a style where oxymora would have been out of place.[b] The third available work, *Autobiography* (1943), is not really an autobiography but a kind of edited poetic diary which contains prose passages of extraordinary density and beauty, built on material collected since the winter of 1939, i.e. about 10 years before her first convulsive seizure. In this work, many oxymora can be found and, interestingly, the author even highlighted some of them by putting them in italics.[c] They include:

- stern kindness
- harsh gifts
- wind. . . fell like a whip and a caress
- the peace of being in the fight
- *dark white* sky
- *swift slowness*
- dark star
- *shaded* by light
- free, even of liberty
- the doublet "murmur of sight, vision of sound"

---

b. Interestingly, *Country Dance* has another epilepsy motive as a baby dies from fits (which is quite a literary topos). Evans had at the time no idea that she suffered from epilepsy herself, and may even not have connected fits of early childhood with epilepsy.

c. *Autobiography* also includes some passages which may more directly refer to the auras. The most suggestive one reads: ". . . to catch that murmur of sight, that vision of sound whose first thrilling even when I was so young seemed to come over immeasurable time and distance. I still have those startling moments, memories from the first instant, which bring through my physical body a spiritual awareness indescribable. Sometimes with a touch they are over: sometimes a day cannot contain them."

There are far too many aspects in *A Ray of Darkness* to be fully analyzed here. Thus, deliberations about death and about God play major roles. One aspect, however, deserves perhaps special attention: the way in which she talks about her aura experiences, which she once characterizes as being "quite literally conscious and unconscious at the same time".[d] The following is a longer quotation from a text of rather unusual structure (the italics are Evans'):

"How can it be described? It came often after I had been stooping—scrubbing the cottage floors perhaps, or planting seeds in our gardens, which was what made me connect it with momentary pressure.

It caused no pain, it lasted a few seconds, I saw and heard and moved while it happened. I have often crossed a room, and, while not losing sight or bearings, not known *how* I crossed it. The sequence of consciousness was so little broken by it, that after it had happened it seemed not an atom of time or myself had been missing, and I only knew it had happened again by the numb sensation in the centre of the brain which followed it. I do not get it now that the major attacks have superseded it; and that makes it still more difficult to be accurate in recollection. I do, however, remember laughing to my husband about my 'little wheel, going off again'. It seemed like a tiny wheel—the wheel, say, of a watch, whirring at blurring speed, quite soundlessly, in my head while I went on with whatever I was doing, guided by *the consciousness left over* rather than the consciousness of the moment.

The wheel would then cease, and there was a loud silence such as follows a blow on a drum, also in my head. A clanging ache followed that. The whole thing took about as long as for a normal person to walk five paces, say.

These spells became more frequent and longer and *darker* during the year 1948 than at any other time in my life. I was then aware of there being at the heart of a second, oblivion of mind and cessation of sight. During the spring and summer of 1949, which I am describing, I had only two of them, both of which strangely enough I remember, and both of which still more strangely occurred at the same spot."

And she will describe this spot, a beautiful place in the wood which she calls "the Cathedral", but before she does this she goes back to the auras once more and formulates another description: "When they have happened to me while crossing a room I have, if I may so illustrate it, left myself on one side and come to myself on the other, while feeling an atom of time divided the

---

d. The Prince's "weird seizures" in Tennyson's *The Princess* are described very similarly. This description is probably based on Tennyson's father's seizures.[12,13]

Table 2. Linguistic peculiarities of aura descriptions.

Abundant reformulations
Externalizing metaphors
Metadiscursive comments
Frequency of:
• Hesitations
• Indicators of vagueness
• Interruptions of sentences

two selves, as the room might divide the figures of myself, supposing any one could create two figures of me."[e]

This is a narrative of experiences which seem to be as difficult to describe as they have fascinated the writer; it is full of digressions; there is a constant urge to reformulate; quite unusual oscillations exist between most trivial facts on one side, and most elaborate abstractions on the other, between the narrative and the metaphoric; metadiscursive comments are interspersed; repeatedly the author works with italics to highlight certain passages such, as the word "darker", which is her quite surprising metaphor for the way these spells have changed in a certain period of time.

What is so fascinating about this is that in the polished, edited literary text of a professional writer we can recognize many elements of a linguistic structure (Table 2) which appeared as typical qualities in spontaneous oral reports of patients with epilepsy who were invited to talk about their seizure experiences.[15]

e. This seems to provide a specific background to Kavanagh's[14] discerning observation that "her real subject is the problem of expressing *this minute* in Margiad Evans' life, not a memory of last minute; it is an attack on the way the immediate seems always to leak away between the words when you try to express it." This is of course to some extent a general experience which, however, fascinated Evans quite unusually.

Similarly, Lloyd-Morgan[11] points out that one of her central themes is the "duality in one person, the idea of crossing over between one state and another", and she relates it to "her practice of transposing adjectives", of which she gives as an example: "As if I'd never tasted corn/Had never seen a field of bread/Ripen.... " Another one is the above quotation from *Autobiography*, with the doublet of what could be called synesthetic oxymora, i.e. "murmur of sight, vision of sound".

The appearance of this characteristic of Evans' style at this particular place seems also to relate it to her aura experiences.

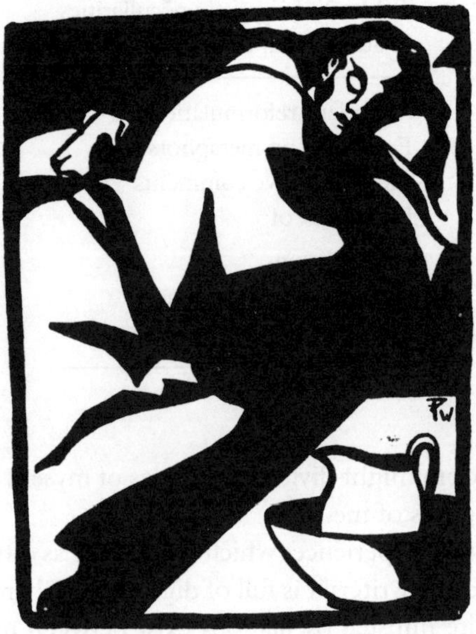

Peggy Whistler (Margiad Evans). Frontispiece for her book *The Wooden Doctor* (1933).

Apart from her descriptions of auras, Evans gives a captivating account of her first grand mal seizure. She was alone in her cottage at night, writing poetry, became tired and decided to make tea and go to bed: "I made the tea, looked up at the clock—a strange chance—saw that is was ten minutes past eleven. The next thing I was still looking up at the clock and the hands stood at five and twenty minutes past midnight. I had fallen through Time, Continuity and Being.... I discovered I was lying on the floor on my back, my head against the rungs of a rocking-chair and my body, full length, crowded between the steel fender and the little table at which I had been writing. The lamp, a tall brass one, on a very slender base, was burning steadily on the table; always cold when sitting still, I had made up a large fire to work by and this was burning hotly in the open fireplace with wood and coal ablaze. It was not until much later on, appalled and shaken, I realized how dangerously I had been placed, unconscious, certainly in convulsions, in a locked cottage alone with my dog at midnight and a quarter of a mile from the village. The space in which I was lying was perhaps a yard wide. My sleeve was charred by an ember, but that was all. Had some special agent of preservation laid me down between lamp and fire it could not have been more dexterously done."

Monika Maron (b. 1941)

The way a first seizure can shatter the notion of life as a matter of course is reflected in a quite different way in the novel *Animal triste* (1997), by contemporary German writer Monika Maron, who has herself had one single seizure (*personal communication*). On one of the first pages, the narrator tells about a "day in April when someone, I don't know who, turned off the electric current to my brain. I was crossing the Friedrichstraße in the early evening to catch the elevated train when my tongue suddenly felt a mysterious numbness, a numbness that soon spread to the rest of my senses. What happened during the next twenty minutes, I know only from the report of a young woman who had stopped to help me as I lay on the asphalt in contortions and foaming at the mouth." A detailed description follows of a generalized tonic–clonic seizure, and how she was brought to a hospital where no causes for the seizure were found, after which the author continues her own experiences: "For several weeks I had at times the impression that something in my head didn't function as it did before the spell—reversed sides, as if someone had switched the poles around. For example, I remembered people's first names after their last names, or I wrote twenty-three when I meant to write thirty-two."

Although the narrator, a natural scientist, is aware that "such symptoms [have] logical, in this case even simple explanations", she becomes increasingly disquieted, and "obsessed with the idea that an alien force had simply switched me off for fifteen minutes... and, for reasons unknown to me, had slightly altered the way my brain functions. I didn't really believe that, but it corresponded well with the state in which this inexplicable incident had left me. However, if this strange event simulated my death in order to resurrect me later with a slight disorientation in my brain as a memento, if it was meant as a scathing demonstration of my mortality, then it was possible to conceive of another force behind all this besides a few neurons gone haywire in the hippocampus or the amygdala."

The seizure clears the way for an invasion of the irrational in this life: "I am ready to believe everything I have ever read about biocurrents and parapsychological phenomena, ever since that time when the currents in my brain were disconnected for about a quarter of an hour." But, more significantly, it influences her encounter with a man whom she meets a year later: "I doubted that I had ever loved a man before Franz, although before I met Franz I was certain I had loved at least two or three men deeply and fervently—even though the suspicion that I had been missing out on love had never left me since that moment when someone had intimated my mortality one early evening in April."

In this way, the seizure experience becomes an announcement and metaphor of the book's central subject, an unconditional, all-consuming love affair, a matter of life and death.

Conclusions

Reflections of writers' experiences of illness in their literary works can be expected to have undergone a process of professional "editing" which may belong to both the creative and discursive, the formal and structural spheres. In this selection of writers who deal with an intimate experience of epilepsy we have seen a wide variety of examples of all these possibilities. The frequent negative social attitudes towards people with epilepsy caused Machado de Assis to try to hide his condition, and refer to it in his work only by a most clandestine and sophisticated allusion. These attitudes are analysed in detail by Muriel Spark, and counterpoised by Siri Hustvedt's empathic description of a seizure, whereas the offence felt by the child on behalf of a beloved father is tangible in the cold rage of Klaus Merz' sarcasm.

Monika Maron turns her experience of a single seizure into the leitmotiv of a story of a deep existential perturbation. The products of Dostoyevsky's literary pursuit of his seizure experiences are famous, unforgettable and should be compulsory reading for everybody with a serious interest in epilepsy; but it is no less fascinating to observe the impact of aura experiences on the literary production of writers like Tryggve Andersen and Margiad Evans at a time when they were naive to their significance, and unaware of the diagnosis. Margiad Evans is unique in giving us an insight into the influence of these experiences on details of her personal literary style. At the same time, some aspects of her writing remain captive of linguistic rules that seem to be determined by the quality of the pathological experience rather than by style.

For Monika Maron, the first seizure marks the invasion, by irrational forces, of a rational mind, used to think along scientific terms. Perhaps the most thought-provoking aspect of this analysis, however, is to see almost all authors in the series who have had seizures themselves take up the theme of death, sometimes appearing as suicide, murder or execution, in more or less close relation to the epilepsy, but usually not directly referring to the seizures.

Unprepared witnesses to convulsive seizures, especially of a first seizure in a close relative, often think first that the person seized by the fit is about to die. On a different level, the epileptic seizure has repeatedly been seen as a symbol of death and resurrection. The literary reflection of epilepsy by writers who suffered seizures themselves tells us that, at least subconsciously, the epileptic experience also subjectively is a matter of life and death.

References

1. P. Wolf, Epilepsy in contemporary fiction: fates of patients, *Can. J. Neurol. Sci.* **27**, 166–72 (2000).
2. S. Hustvedt, Gesprenkeltes chaos, *Die Zeit – Magazin*, 3 May 1998, pp. 32–8.
3. N.H. Platz, *Epilepsie im Leben und Werk von Janet Frame.* In: D. v. Engelhardt, H. Schneble and P. Wolf (Hrsg.), "*Das ist eine alte Krankheit*"*–Epilepsie in der Literatur* (Schattauer, Stuttgart, 2000), pp. 197–207.
4. P. Wolf, *Epilepsie als Metapher in der zeitgenössischen Literatur. Epilepsie-Blätter* 7, Suppl. 2, 31–5 (1994).
5. H. Gastaut, Y. Gastaut and R. Broughton, Gustave Flaubert's illness: a case report in evidence against the erroneous notion of psychogenic epilepsy, *Epilepsia* **25**, 622–37 (1984).
6. C.A.M. Guerreiro, Machado de Assis's epilepsy, *Arquivos de Neuro-Psiquiatria (São Paulo)* **50**, 378–82 (1992).
7. P. Vogel, *Von der Selbstwahrnehmung der Epilepsie. Der Fall Dostojewski. Nervenarzt* **32**, 438–41 (1961).
8. D. Janz, *Anmerkungen zu Epilepsiegestalten bei Dostojewskij, Epilepsie-Blätter* 7, Suppl. 2, 15–17 (1994).
9. W.R. Gowers, *Epilepsy and Other Chronic Convulsive Diseases: Their Causes, Symptoms & Treatment* (Churchill, London, 1881).
10. J. Aarli, Epilepsy in Tryggve Andersen: epileptic hallucinations in the 1890s, fact or fiction?, *Epilepsia* **36**, 308–15 (1993).
11. C. Lloyd-Morgan, *Margiad Evans* (Poetry Wales Press, Bridgend, Wales, 1998).
12. P. Wolf, Epilepsy and catalepsy in Anglo-American literature between romanticism and realism: Tennyson, Poe, Eliot and Collins, *J. Hist. Neurosci.* **9**, 286–93 (2000).
13. B.H. Wright, Tennyson, the weird seizures in The Princess, and epilepsy, *Literature and Medicine* **6**, 61–76 (1987).
14. P.J. Kavanagh, Margiad Evans. In *Evans M. Autobiography*, revised ed. (Calder and Boyars, London, 1974), pp. i–vii.
15. P. Wolf, M. Schöndienst and E. Gülich, Experiential auras. In: H.O. Lüders and S. Noachtar (eds.), *Epileptic Seizures: Pathophysiology and Clinical Semiology* (Churchill Livingstone, New York, 2000), pp. 336–48.

List of Discussed Books

(with year of appearance and available editions; for Dostoyevsky see text)

Andersen, Tryggve:
Mot kvæld (1900); Eide, Bergen, 1970

Evans, Margiad:
Country Dance (1932); Calder, London, 1978
Autobiography (1943); Calder and Boyars, London, 1974
A Ray of Darkness (1952); Calder, London, 1978

Frame, Janet:
Owls Do Cry (1957); The Women's Press, London, 1985
The Edge of the Alphabet (1962); Braziller, New York, 1995

Hustvedt, Siri:
The Blindfold (1992); Norton, New York, London, 1993

Machado de Assis, Joaquím María:
Quincas Borba (1891)
English edition: *Quincas Borba* (transl. Gregory Rabassa), Oxford University Press, Oxford, 1999

Maron, Monika:
Animal triste (1996); Fischer, Frankfurt, 1997
English edition: *Animal Triste* (transl. Brigitte Goldstein), University of Nebraska Press, Lincoln, London, 2000

Merz, Klaus:
Am Fuß des Kamels (1994); Haymon, Innsbruck, 1994 (includes short story "*Im Schläfengebiet*")
Jakob schläft (1997); Haymon, Innsbruck, 1997

Spark, Muriel:
The Bachelors (1960); Penguin, London, 1981

Chapter 19

The Aetiology of Dostoyevsky's Epilepsy

Halfdan Kierulf

Dostoyevsky is the writer who has had the greatest significance for me, and the fact that he suffered from epilepsy and haemorrhoids, and perhaps tuberculosis and venereal diseases, simply serves to increase my respect for him. This is something I share with many others who have worked in depth on his life and works, such as A. Gide,[1] J. Catteau[2] and J. Rice.[3] My own contributions to this not insignificant part of Dostoyevsky research have been made over the past 30 years and have among other things resulted in

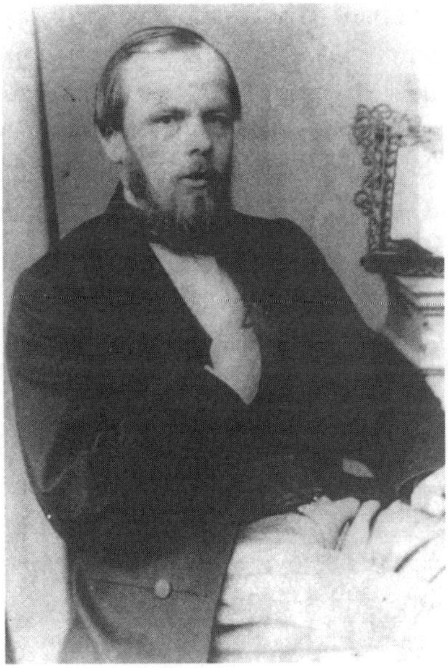

Dostoyevsky

a French doctoral degree in medicine in 1971,[4] articles in the journal of the Norwegian Medical Association,[5,6] and a presentation at the 8th International Dostoyevsky Congress in Oslo in 1992.[7] During these years, research on epilepsy in general and Dostoyevsky's epilepsy in particular has undergone great changes, but the major motive for going through this complex of problems again arises from the articles by Moiseeva and Nikitina from 1993–96.[7]

My main thesis is that from the second half of the 1840s Dostoyevsky suffered from a form of epilepsy that we would today classify as"partial complex seizures with secondary, most often nightly, generalisation". The cause of this epilepsy is in my opinion syphilitic meningo-encephalitis, which Dostoyevsky contracted in the middle of the 1840s.

The arguments for these claims are as follows:

In spite of the resounding success of *Poor Folk* in May 1845, the time both before and afterwards was tumultuous for the author. The first note that we have of a loss of consciousness, which might have been an epileptic seizure, comes from his friend Grigorovitch: in January 1845 Dostoyevsky collapsed in the street as a funeral procession was passing.

There is no doubt that the young and vital writer had an active sex life during this period. This is confirmed in his letter to his brother Mikhail dated 16 November 1845: "The Minnas, the Klaras, the Mariannas, etc., have grown so much prettier that it is hard to believe, but they cost a frightful lot of money. A few days ago, Turgenev and Belinksy gave me hell for my disorderly life." There is reason to believe that among these female acquaintances there was a possibility of transmission of a venereal infection to the writer.[8]

On 26 April 1846 he writes again to his brother that he has been unable to hold a pen in his hand since the last time he wrote, and the reason is: "I have been sick and near death in the full sense of the word. I was ill in the most intense degree with an irritation of my entire nervous system, and the illness rushed to my heart, caused a rush of blood and an inflammation in the heart, which was barely checked by leeches and two bleedings. Besides I've been ravaged by decoctions, drops, powders, mixtures, and such abominations. Now I am out of danger. But just barely, because the illness has stayed with me, and according to my doctor it is because it has been accumulating for three or four years; so it will not be healed in a short time. My treatment must be physical and moral [*nravstvennoe*]—the former by diet and constant physical deprivations prescribed for me. . . . "[9]

By physical deprivation I understand him to mean sexual abstinence. This tells me that in April 1846 Dostoyevsky had a venereal, probably syphilitic, infection that had reached its secondary stage and caused symptoms from both the central nervous system and the cardio-vascular system.

We know that at the end of May the writer went to a new doctor, Dr S. Janovsky, who began treating him and remained his friend for the rest of his life. Janovsky relates in his memoirs (1881 and 1885), written after Dostoyevsky's death, that in May 1846 he was treating the writer for a "local ailment that it took several months to cure". J. Frank writes: "Such discretion leads one to suspect that the ailment might have been venereal."[10]

The temporal perspectives may cause confusion: if Dostoyevsky contracted his primary syphilitic infection in the autumn of 1845 or earlier, and his secondary infection in the spring of 1846, it may be difficult to explain what "local ailment" he was being treated for by Janovsky in May 1846. Even though a continuing syphilitic chancre cannot be excluded, a gonorrhoeal infection is perhaps more probable. Indeed, an argument against my hypothesis here is that he was quite simply thinking of haemorrhoids!

With regard to the natural course of these two venereal diseases, a gonorrhoeal infection nearly always cures itself while a syphilitic infection does not cause permanent damage in more than 60–70% of those infected. Syphilis was a fatal disease for many of the greatest artists, and T. Gjestland, a Norwegian epidemiologist, showed this on the basis of data including 1000 untreated syphilis patients between 1891 and 1927.[11] Is Dostoyevsky's history of illness compatible with syphilis (and gonorrhoea), and could syphilis have caused his epilepsy?

Syphilis is a venereal disease caused by the micro-organism (spirochete) *Treponema pallidum*,[12] which develops in three stages:

Stage 1: Approximately three weeks after infection a painless sore (chancre) appears, which without treatment lasts for between two and eight weeks.

Stage 2: During the following weeks this is followed in a third of the patients by an invasion of the central nervous system that may produce symptoms like those of encephalitis or meningitis. In approximately 60–70% of cases the infection is arrested but may have left a scar on the surface of the brain. As with any other scar on the brain, this could produce epileptic seizures for the rest of a person's life.

Stage 3: Tertiary syphilis, which can develop during any time up to 30 years, usually leads to the disastrous and well-known conditions of GPI (general paralysis of the insane) and tabes dorsalis. It was these forms that claimed the lives of so many people, both famous and unknown.

It is my opinion that Dostoyevsky contracted secondary syphilis due to infection of the meninges or the cerebrum, and that this caused his lifelong epilepsy. I have no doubt that he had geniune epileptic seizures. These were described by friends and especially by his wife, Anna, who writes: "On the last day of Carnival we dined at the home of relatives and then went to spend the evening at my sister's. Supper was gay (and accompanied again by champagne). The other guests left, but we stayed on for a while. Fyodor Mikhailovich was extremely animated and was telling my sister some interesting story. Suddenly he broke off in mid-syllable, turned white, started to get up from the couch and began leaning over toward me. I looked in amazement at his changed face. And suddenly there was a horrible inhuman scream, or more precisely a howl—and he began to topple forward. At the same moment my sister, who had been sitting alongside of him, let out a piercing scream, jumped up from her chair and ran out of the room with hysterical sobs. My brother-in-law rushed after her. In later years there were dozens of occasions when I was to hear that inhuman howl....[13] This cannot have been anything but a genuine epileptic seizure, particularly when compared with the description of a typical epileptic seizure taken from one of the standard textbooks of neurology in Western Europe[14]: "Grand Mal Epilepsy, Clinical aspects. This is the classic form, familiar to the layman, typified by severe and generalised convulsions and unconsciousness. The attack may be preceded by a premonitory subjective sensation, the so-called aura. Suddenly, a generalised tonic convulsion occurs with respiratory arrest, the patient falls to the ground and may utter a cry: after 10 s, clonic convulsions follow. The patient may foam at the mouth, bite his tongue, and be incontinent of feces and urine. The clonic convulsions may last for several minutes, and they are followed by a period of unconsciousness which passes into a state of postictal confusion. Finally normal consciousness returns. Amnesia lasting 10 min or longer is present for the attack and the postictal phase."

That Dostoyevsky's type of epilepsy exists has been confirmed by recent research and has fascinated many epileptologists.[15–17] There is agreement that sources of the author's epilepsy were to be found in the area of his left temple. This accounts for the difficulty in speaking he experienced before and after the convulsions and also the ecstatic feeling he felt on certain rare occasions and mentioned among other things to his friend Strakhov and his lady friend Kowalewskaya. This ecstatic aura, which he also described as affecting Prince Myshkin, he certainly experienced, albeit rarely, but then most of his seizures were nocturnal and quite undramatic.

What then of the arguments put forward by Moiseeva and Nikitina? These concern the disease itself as if it had been taken out of a textbook from Dostoyevsky's own time, in which observations most often concerned the most severely affected epileptic patients who were detained in psychiatric institutions. By far the great majority of epileptic patients would, also at that time, live approximately normal lives—like Dostoyevsky himself. Most epileptic patients lead normal lives physically and mentally apart from their seizures: they are not particularly egoistic, dishonest or lacking in the capacity for deep and unselfish love. The terms introduced for acute cerebral vascular crises are foreign to modern medical terminology. Had he had marked changes in blood pressure, this would probably have led to myocardial infarction or strokes, and Dostoyevsky might not have reached the age of 60. The notion of sudden changes in blood pressure as the cause of Dostoyevsky's seizures is difficult to accept. Similarly is the argument that Dostoyevsky's seizures lasted too long for them to be of an epileptic nature: if we consider the whole seizure with aura, and the tonic and clonic movements, each of which seldom lasted more than 5–10 minutes. The postictal phase with unconsciousness and confusion before consciousness gradually returns can last between 30 and 60 minutes.

Recognition must be given to the rejection of hereditary factors put forward in the article. The criticism of Dr Ermakov's medical certificate of 16 December 1857 is quoted in practically all biographies of Dostoyevsky but, according to Moiseeva and Nikitina, the certificate may have been a fake—that it could have been obtained to order or by bribery is without any basis in fact. Until this paper, Dostoyevsky's biographers had accepted the validity of the certificate, and those familiar with the Russian bureaucracy of the 1850s could discuss the problem in greater depth, but it can hardly be denied that at that time there could have been a discrepancy between reality and bureaucracy. I think my colleague Ermakov wrote the certificate on the basis of his honest conviction and to help Dostoyevsky out of an untenable situation in Semipalatinsk—and in this he was indeed successful!

Finally, a detail taken from Ermakov's certificate that makes a syphilitic brain infection even more probable, reads: "... he often suffers from nervous pain in his face due to organic sufferings of the brain." This must be trigeminal neuralgia—one of the most common complications of neuro-syphilis. However, the fact that he died after a haemoptysis at the age of 60 hardly had anything to do with his syphilis—here we must point to his chain-smoking, which gave him emphysema, and perhaps to a tuberculous infection.

The fact that our author's special type of epilepsy—especially the ecstatic aura—was presented by some writers as a poetic fiction right up to a century after his death is very strange. That his aura type has been not completely unusual has been confirmed by Italian, Japanese and Spanish colleagues recently.[19–21]

In the international epilepsy literature, epileptologists wrote of "the so-called Dostoyevsky epilepsy" until recently. During the past decade scholars have spoken of "Dostoyevsky's epilepsy" as a separate form of epilepsy. And right they are!

References

1. A. Gide, *Dostoievski* (Librairie Plon, Paris, 1923), p. 23.
2. J. Catteau, *La Création litteraire chez Dostoievski* (Institut d'études slaves, Paris, 1978).
3. J. Rice, *Dostoevsky and the Healing Art* (Ardis, Ann Arbor, 1985).
4. H. Kierulf, *L'epilepsie dans la vie et l'oevre de Dostoievski. Thèse pour le doctorat en médicine* (Univ. Louis Pasteur de Strasbourg, 1971).
5. H. Kierulf, *Dostojevskij og epilepsien, Tidsskrift for Den Norske Lægeforening* **92**, 1303–7 (1972).
6. H. Kierulf and G. Kjetsaa, *Dostojevskijs epilepsi: Et nytt syn på en stor dikters sykdom, Tidsskrift for Den Norske Lægeforening* **119**, 2474–6 (1999).
7. H. Kierulf, "Dostoevsky's epilepsy: status praesens", presentation at the 8th international Dostoevsky congress, Oslo, 1992.
8. N.N. Moiseeva and L.N. Nikitina, Falsity of stamp concept of F.M. Dostoevsky's epilepsy, *Vestnik gipnologii i psichoterapii.* **2**(5), 91–105 (1993).
9. J. Frank and I. Goldstein, *Selected Letters of Fyodor Dostoevsky* (Rutgers, London, 1987), p. 4.
10. J. Frank, *The Seeds of Revolt, 1821–49: Dostoevsky* (Princeton University Press, 1976), p. 165.
11. T. Gjestland, The Oslo study of untreated syphilis, *Acta dermato-venerologica* **34**, suppl. 35, Oslo (1955).
12. M.A. Samuels and S. Feske, *Office Practice of Neurology*, N. 4 (Churchill Livingstone, 1996), p. 381.
13. Anna G. Dostoievskaia, *Reminescences*, Eng. transl. (Liveright, New York, 1975), pp. 79–80.
14. M. Mumenthaler, *Neurology* (G. Thieme Verlag, Stuttgart, 1990), p 262.
15. T. Alajouanine, Dostoievski's epilepsy, *Brain* **86**, 209–18 (1963).
16. H.F.M. Gastaut, Dostoievsky's involuntary contribution to the symptomatology and prognosis of epilepsy, *Epilepsia* **19**, 186–201 (1978).
17. P.H.A. Voskuil, The epilepsy of F.M. Dostoevsky (1821–81), *Epilepsia* **24**, 658–67 (1983).
18. H. Gastaut, New comments on the epilepsy of F. Dostoevsky, *Epilepsia* **25**(4), 408–11 (1984).
19. F. Cirignotta *et al.*, Temporal lobe epilepsy with ectstatic seizures (so-called Dostoevsky epilepsy), *Epilepsia* **I, 21**, 705–10 (1980).
20. F. Cabrera-Valdivia, Dostoevsky's epilepsy induced by television, *J. Neurol. Neurosurg. Psychiatry* **61**, 653 (1996).
21. H. Naioto and N. Matsui, Temporal lobe epilepsy with ictal ecstatic state, *The Journal of Nervous and Mental Disease* **176**(2) (1988).

Chapter 20

Neurology and Sherlock Holmes

E. Wayne Massey

Discussing Dr Arthur Conan Doyle's famous detective, Sherlock Holmes, and the neurologic diseases he encountered during his escapades is exciting. There have been, of course, many physician writers of fiction, but Sherlock Holmes remains prominent among literary characters. Conan Doyle was a physician who practiced medicine for several years. Interestingly, Dr James Watson is the chronicler of Holmes' exploits, hence the record of multiple medical—specifically neurologic—diseases which occur during the stories. This is a fascinating study of medical history. Beyond the extraordinary history behind Conan Doyle's medical experiences lay the influences on him from Dr Joseph Bell. The possible effects from other physician acquaintances are also intriguing.

Arthur Conan Doyle (1859–1930) (Figure 1) practiced medicine for about ten years after graduation. As a medical student, he served as a surgeon on an Arctic whaler for seven months and was also a student clerk for the surgeon Joseph Bell. He spent time as a student assistant to general practitioners and, after graduation, for the first year, he was again a ship's surgeon, for three months on a steamer to West Africa and later as a medical assistant to two physicians in Birmingham and Plymouth. In July 1882, he became a general practitioner at Southsea, near Portsmouth, where he remained for over eight years. He was also a civilian doctor to the local unit of the British Army and performed eye refractions at the Portsmouth Eye and Ear Infirmary. In 1890, he spent three months in Vienna attending ophthalmologic lectures, after which he opened an office in London as an ophthalmologist. However, by 1891 he had become a full-time writer of fiction. His many literary works had already begun, specifically the mystery stories for which he is famous, and

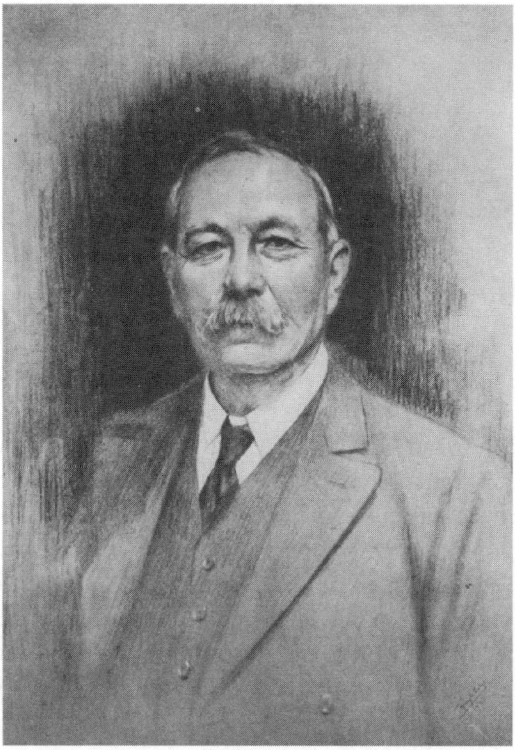

Fig. 1. Arthur Conan Doyle.

subsequently many more followed. In 1900, during the Boer War, he served as a voluntary physician at the Military Hospital in South Africa.

Conan Doyle's writings are an example of the influence of medical knowledge and experience upon an author who is a physician by profession. He became a writer of novels, short stories, poetry, plays, science fiction, histories, and works on spiritualism. He even wrote a comic opera titled *Jane Annie* with his friend and collaborator Sir James Barrie.

Dr Conan Doyle has described his experiences in his autobiography of 1924, as well as in personal letters.[10] He was a prolific author whose stories often used cases involving his personal experiences, as well as information from medical journals. Fictional counterparts of his own patients occur in a variety of his writings, both in Sherlock and in non-Sherlock stories. Dr Rodin and Mr Key have described how the author's literature was greatly influenced by his life experiences.[19,20]

Who Was Sherlock Holmes?

Although Dr Joseph Bell (1837–1911) of Edinburgh wrote few medical works, one of his students, Arthur Conan Doyle, seems to have based his famous character, Sherlock Holmes, on Bell's abilities. Arthur Conan Doyle, N.B.C.N., N.D., LLD. (Hon.), was a student clerk for Joseph Bell, M.D., F.R.C.S. (Figure 2), consulting surgeon to the Royal Infirmary and Royal Hospital for Sick Children, and a member of the University Court, Edinburgh University. He was one of many physicians named Bell who were famous surgeons in Edinburgh.[13]

Dr Bell has been described as a wiry, dark man with penetrating gray eyes and acute features, who had the amazing ability to sit in his receiving room and diagnose people as they came in before they opened their mouths. He apparently could recite their symptoms and give them details of their past life and would hardly ever make a mistake. Conan Doyle in his memoirs and adventures stated that he thought of his old teacher when he considered the essential character for his detective stories: "If he were a detective, he would

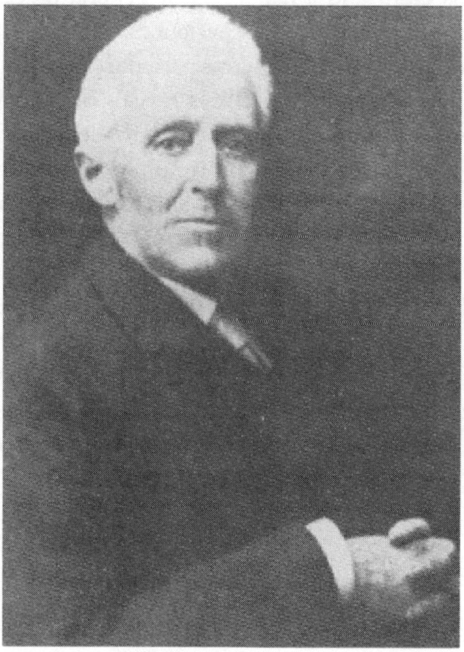

Fig. 2. Joseph Bell.

surely reduce this fascinating business to something near an exact science." Conan Doyle wrote to Dr Bell in May 1892: "It is most certainly to you that I owe Sherlock Holmes." Later he stated: "I do not think that his analytical work is in the least an exaggeration of similar effects which I have seen you produce in the outpatient ward."[13]

When his friend Robert Lewis Stephenson wrote to Conan Doyle in 1893, he asked about Sherlock Holmes: "Can this be our old friend Bell?" Being a humble man, Dr Bell later stated that Conan Doyle had made a great deal out of very little and proceeded to credit Sherlock Holmes' genius to Doyle's own gifts.[13]

How the names Sherlock and Holmes were derived is also interesting and revealing.[2]

Medical Conditions

Sir Conan Doyle did extensive reviews and studies of tabes dorsalis in his doctoral thesis as a medical student.[20] In addition, he saw many patients, particularly during his eight-and-a-half years of general practice, and recorded many observations regarding these experiences. His descriptions of the diseases he saw include comments on doctor–patient relationships. His discussion of medical experiences in all of his stories reveals obvious knowledge about these disease states during the latter half of the 19th century. Sometimes Conan Doyle uses diseases in patients to introduce philosophical themes.[19]

General diseases referred to in both Sherlock and non-Sherlock literature (Tables 1 and 2) are numerous, but we will review only those occurring in Sherlock Holmes stories that are neurologic. However, in Sherlock Holmes stories, there are discussions about infections, cancer, gout, lung disease, ophthalmologic diseases, heart disease (congestive heart failure), chronic alcoholism and insanity, closed head injury and wounds inflicted by bullets (Table 3). Holmes describes aging in an elderly man, Professor Presbury, who had "dabbled in" injections of monkey serum for rejuvenation, popular during that period.[2]

Neurology and Holmes

There are numerous neurologic diseases that Sherlock Holmes experiences or deals with during his 56 short stories and 4 novels about him (Table 4). Many of them have been discussed previously.[4,8,14]

Table 1. Medical conditions in Arthur Conan Doyle's books.

Trauma
Wounds (bullet)
Infections
Cancer
Gout
Asthma
Eye disease
Gynecologic/obstetric
Neurologic
Psychiatric
Geriatric

Table 2. Medicine in Sherlock Holmes stories.

Malaria	"The Sign of Four"
Typhoid	"The Valley of Fear"
Coolie disease (Sumatra)	"The Dying Detective"
Tuberculosis	"The Missing Three-Quarter"
Gout	"The Missing Three-Quarter"
Blindness	"The Dying Detective"
Cataract	"The Adventure of Silver Blaze"
Asthma	"The Norwood Builder"
	"The Three Gables"
Heart failure	"The Sign of Four"
Rejuvenation	"The Creeping Man"
Leprosy	"The Blanched Soldier"
Ruptured aneurysm	"A Study in Scarlet"

Dr John Watson describes his friend and colleague as the "most perfect reasoning and observing machine that the world has ever seen" ("A Scandal in Bohemia"), so it is not surprising that the Sherlock Holmes canon demonstrates the value of history taking, observation, and deductive reasoning.[5]

Holmes considers the brain the most important organ: "Surely, as a doctor, my dear Watson, you must admit that what your digestion gains in the way of blood supply, is so much lost to the brain. I am a brain, Watson. The rest of me is a mere appendix. Therefore, it is the brain I must consider." ("The Adventures of the Mazarin Stone") Several of his stories have to do with intelligence and the decline of it, i.e. dementia. Toxic-metabolic encephalopathies

Table 3. Arthur Conan Doyle's medical writing other than Sherlock Holmes stories.

Measles	"The Stark Munro Letters"
Typhoid	
Tuberculosis	
Syphilis	"The Surgeon Talks"
Tabes dorsalis	
Meningoencephalitis	"A Medical Document"
Congenital	"The Third Generation"
Cancer	"His First Operation"
	"A Medical Document"
Gout	"A Question of Diplomacy"
	"The End of Devil Hawker"
Asthma	"A Straggler of '15"
Heart failure	"Sweethearts"
Trauma	"The Stark Munro Letters"
	"Songs of the Road"
Bullet Wounds	"The Mystery of Cloomber"
Delivery	"A Duet"
	"The Curse of Eve"
	"A Medical Document"
Aging, atherosclerosis	"The Mystery of Cloomer"

are seen in several settings, including the men in the Tregennis family in the "The Adventure of the Devil's Foot." In "The Adventure of the Dying Detective," when Holmes feigns a tropical illness, he is thought to be delirious by Dr Watson (Table 5).

Seizures occur on several occasions in "The Study in Scarlett." A dog has a terminal seizure after ingestion of a toxin. Julia Stoner, in "The Adventure of the Speckled Band," is described as having an agonal seizure due to snake venom. Percy Phelps, in "The Naval Treaty" has a seizure associated with brain fever. Von Straker has problems with convulsive struggles which follow brain injury.[3]

In "The Resident Patient" (Figure 3) Dr Percy Trevelyan describes his patient: "Suddenly, however, I sat writing, he ceased to give any answer to all my inquiries and on my turning towards him, I was shocked to see that he was sitting bolt upright in the chair staring at me with a perfect blank and rigid face." Although this sounds like a complex partial seizure, the patient was feigning an illness to gain entry into the doctor's office. Catalepsy has been suggested, but this term is certainly vague as to its medical meaning.[4]

Table 4. Sherlock Holmes and neurology.

Intelligence
Henry Baker: "The Adventures of the Blue Carbuncle"
Sir Charles Augustas Milverton: "The Adventures of Charles Augustas Milvertin"
Professor Moriarity: "The Final Problem"
Delirium/encephalopathy
George and Owen Tregennis: "The Adventure of the Devil's Foot"
Sherlock Holmes: "The Adventure of the Dying Detective"
Edward Rucastle: "The Adventure of the Copper Beeches"
Brain fever
Alice Rucastle: "The Adventure of the Copper Beeches"
Percy Phelps: "The Naval Treaty"
Sarah Cushing: "The Adventure of the Cardboard Box"
Nancy Barclay: "The Crooked Man"
Rachel Howells: "The Musgrave Ritual"
meningitis: "The Sussex Vampire"
Seizures
Jefferson Hope: "A Study in Scarlet"
John Straker: "Silver Blaze"
Julia Stoner: "The Adventure of the Speckled Band"
Percy Phelps: "The Naval Treaty"
patient: "The Resident Patient"
Pseudoseizure (catalepsy?)
Sherlock Holmes: "The Reigate Squires"
Dr Trevelyan's patient: "The Resident Patient"
Syncope
John Horner: "The Adventure of the Blue Carbuncle"
Hattie Doran: "The Adventure of the Noble Bachelor"
Dr Watson: "The Adventure of the Empty House"
Movement disorder
Henry Baker: "The Adventure of the Blue Carbuncle," tremor
Mr Farquhar: "The Stockbrokers Clerk" (chorea?), twitch (St Vitus' dance?)
"The Greek Interpreter" (St Vitus' dance?)
Stroke
Mr Trevor, Sr: "The Gloria Scott"
Colonel Barkley: "The Crooked Man" (cerebral hemorrhage)
carotid artery: "The Adventure of the Golden Pince-Nez"
Alcoholism
Henry Baker: "The Adventure of the Blue Carbuncle"
Captain Peter Carey: "The Adventure of Black Peter"
Jim Browner: "The Adventure of the Cardboard Box"

Table 4. Continued.

Malingering
Sherlock Holmes: "The Adventure of the Dying Detective"
Lady Hilda Trelawney Hope: "The Adventure of the Second Stain"
Bannister: "The Adventure of the Three Students"
Craniocervical deformities
Henry Wood: "The Crooked Man"
Mr Culverton Smith: "The Adventure of the Dying Detective"
Hereditary
Monographs: *Variability of Human Ears* "The Adventure of the Cardboard Box"
EEG
"The Valley of Fear," 1888
Pupillary abnormality
Isa Whitney: "The Man with the Twisted Lip"
Miss Burnett: "The Adventure of Wisteria Lodge"
Sherlock Holmes: "The Adventure of the Dying Detective"
Trauma
"The Boscomle Valley Mystery"
"The Solitary Cyclist"
"The Priory School"
"The Crooked Man"
"The Hound of the Baskervilles"
"Silver Blaze"
"The Asby Grange"
Toxins
Tetanus: "The Sign of Four"
Curare: "The Sussex Vampire"
Strychnine: "The Sign of Four"
Automic neuropathy
"The Adventure of the Dying Detective"

Table 5. Conan Doyle's contemporaries.

Oliver Wendell Holmes
S. Weir Mitchell
William Osler
Robert Bentley Todd
J. Hughlings Jackson
Frederick Treves

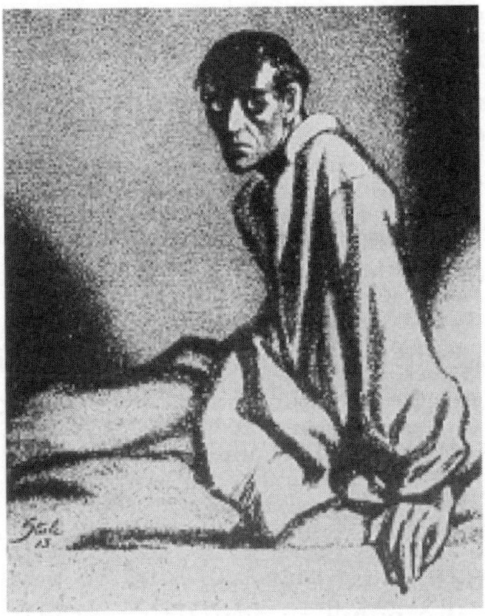

Fig. 3. Pseudoseizure: Sherlock.

Pseudoseizures, as well as complex "temporal lobe" seizures, were beginning to be recognized in the medical literature at that time.[10] Clearly, however, Holmes feigns a seizure in "The Reigate Squires," producing a pseudoseizure. Of course, he tells us in the "The Adventure of the Dying Detective" that "malingering is a subject upon which I have sometimes thought of writing a monograph." Other spells suggesting syncope also occur.[4,19,20]

Movement disorders, such as tremor possibly related to alcoholism, occur in Henry Baker in "The Adventure of the Blue Carbuncle." St Vitus' dance is mentioned in "The Greek Interpreter" as Wilson Kent is described, and it also mentioned in "The Stockbroker's Clerk" with Mr Farquhar. If the movement came on in older age, it could represent senile chorea, Huntington's chorea (no family history) or parkinsonism (plus), or perhaps focal vascular disease. If he had the chorea for many years we would include Sydenham's chorea.

Cerebrovascular disease is described in two situations: Mr Trevor, Sr, upon receiving a threatening letter, suddenly grasps his head and has a stroke ("The Gloria Scott"); his paralysis spreads, with subsequent loss of consciousness. This suggests that it may have been an intracerebral bleed that spread to the ventricle and subsequently produced secondary brainstem herniation (Duret hemorrhage?). Another possibility is pontine tegmental infarction from a progressive basilar artery syndrome. Col. Barkley, in "The Crooked Man," also develops a stroke associated with an emotional situation.

Brain fever appears in several stories, but is not well described. Whether this represents encephalitis, meningitis, acute reaction to stress, or perhaps even psychosis, is not clear; this illness seemed to be self-limited, lasting for only days to weeks.[4,6]

Autonomic dysfunction seems to be prevalent in several situations. Holmes has autonomic dysfunction in "The Dying Detective" (Figure 4). Dr Watson, upon seeing Holmes after believing him dead for three years, says: "A gray mist swirled before my eyes and when it cleared, I found my collar ends undone and a tingling aftertaste of brandy upon my lips." ("The Adventure of the Empty House.") Holmes loses consciousness after inhalation of fumes in "The Devil's Foot Root," as well as his experiences in "The Dying Detective" where he simulates a rare tropical fever.[17]

Small pupils are described as being associated with opium intake by Isa Whitney ("The Man with the Twisted Lip") and Ms Burnett ("The Adventure of Wisteria Lodge"); also pupillary dilatation secondary to belladonna self-administered by Holmes occurs.

Several traumatic injuries occur. Dr Watson is struck by a Jezail bullet, perhaps involving his brachial plexus, while in the disastrous Maiwand

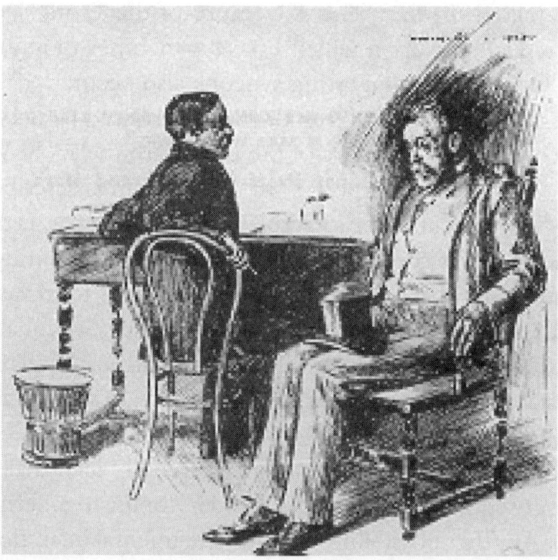

Fig. 4. Sherlock Holmes in "The Dying Detective."

field in Afghanistan ("Study in Scarlet"). Jackie Ferguson, in "The Adventure of the Sussex Vampire," has a crippling illness due to a spinal problem, as does his dog, Carlo, with weakness of the hind legs. Professor Presbury, in "The Adventure of the Creepy Man," is diagnosed with lumbago by Dr Watson. He also demonstrates unusual behavior, as he is using monkey serum in his search for the elixir of youth; neurologists such as Brown-Séquard had similar experiences during their lifetime.[20] Spinal deformities were described in "The Crooked Man" and "The Adventure of the Dying Detective" and may represent either myelodysplasia, Pott's or Paget's disease.[17]

Toxic effects from alcohol and other medications are described in several characters, including Henry Baker with a tremor in "The Adventure of the Blue Carbuncle," as well as the pathological intoxication of Captain Peter Carey in "The Adventure of Black Peter" and Jim Growner in "The Adventure of the Cardboard Box."

Neurologically associated descriptions include electroencephalography in "The Valley of Fear," where the brainwave is described.[7] Various postulated neurologic problems occur in both Watson and Holmes.[22,24,25,27] Holmes had a problem with cocaine addiction and some have thought that he had classical paranoia.[1,9,22]

Sir Arthur Conan Doyle and His Colleagues

Oliver Wendell Holmes

Undoubtedly, physician authors may be influenced by the experiences of their colleagues. Conan Doyle was a fan of Oliver Wendell Holmes and his writings. Although he had never met the Boston physician, he often spent his medical school lunch hours reading Holmes' works.[14] There is some possibility that the name "Sherlock Holmes" was influenced by the fact that Conan Doyle thought a great deal of Oliver Wendell Holmes.

A famous statement of Oliver Wendell Holmes is "Science is a first rate piece of furniture for a man's upper chamber if he has common sense on the ground floor." It is interesting that Sherlock Holmes quotes to Dr Watson in "The Sign of Four" that "the brain is like an attic; to store additional furniture, one must first clean out the old furniture."[14] Professor Oliver Wendell Holmes was well recognized for his work *Nature and Treatment of Neuralgias.* Conan Doyle suffered from neuralgia,[20] but we do not know if the two men ever corresponded with each other.

S. Weir Mitchell

Another American neurologist, S. Weir Mitchell, also a novelist and poet, who was credited with being the most versatile American since Benjamin Franklin, was a friend of Oliver Wendell Holmes. He was well known for his work with toxicology, particularly snakes and snake venom. We have no evidence that he ever met Conan Doyle. Oliver Wendell Holmes, S. Weir Mitchell and Conan Doyle, as physician writers, all use their snake venom interest in fictional literature.[21]

William Osler

William Osler and Conan Doyle both had extensive interest in antivivisection, which was so prominent in their respective countries during the latter part of the 19th century, and their involvement has previously been chronicled.[11] Both men gave medical class addresses, such as Doyle's "The Romance of Medicine" in 1910.[18] Osler extolled the value of vivisection to humanity in the London newspapers, in his articles, and even in political arenas.[11]

Robert Bentley Todd and John Hughlings Jackson

The doctoral thesis of Conan Doyle was on tabes dorsalis. The major physician who had influenced the study of tabes dorsalis in the world, specifically in London, was Robert Bentley Todd of King's College Hospital. Now he is best known in neurology for descriptions of postseizure paralysis. During his lifetime he was known for work on tabes dorsalis, studies in epilepsy, the use of alcohol as a therapy, and his description of mononeuropathies.[12] In the latter half of the 19th century, John Hughlings Jackson performed studies in evaluating the various characteristics of complex partial seizures. These two individuals may have influenced Conan Doyle's ability to describe the patient of Dr Trevelyan in "The Resident Patient" as having either a complex partial seizure or a pseudoseizure.[14,15] Hughlings Jackson and Conan Doyle both received honorary degrees from King's College in 1908.

Frederick Treves

In "The Resident Patient," the physician Dr Trevelyan is known for his work on "rare and complex neurologic diseases." If the authorship occurred in 1886, as Dr William S. Barring-Gould suggests, the story was written shortly after the famous description of the elephant man by Sir Frederick Treves (1884).[2] Conan Doyle, as a physician in London during those years, almost certainly knew of that famous case.[15] In 1884, Treves wrote an extensive monograph on his evaluation of John (*sic*) Merrick, describing a "case of congential deformity" in the *Transactions of the Pathological Society of London*. Dr. Percy Trevelyan was the author of "obscure nervous lesions" and was known for writing on catalepsy.[15]

Summary

This chapter describes the very interesting characteristics of neurology demonstrated in Sherlock Holmes stories from Conan Doyle's personal experiences, the influences of the surgeon Joseph Bell and other colleagues, as well as the medical advances at that time. Sherlock Holmes' adventures have entertained many for over a century with exhilarating mystery; knowing the medical background will entertain us even more.

References

1. F.A. Allen, Devilish drugs: part one, *Sherlock Holmes Journal* **3**, 12–18 (1957).
2. W.S. Baring-Gould, *The Annotated Sherlock Holmes*, 2 vols. The 4 novels and 56 short stories (complete) by Sir Arthur Conan Doyle. New York Clarkson N. Potter, 1967.
3. C.B. Brell, Sherlock Holmes: neurologist, *Neurology* **37**(11), 1821 (1987).
4. R.F. Brenner, Holmes, Watson and neurology, *J. Clin. Psychiatry* **41**(6), 202–5 (1980).
5. H.S. Carter, Medical matters and the Sherlock Holmes stories: from the records of John H. Watson, M.D., *Glasgow Medical Journal* **28**, 414–26 (1947).
6. L. Cassamajor, Brain fever, *JAMA* **149**, 1443–6 (1952).
7. R. Caton, The electric currents of the brain, *Brit. Med. J.* **5**, 278 (1875).
8. M. Cherington, Sherlock Holmes: neurologist, *Neurology* **37**, 824–5 (1987).
9. B.S. Clark, The pathological Holmes. In *The Best of the Pips* (The Five Orange Pips, Westchester County, NY, 1955), pp. 104–14.
10. A.C. Doyle, *Memories and Adventures* (Hodder & Stoughton, London, 1924).
11. J.D. Key and A.E. Rodin, William Osler and Arthur Conan Doyle versus the antivivisectionists: some lessons from history for today, *Mayo Clinic Proc.* **59**, 189–96 (1984).
12. J.B. Lyons, The neurology of Robert Bentley Todd, *Historical Aspects of the Neurosciences*, eds. F.C. Rose and W.F. Bunun (Raven, New York, 1982), pp. 137–50.
13. E.W. Massey, Joseph Bell, M.D., F.R.C.S.—Mr Sherlock Holmes, *Southern Medical Journal* **73**(12), 1635–6 (1980).

14. J. Massey and E.W. Massey, Sherlock Holmes and neurology, *Neurology* **32**(2), 193 (1982).
15. J. Massey and E.W. Massey, Dr Trevelyn and Mrs. Treves, Sherlock Holmes and the Elephant Man, *Southern Medical Journal* **78**(7), 854–7 (1985).
16. D.F. Musto, Sherlock Holmes and heredity, *JAMA* **196**, 45–9 (1966).
17. W.B. Ober, Conan Doyle's "dying detective": problems in differential diagnosis, *N.Y. State J. Med.* **67**, 2141–5 (1967).
18. A.E. Roden and J.D. Key, Arthur Conan Doyle's thesis on tabes dorsalis, *JAMA* **247**(5), 646–50 (1982).
19. A.E. Roden and J.D. Key, Dr Arthur Conan Doyle's patients in fact and fiction, *Medical Heritage*, Mar./Apr. 1985, pp. 80–98.
20. A.E. Roden and J.D. Key, *Medical Casebook of Dr Arthur Conan Doyle* (Malaber, Fl. Robert E. Krieger, 1984).
21. J.M. Schneck, S. Weir Mitchell and Oliver Wendell Holmes, *JAMA* **246**(9), 974–8 (1981).
22. D.C. Shannon, Poor devil, *The Pharos* **41**, 4–9 (1978).
23. Frederick Treves, A case of congenital deformity, *Transactions of the Pathological Society of London* **36**, 494–8 (1885).
24. G. Vash, The states of exhaustion of Mr Sherlock Holmes, *JAMA* **197**, 664–5 (1966).
25. E.J. Van Liere, Doctor Watson and nervous maladies, *Baker Street Journal* **4**, 100–8 (1954).
26. E.J. Van Liere, Brain fever and Sherlock Holmes, *W. Va. Med. J.* **49**, 77–80 (1953).
27. E.J. Van Liere, Dr John H. Watson and the subclavian steal, *Arch. Intern. Med.* **118**, 245–8 (1966).

Chapter 21

James Joyce in a Clinical Context

J.B. Lyons

Born in a well-to-do Dublin suburb on 2 February 1882, the eldest surviving son of a spendthrift, intemperate father and a devout Catholic mother (she succumbed to cancer in 1903), James Joyce died unexpectedly in Zurich on 13 January 1941 following perforation of a duodenal ulcer.[1] His literary reputation as author of *Dubliners*, *A Portrait of the Artist as a Young Man*, *Ulysses*, *Finnegans Wake*, etc., was already established; it continues to increase, encouraged by a torrent of secondary publications from academe—but, to borrow a comment from the late Augustine Martin, "One senses a certain

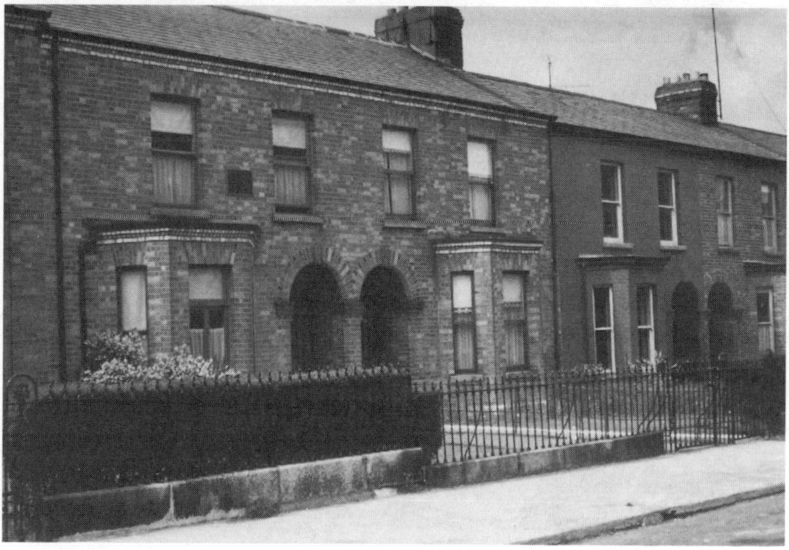

Fig. 1. Birthplace, with plaque; 41 Brighton Square, Rathgar, Dublin.

exegetical desperation creeping in."[2] Being amply forewarned, I shall confine my observations to matters linking Joyce with medicine.

Joyce is spoken of as an ex-medical-student although in Dublin the connection was limited, in Paris tentative: he never "walked the wards". At the Catholic University Medical School mentioned in *Finnegans Wake*—"Then he went to Cecilia's treat on his solo to pick up Galen"[3]—he wrote 13 pages of notes on anatomical terminology.[4] In company with "cervix" and "cilia" we encounter "chiasma" ("crossing of fibres like limbs of X") and it may be correct to link Joyce's introduction in 1902 to the optic chiasma with his later use of chiasmus as a literary device.[5]

His guarded behaviour while at the Sorbonne, where as we learn from *Ulysses* that he had read in the library of Saint Genevive, "sheltered from the sin of Paris, night by night",[6] probably owed as much to the unfamiliarity of his surroundings as to the prudence enjoined by his elders against dangers pictured luridly in Dublin by his friend Oliver St John Gogarty, a future E.N.T. surgeon:

There once was a solar eclipse
Which could only be seen from the Kips,

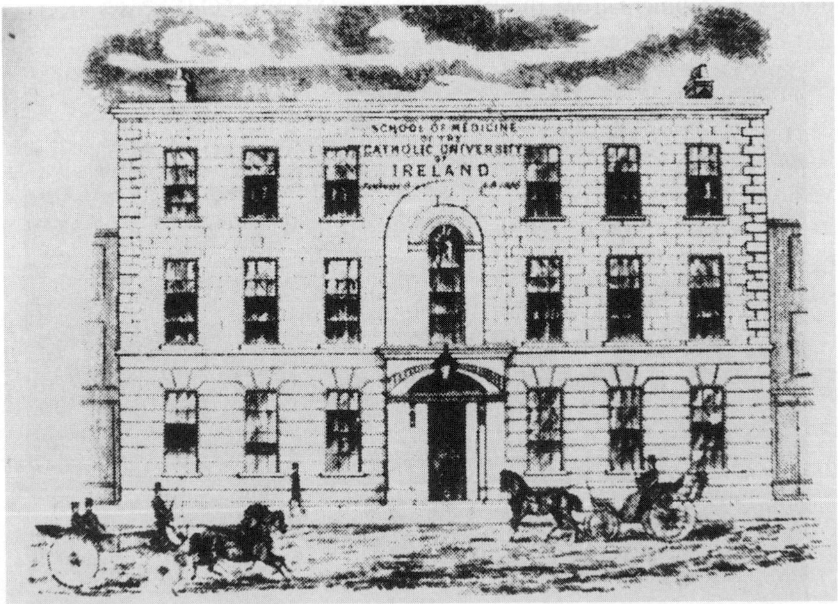

Fig. 2. Catholic University Medical School, Cecilia Street.

As the daylight grew darker
I thought I saw Parker [an anatomy "crammer"]
Astride on a prostitute's hips.

Less cautious in the company of his familiars, Joyce did not emerge unscathed from Nighttown. Seeking the opinion of his medical-student friend, then in Oxford competing for the Newdigate Prize, he was told that he probably had a relapse of a venereal infection. "As it would be absurd and pernicious for me [Gogarty continued] to prescribe for a penis in a poke, so to speak, I enclose a letter for you to hand to my old friend Dr Walsh, one of the best." And to Dr Michael Walsh, a local GP, he wrote: "Mr Joyce is the name of the tissues surrounding the infected part; if you will cure him you will delight me. He may have waited too long and got gleet."[7]

Nora Barnacle

Evidently progress was satisfactory. Within a matter of months Joyce was courting Nora Barnacle, the young Galway girl who quickly agreed to accompany him to the continent, and live with him unwedded on his meagre earnings as a language teacher.[8] He had written plainly to her so that she should not misunderstand him.

> "My home was simply a middle-class affair ruined by spendthrift habits which I have inherited. My mother was slowly killed, I think, by father's ill-treatment, by years of trouble, and by my cynical frankness of conduct. When I looked on her face as she lay in her coffin—a face grey and wasted with cancer—I understood that I was looking on the face of a victim and I cursed the system which had made her a victim."[9]

On 8 October 1904 the couple went via London to Zurich, from which he wrote to Stanislaus, his brother and confidant "*elle n'est pas encore vierge*", and on to Trieste and Pola, returning to Trieste when a post was available in its Berlitz School. Soon Nora was pregnant and Joyce asked his brother "to study... some midwifery and embryology and to send me the results of your study" (*Letters*, II, p. 73).

Apart from a spell in Rome (where he worked in a bank), the Joyces remained for many years in Trieste, where they were joined by Stanislaus, moving to neutral Zurich during World War I, and settling in Paris in 1920. The final step in the hegira was the wartime return to Zurich in 1940.

Dubliners

At Belvedere, his Jesuit school, Joyce had excelled at the weekly English composition; in University College, reading English, French and Italian and known as "the bard" or "the [mad] hatter", he had starred in the debating society. His article "Ibsen's New Drama" was published by the *Fortnightly Review*. Add to this a handful of book notices, a few light lyrics and some stories in the *Irish Homestead*... a literary career beckoned. He had not, however, counted on refractory publishers, or on the hazards of illness. The former objected to certain things in *Dubliners*, a book of short stories which initially they rejected. Nature undermined him physically with polyarthritis and iritis, leaving him partially blind, and dependent on others during the preparation of his complicated texts.

On its eventual publication in1914, *Dubliners* was widely reviewed. Ezra Pound wrote: "He gives us Dublin as it presumably is.... He gives us things as they are, not only for Dublin, but for every city."[10] Pound was not to know that Joyce had a private agenda, nurturing an ambivalence towards his native city, which he intended to depict as a centre of paralysis, an intention not apparent to the first wave of reviewers.

I should explain that writing to a friend, Constantine Curran, about his short stories in July 1904, Joyce had said: "I call the series *Dubliners* to betray the soul of that hemiplegia or paralysis which many consider a city." (*Letters*, I, p. 55). This curious intention, undetected by the early critics, was to earn the enthusiastic and profitable approval of later commentators, apparently unaware of Curran's dissent: "Nothing seemed to me [Curran has written] more inept than to qualify the focus of this activity as a hemiplegia or paralysis, however much one might quarrel with its exuberances or fanaticisms." He attributed it to his friend's "ardour and youthful impatience".[11]

"How sick, sick, sick I am of Dublin! [Joyce wrote when visiting the city in 1909]. It is the city of failure, of rancour and of unhappiness. I long to be out of it." (*Selected Letters*, p. 163). Presumably this was a personal reaction to the dysfunctional and penurious environment of his youth, for he was to praise it ecstatically in *Finnegans Wake*—"the cornflowers have been staying at Ballymun, the duskrose has choosed out Goatstown's hedges, twolips have pressed togatherthem by sweet Rush, townland of twinedlights, the whitethorn and the redthorn have fairygeyed the mayvalleys of Knockmaroon" (015.04).

Close contemporaries, too, other than Con Curran, disapproved of *Dubliners*: "It is interesting but unpleasant [wrote James Stephens] and must be counted among his many wild oats, that man's crop seems interminable."[12]

Speaking of the Irish capital in the House of Commons, T.M. Kettle, M.P., said: "In spite of the many reverses with which we have to deal Dublin does not stand still but progresses."

The most prevalent disease in *Dubliners* is alcoholism; the book, indeed, could serve as a temperance tract.[13] I do not wish to imply that Joyce intended his work as a corrective to this social problem, but his pages reflect the community's attitudes to alcohol and present object lessons of increasing gravity. John Stanislaus Joyce, the author's father, a severe chronic alcoholic, ran through a fortune, gradually moving from Dublin's affluent Southside to rent meaner dwellings in Dublin North.

Joyce focuses on paralysis in "The Sisters", which discusses the case of Father Flynn, an old priest who has died from a third stroke, having for years been subject to mental problems. This is the most clinical of Joyce's stories—not, indeed, that he was interested intrinsically in medicine. Had he not been excluded from the profession by lack of funds, his intention was to practise for a few years and accumulate a financial competency which would enable him to write independently of editorial whims.

Polyarthritis

Joyce was 25 when taken acutely ill in 1907 in Trieste, with what was miscalled "rheumatic fever". According to Ellmann, "he had to be put in the city hospital";[14] John McCourt, on the other hand, points out that in his diary Stanislaus "makes absolutely no mention of Joyce being hospitalized".[15] McCourt insists that Joyce was treated at home by the family doctor, Dr Sinigaglia.

It hardly matters whether or not Joyce was an inpatient. This certainly could affect his comfort, and might influence the accuracy of the diagnosis. The latter, however, is already suspect, for iritis (uveitis) is unlikely to occur as a complication of rheumatic fever. The arthritis prevented him from writing to Elkin Mathews, publisher of *Chamber Music*, and to Geoffrey Palmer, who wished to set Joyce's verses to music, tasks undertaken by Stanislaus. Genito-urinary involvement is not mentioned, but tactful silence on this point would be understandable. There was, in any case, a previous history of such involvement—and there were to be future puzzling allusions to genital lesions which remain unclarified, and may indicate the occurrence of a relevant development, circinate balanitis.

Whether Joyce would have been altogether frank with the doctors is open to question. Prior to leaving Rome a few weeks previously, he was drinking heavily, and he brought his visit "to an orgiastic close".[16] Accompanying two mailmen he went to dance on the Pincio; on another night he was mugged and robbed. His return to Trieste gave abundant cause for celebration: his first book, *Chamber Music*, was about to be published. Nora was then at an advanced stage of pregnancy; it is possible that Joyce looked elsewhere for sexual gratification, with disastrous consequences. If so, he may have developed "Reiter's syndrome", an entity not then included in the repertoire of clinical medicine. This would explain persisting rheumatic symptoms, and the low-grade ocular conflagration that had been ignited—then or later Joyce was under the care of Dr Oscar Oblath, a local eye specialist.[17]

Reiter's Syndrome

At the date of Joyce's illness this intriguing syndrome was unknown. Hans Reiter of the German Army Medical Corps described it in 1916 in a German lieutenant serving on the Balkan front, but new ideas are taken into the general body of medicine at the pace of a tortoise. Reiter's syndrome is not featured in Price's *Practice of Medicine* (1930); it gained a mention in the 7th edition (1947) of Cecil's *Medicine*, and had become a common research subject only in the 1950s and 1960s. It is characterised by arthritis, such ocular manifestations as conjunctivitis and/or iritis, and urogenital involvement in the form of urethritis and/or prostatitis. The urethritis may be copious and purulent, or barely detectable following prostatic massage.[18]

The acute manifestations of Joyce's rheumatism gradually resolved. By September 1907 he was active again but prone to recurrences. He resumed correspondence with Gogarty, then a graduate student in Vienna, the latter commiserating with him towards the end of October. He had obtained his address from Joyce's Auntie Josephine: "I think he is sorry for his past rudeness [Mrs Murray assured her nephew] and would like to say so to you. He still seems to retain the "old gra" [friendship] for you".[19]

> "I heard you were stricken with a grievous distemper [Gogarty wrote], and that you were paralysed. You can understand that the sight of your handwriting rejoiced me, as it disproved the statement that your right arm was paralysed."[20]

Understandably, in view of the urethritis in 1904, Gogarty had worried in case Joyce had actually then contracted a dual infection and now had meningo-vascular syphilis. But Joyce's uncle had assured him that the disease was "altogether ethical", and lo and behold the present evidence that Joyce was "miraculously made whole again".

Writing to his sister on 8 December 1908, Joyce remarked: "I feel a little better of the rheumatism and am now more like a capital S than a capital Z." (*Letters*, II, p. 226). Flare-ups of the iritis were exacerbated by alcohol. "Do you want to go blind?" scolded Stanislaus. "Do you want to go about with a little dog?" [21]

Naturally, the differential diagnosis of iritis includes syphilis, a possibility which Joyce himself mentioned in a letter to Harriet Shaw Weaver in 1930. He explained that congenital syphilis was suggested as being accountable for his eye troubles by Dr Hartmann, a Paris ophthalmologist, but Dr Borsch and Dr Collinson had already considered this and excluded it. The death of Joyce's elder sibling might, indeed, add some credence to syphilis in congenital form—but John Stanislaus Joyce's infection, admitted boastfully to a group of medical students, had occurred more than ten years before his marriage to Mary Jane Murray on 5 May 1880, and was most unlikely to have been transmitted. Had she actually contracted a luetic infection an abortion or miscarriage would have resulted, whereas her ill-fated infant was fully formed but premature.

Selected Letters

Joyce and Nora were sexually passionate. Their temporary separation during his visits to Dublin in July and November 1909 resulted in an erotic correspondence consisting of fantasies, amounting to what Mark Shechner has called "improvised coitus at a distance".[22] Joyce's sexual repertoire, according to Shechner, was extensive: "No part of the body, no human function, nor any variety of orificial contact seems to have lacked its libidinal valence."[23] His imagination, a powerful aphrodisiac, was onanistic in intent.

Joyce returned to Dublin in the guise of a businessman towards the end of October 1909, his task to open the Volta Cinema for some Triestian associates. Secretly nursing what Richard Ellmann (*Letters*, II, p. 259, fn) refers to rather casually as "a minor complaint possibly contracted from a prostitute," Joyce found it a relief to be assured by Nora that she was quite well. It seems unlikely that his nasty lesion was either a chancre or urethritis or was recently acquired. It may have been the circinate balanitis referred to above, now recognised as a not uncommon feature of Reiter's syndrome.

He had been so active in his private orgy (he explained in a letter to Nora) that he hardly dared look to see what had become of his unsightly lesions.

Family

Joyce's love for Giorgio and Lucia, his children born in Trieste, shines in his poems, which, to favour the conservation of space, should be consulted directly by the reader. The boy is the subject of "On the Beach at Fontana", written in 1914. Endowed like his father and grandfather with a fine voice, Giorgio failed to establish himself on the concert platform. He married an American lady some years older than himself, remarrying after their divorce. In middle age and later he was alcoholic, and on bad terms with Stephen, the son born of his marriage.

Simples, featuring Lucia (ironically fated to develop schizophrenia), was written in 1915. Lucia Joyce died at St Andrew's Hospital, Northampton, in 1982.

The tender and guilt-ridden *Ecce Puer*, inspired by the birth of Stephen Joyce little more than a month after the death of his great-grandfather in Dublin, has an ineffable note of piety and regret.

Ulysses

Ulysses was banned in the UK and the USA. F.R. Leavis was refused permission to import a copy which he needed for a lecture on modern literature. On pressing the point he was dismissed as "a crank—or worse". The censorship was not enforced in Ireland, where the book stores did not bother to stock it. There is, however, a further example in the Joyce/Léon papers of its hostile reception in Dublin: an assistant librarian at Trinity College confirmed to a relative of Joyce in March 1922 that it had been ordered and received—but "it was nothing but a *disconnected* story of gross obscenity". Reviewers highlighted the novel's unusual features. Shocked by Molly Bloom's soliloquy (which fascinated Jung), the British DPP decreed that customs officials should impound and destroy it. A consignment of 499 copies was seized in Folkestone and dealt with accordingly.

A big blue book vaguely reminiscent of a telephone directory, *Ulysses* has 18 sections, each with its Homeric parallel, its anatomical organ (there are no organs for the first three sections), its colour, art, etc. The brain is the disappointing organ of "Scylla and Charybdis". Medicine is the art of the

"Oxen of the Sun" episode, with the womb as organ, the scene the hospital, The National Maternity Hospital, Holles Street, where the Master is Dr Andrew Horne—a name ripe for a *double entendre*: "Of that house A. Horne is lord." Joyce's playful use of "Purefoy" (Dr Purefoy was an ex-Master of the Rotunda Hospital, the rival establishment) as a surname for a patient with a protracted labour may have escaped general attention. The locomotor apparatus is the organ of "Circe", the rhythm of which, as Joyce told Frank Budgen, is that of locomotor ataxia, a form of neurosyphilis; nerves supply an organ for "Eumeus".

The action, such as it is, takes place on a single day, 16 June 1904, opening in the Martello Tower in Sandycove: "Stately, plump Buck Mulligan came from the stairhead, bearing a bowl of lather on which a mirror and a razor lay crossed. . . . "

In addition to many well-known Dublin citizens, the novel features Stephen Dedalus, Joyce's surrogate (and his father, Simon); Leopold Bloom and his wife, Molly, who is having an affair with Blazes Boylan; Buck Mulligan, who is a caricature of Oliver St John Gogarty, Joyce's erstwhile friend and future enemy. From the Tower we move to the 40-foot bathing place, to a school in Dalkey where the headmaster is writing a letter to a newspaper about foot and mouth disease. We spend the day in the company of Leopold Bloom and others, ruminating in odd corners of Dublin.

Dr Joseph Collins, a New York City neurologist, said in an early review (1922) of *Ulysses* that he had "learned more psychology and psychiatry from it than [he] did in ten years at the Neurological Institute".[24] C.G. Jung, attempting to read *Ulysses* in 1922, was obliged to put it down. "You read and read and read [he complained] and you pretend to understand what you read." Incorporating the stream-of-consciousness technique, "the stream begins in the void and ends in the void". One fails to encounter a resting place from which to look back and contemplate the ground covered. "This utterly hopeless emptiness [Jung continued] is the dominant note of the whole book. It not only begins and ends in nothingness, it consists of nothing but nothingness".[25]

Falling asleep over *Ulysses*, Jung awoke and continued his reading, *backwards*. "This method [he said] proved as good as the usual one; the book can just as well be read backwards, for it has no back and no front, no top and no bottom."[26] Joyce hit the nail on the head, however, when he said that Jung read *Ulysses* from beginning to end without a smile. Be that as it may, Jung, like Dr Collins, was impressed by the novel's psychological content. Writing privately to the author, he admitted uncertainty as to whether or not he had enjoyed *Ulysses*—"because it meant too much grinding of nerves and of grey matter". He selected the 40 pages of Molly Bloom's unpunctuated ruminations as "a string of veritable psychological peaches". He was unlikely, on the other hand, to have spotted the passages concealing Joyce's representation of anatomy, the most striking of which is "Sirens" dealing with the ear.

Anatomy

Joyce's brief contact with academic anatomy has been referred to above. He never actually dissected. Needing to learn some anatomy when writing *Ulysses*, he fell back on a literary source by Fletcher, which, with supreme confidence, he felt he had managed to surpass. "Among other things," he told Frank Budgen, "my book is the epic of the human body. The only man I know who has attempted the same thing is Phineas Fletcher. But then his Purple Island is purely descriptive.... In my book the body lives in and moves through space and is the home of a full human personality."[27] Many basic functions are accommodated—defecation, menstruation, parturition, masturbation, coitus.

The organ nominated for representation in a particular episode is mentioned repetitively but unobtrusively in that context. With a little concentration, the attentive reader catches on. The *brain*, the organ of "Scylla and Charybdis", is mentioned only three times in the episode where we also find "mystic mind", "myriadminded", "dullbrained", "soul", "skull" and "pineal glands".

The *heart*, the organ of Hades, is mentioned at least 40 times: "he took it to heart", "wear the heart out of a stone", "good-heartedness", "the Sacred Heart", "heart on his sleeve", etc. The author is just as detached as a modern cardiologist: "Seat of affections. Broken heart. A pump after all, pumping thousands of gallons of blood every day. One fine day it gets bunged up and there you are. Lots of them lying around here: lungs, hearts, livers. Old rusty pumps: damn the thing else."

"Sirens", the most melodious episode, has the *ear* as its organ, substantively or embedded in other words ("n*ear*", "an*ear*", "an*ear*by", "h*ear*d", "c*rea*m", "b*rea*th"), synonyms ("red lugs", "lugugugubrius", "purple lobes", "peeping lobe"), and, by implication, in the imperative "Listen!", as well as negatively, in "deaf Pat", "Pat doesn't hear".

The following passage illustrates his method:

> Ah, now he heard, she holding it to his ear. Hear! He heard. Wonderful. She held it to her own and through the sifted light pale gold in contrast gilded. To hear.

Tap.

Bloom through the bardoor saw a shell held at their ears. He heard more faintly that that they heard, each for herself alone, then each for other, hearing the plash of waves, loudly, a silent roar.

Bronze by a weary gold, anear, afar, they listened. [U 280]

A Bad Press

In maturity Joyce got rather a bad press. H.G. Wells spoke of the "cloacal obsession" of *Ulysses*. According to Sir Edmund Gosse, the book was anarchical, "infamous in taste, in style, in everything.... He is a sort of Marquis de Sade, but does not write so well. He is the perfect type of the Irish *fumiste*, a hater of England, more than suspected of partiality for Germany...."[28] Aldous Huxley found it dull and insignificant. Cyril Connolly said Joyce was "resented in Ireland, neglected in England, admired by a set in America, and idolized by another in France". (Deming, *Critical Heritage*, p. 401).

Among his friends and most appreciative admirers in Paris was Louis Gillet of the Academie Française, who approached *Ulysses* as a novel, only to find that it was a poem. "I can still see the spectre of the author of *Ulysses*—[Gillet recalled] gaunt and as if disincarnated, his profile like a crescent under his thick lenses, eye vexed and obstructed by a black felt patch—slide gropingly, with a step at the same time hesitant and lordly, among respectful people ready to make room for him."[29]

"I have great difficulty in coming to any understanding with the English [Joyce told Gillet]. I don't understand them no more than they understand me." ("But I don't write in English," he used to say.)[30]

Blindness

With the passage of time further intraocular deterioration was unavoidable. An iridectomy was performed in Zurich on 24 August 1917 by Ernest Sidler Huguenin (paid for by Edward Marsh). A disabling attack of acute glaucoma occurred in 1918 in Zurich and is commemorated in the poem "*Bahnhofstrasse*".

Ezra Pound felt as competent to advise on health matters as on literary affairs. He urged Joyce to consult Dr George Milbry Gould, who had treated Lafcadio Hearn. But Gould practised in Baltimore, Maryland; he advised Joyce, who communicated with him, to consult someone reliable closer to home. Prof. Alfred Vogt of Zurich was recommended by friends in that city.

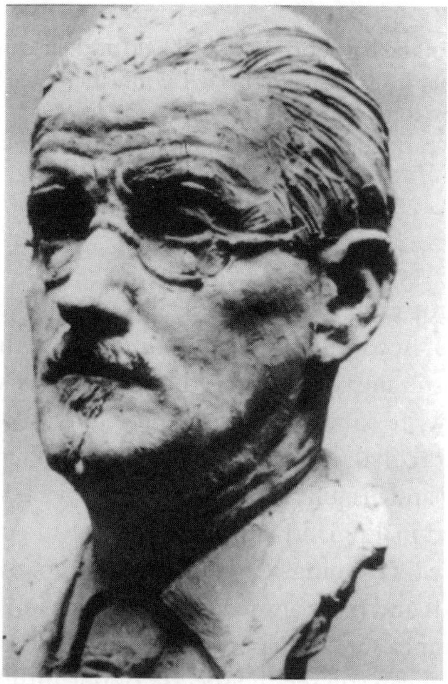

Fig. 3. Sculpture by Jo Davidson. "This is certainly one of the best and most faithful images of my grandfather. . . . "—Stephen James Joyce.

Vogt operated (this was the ninth operation) on the left eye for tertiary cataract on 15 May 1930, waiving his fee and accepting instead a copy of *Ulysses* signed for his daughter. Joyce experienced a decided improvement. Keeping this secret he attended the Paris Opera, where his friend Sullivan was singing in *Guillaume Tell*—during an interval Joyce stood up, leaned forward and, taking off his dark glasses, exclaimed loudly: "*Merci, mon Dieu pour ce miracle! Après vingt ans je revois la lumiere!*"

Mr Oliver Gogarty, FRCSI

Oliver St John Gogarty's *As I Was Going Down Sackville Street* was awaited impatiently by the Joyce brothers in the early months of 1937. Stanislaus wrote to James from Trieste on 27 March: " 'As I was walking down Sackville St':—or was it Tyrone St?—is sure to be full of 'The mockery of it'. No doubt Oliver St Jesus will get his own back on the author of 'U' ." (*Paul Léon Papers*, NLI).

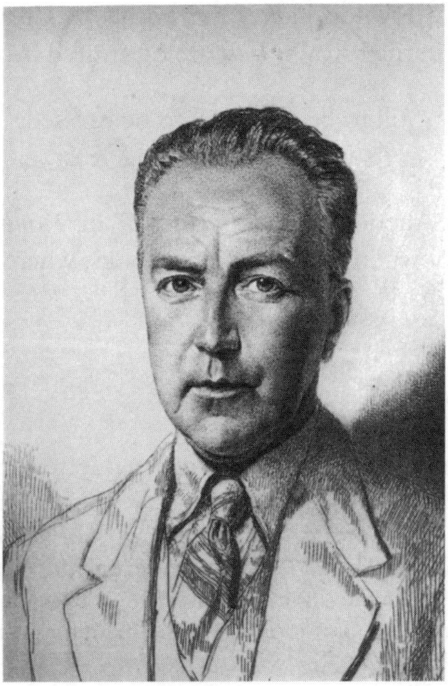

Fig. 4. Oliver St John Gogarty, MD, FRCSI, 1878–1958.

The elder brother commissioned Paul Léon to procure a copy; the latter was in touch with Harriet Shaw Weaver, who wrote on 9 February to say that Rich and Cowan had not yet published the book "but have announced it for the coming spring. Unless I hear to the contrary I will order a copy for Mr Joyce on publication". Ben Huebsch, too, wrote from the SS *Queen Mary* to tell Léon that he had ordered "Gogarty's memoirs" for Joyce but was unable to get him Gogarty's poems, *Wild Apples.*

Joyce sent a postcard to Léon from Zurich (*Paul Leon Papers*, 6 April 1937) asking him to buy *The Observer*, which had reviewed *Sackville Street.* "Also look to see is there a review of O.G. book in *N. Statesman* and *Spectator*. Where is the book itself. Better order one copy." A week later another postcard was dispatched: "As I have not had the promised wire I presume Transition has not come. And the O.G. book has been nicely bungled too."

Whether and when the book was received has not been recorded but Joyce's persisting interest in his former boon-companion's literary career is illuminating. *As I Was Going Down Sackville Street* did not pillory Joyce. He drinks with his friends in "The Bleeding Horse" and slips into the lavatory to record an "epiphany". John Elwood judges him to be "A Great Artist!" and three "auld ones" attired in their frowsy best are captivated by Ben Johnson's lines:

Still to be neat, still to be dressed,
As you were going to a feast.

There is a less sympathetic portrait of "Kinch" in *Tumbling in the Hay* and Joyce bobs up and down in Gogarty's later books, where repetition and inaccuracy are major faults.[31]

Finnegans Wake

Stanislaus Joyce sent his brother an ill-tempered letter on 7 August 1924:

> "I have received [he wrote] one installment of your yet unnamed novel in the *Translantic Review*. I don't know whether the drivelling rigmarole. . . is written with the deliberate intention of pulling the reader's leg or not. . . . Or perhaps—a sadder supposition—it is the beginning of softening of the brain." (*Letters*, III, 102)

Stannie evidently found *Finnegans Wake* "unspeakably wearisome". Others, too, were dismayed by the direction and form Joyce's writing was taking. Ezra Pound said that were it to conceal a "cure for the clap" this would hardly justify the labour of reading it. But this book caused "a new tumult in the world".[32] It rapidly gave origin to an entire library of secondary works which include *Our Exagmination Round His Factification for Incamination of Work in Progress* by Samuel Beckett and others, James Atherton's *The Books at the Wake*, Adaline Glasheen's *A Census of Finnegans Wake*, *A Second Census of Finnegans Wake*, etc.

"Fruit of loneliness, bitterness, wrath, regret and nostalgia," wrote Louis Gillet of the Academie Française, "this peculiar book was shaped by them little by little. It is made of bile and sorrow, of love contradicted and turned into irony. . . ." *Finnegans Wake*, according to this interpreter, "is a sort of woven tapestry, an illiad of puns, an amazing verbal fantasia, a game in the true meaning of the French *jeu de mots. Words, words, words*, says Hamlet, *Camelot Prince of Dinmurk*, as the author calls him with irreverence." Some of these pranks are excellent, others unintelligible.[33]

Finnegans Wake was reviewed by Gogarty in *The Observer* on 7 May 1939. He dismissed it as "the most colossal leg pull in literature since McPherson's Ossian", but he also had generous things to say (Deming, *Critical Heritage*,

II, 673). "The immense erudition employed [he wrote], and the various languages ransacked... is almost incredible to anyone unaware of the superhuman knowledge the author had when a mere stripling".

Gogarty saw the book as "an attempt to get at words before they clarify in the mind"; he said that Yeats found "this kind of prose made any other colourless". He wished to grant the work meaning and coherency but wondered if it was "wrong to look for meaning where there is every meaning".

My own progress through *Finnegans Wake* has been slow, intermittent and recurring. I am obliged to admit that I have not ventured beyond the nursery slopes. Yet I did shed light on "the ogry Osler" (317.16), whose readiness to "oxmaul us all" remained unclarified in the first edition of Adaline Glasheen's *Census.*[34] It was a by-product of Sir William Osler's "Fixed Period" address delivered on the occasion of his departure from Baltimore. He suggested jocosely that as the real work of life is done by the 40th year, men should be painlessly eliminated at 60 after a period of contemplation, but the joke misfired and was taken seriously by the newspapers.

In the sphere of anatomy there are numerous references, the most amusing of which is a description of deglutition: "the faery pangeant fluwed down the hisophenguts, a slake for the quicklining, to the tickle of his tube and the twobble of his fable" (319.12); the most ingenious a detailed account of the ear already featured in the "Sirens" episode of *Ulysses*:

> (to) pinnatrate inthro an auricular forfickle (known as the Vakingfar sleeper, monofractured by Piaras UaRhuamhaighaudhlug, tympan founder, Eustache Straight, Bauliaughacleeagh) a meatous conch culpable of cunduncing Naul and Santry... up his corpular fruent and down his reuctionary buckling, hummer, enville and cstorrap (the man of Iren, thore's Curlymane for you!), lill the lubberendth of his otological life. (310.9)

The folk at the wake include Max Planck ("Let's hear what science has to say, pundit-the-next-best-thing. Splanck!"), while by borrowing from *Three Quarks for Muster Mark!* (383.1) to name "the quark", his postulated subunit of the neutron and proton, Professor Murray Gell-Mann neatly bridged the gap between "the two cultures".

Only a minority can attain familiarity with this book, though there is probably something there for everyone: medical readers will find hospitals, diseases, literary figures and much more besides.

> Brimgem young, bringem young, bringem young!: in my bethel of Solyman's I accouched their rotundaties and I turnkeyed most insultantly over raped

lutetias in the lock: I gave bax of biscums to the jacobeaters and pottage bakes to the esausted. (542.27)

Giacomo Joyce

There is a slim, elegantly produced book, *Giacomo Joyce* (1968), to which I turn for a closing sentence, Joyce's presumed acknowledgement of the exquisite texture of the eye so recklessly endangered—"The long eyelids beat and lift: a burning needleprick stings and quivers in the velvet iris."[35]

Acknowledgement

Permission to include quotations from *Ulysses*, *Finnegans Wake*, *Giacomo Joyce* and *Letters of James Joyce* has been given on behalf of the James Joyce Estate by Stephen James Joyce.

References

1. R. Ellmann, *James Joyce*, 2nd ed. (OUP, New York, 1982), passim.
2. A. Martin, ed., *James Joyce: The Artist and The Labyrinth* (Ryan, London, 1990), p. 14.
3. J. Joyce, *Finnegans Wake* (Viking, New York, 1967), p. 424.06. Further references to *FW* are given in parentheses in the text.
4. J.B. Lyons, Picking up Galen: James Joyce in Cecilia Street, *J. Irish Colls. Phys. Surg.* **26**, 215–8 (1997).
5. H. Kenner, *A Colder Eye* (Penguin, Harmondsworth, 1984), p. 196.
6. J. Joyce, *Ulysses* (Bodley Head/Penguin, Harmondsworth, 1960), p. 31.
7. J.B. Lyons, *James Joyce & Medicine* (Dolmen, Dublin, 1973), p. 60.
8. Brenda Maddox, *Nora* (Hamish Hamilton, London, 1988), passim.
9. *Letters of James Joyce*, Vol. II, ed. Richard Ellmann (Faber, London, 1966), p. 48. Subsequent quotations from letters are given in parentheses in the text: Vol. I, ed. Stuart Gilbert; Vols. II, III, and *Selected Letters*, ed. R. Ellmann; *Paul Léon Papers*, ed. C. Fahy (National Library of Ireland, Dublin, 1992).
10. Ezra Pound; see *The Critical Heritage*, ed. R.H. Deming, Vol. I (Routledge, London, 1970), p. 67.
11. C.P. Curran, *James Joyce Remembered* (OUP, New York, 1968), p. 55.
12. R.J. Finneran, ed., *Letters of James Stephens* (Macmillan, London, 1974), p. 138.
13. J.B. Lyons, "Diseases in Dubliners: tokens of disaffection", in *Irish Renaissance Annual II*, ed. Zack Bowen (University of Delaware Press, Newark, 1981), pp. 185–94.

14. R. Ellmann, *James Joyce* (OUP, New York, 1982), p. 262.
15. J. McCourt, *The Years of Bloom* (Lilliput, Dublin, 2000), p. 122.
16. R. Ellmann, *James Joyce* (OUP, New York, 1982), p. 241.
17. J. McCourt, *The Years of Bloom* (Lilliput, Dublin, 2000), p. 113.
18. A.J. King and Mason, R.M. Reiter's disease, *Textbook of the Rheumatic Diseases*, ed. W.S.C. Copeman (Livingstone, Edinburgh, 1969), pp. 366–83.
19. Ms Cornell, ALS Josephine Murray/J. Joyce, 4 June 1907.
20. J.B. Lyons, *James Joyce & Medicine* (Dolmen, Dublin, 1973), p. 65.
21. R. Ellmann, *James Joyce* (OUP, New York, 1982), p. 267.
22. M. Shechner, *Joyce in Nighttown* (University of California Press, London, 1974), p. 88.
23. M. Shechner, *Joyce in Nighttown* (University of California Press, London, 1974), p. 89.
24. J. Collins, James Joyce's amazing chronicle, *New York Times Book Review*, 28 May 1922, pp. 6, 17.
25. C.G. Jung, *The Spirit in Man, Art, and Literature: Collected Works*, Vol. 15 (Routledge, London, 1966), p. 110.
26. C.G. Jung, *The Spirit in Man, Art, and Literature: Collected Works*, Vol. 15 (Routledge, London, 1966,), p. 111.
27. F. Budgen, *James Joyce and the Making of Ulysses* (Indiana University Press, Bloomington, 1960), p. 21.
28. E. Gosse, Letter to Louis Gillet, 7 June 1924, in: L. Gillet, *Claybook for James Joyce* (Abelard-Schuman, London, 1958), p. 31.
29. L. Gillet, *Claybook for James Joyce* (Abelard-Schuman, London, 1958), p. 27.
30. L. Gillet, *Claybook for James Joyce* (Abelard- Schuman, London, 1958), p. 18.
31. J.B. Lyons, *Oliver St John Gogarty—The Man of Many Talents* (Blackwater, Dublin, 1980).
32. L. Gillet, *Claybook for James Joyce* (Abelard-Schuman, London, 1958), p. 21.
33. L. Gillet, *Claybook for James Joyce* (Abelard- Schuman, London, 1958), p. 71.
34. A. Glasheen, *A Census of Finnegans Wake* (Faber, London, 1957).
35. J. Joyce, *Giacomo Joyce: With an Introduction and Notes by R. Ellmann* (Viking Press, New York, 1968), p. 1.

Chapter 22

Neurology in the Nordic Sagas

Ragnar Stien

The archaic Nordic language was in medieval times spoken in Iceland, Norway, Sweden, Denmark, Greenland, the Faroe Islands, the Shetland Islands, the Orkney Islands and the Hebrides. In that period (1100–1350), when learned men from the rest of Europe were writing in Latin, a rich literature was created in the Nordic countries in their own language. Most of the writing was done in Iceland, the rest mainly in Norway, and very little in Greenland and the other Atlantic islands; events in Denmark and Sweden are dealt with on a smaller scale.

The dominant role of Iceland and Norway is best explained by the way Iceland was inhabited: influential families from the west coast of Norway fled the country from 870 to 950 to avoid the power of the new, strong kingdom of Harald 1 Fairhair. They settled in Iceland, and for centuries the Iceland colony preserved and fostered the cultural traditions of western Norway. This oligarchy of families were intensely proud of their ancestry. Jealous of their cultural heritage, they were very eager to keep traditions and language unchanged. In this setting the old orally transmitted sagas and poems were written down and kept until collectors started to hunt down manuscripts in the17th and 18th centuries. The most important of these manuscripts were given to the Danish–Norwegians kings or to the University of Copenhagen.

Both the sagas and the poems describe very dramatic events connected with well-known persons or families. Very little deals with medical matters, and neurology as such is naturally not mentioned. I will give some examples of medical reports in the literature and discuss the possible sources of medical knowledge.

The Nordic literature is often divided into three different groups: (1) religious prose, laws and commentaries on the laws; (2) poems; (3) sagas.

Religious Prose

The first group is not very interesting from a medical point of view. Some of the stories about the early bishops of Iceland (*Biskuppasogur*) report on miracles done by the later holy men. Particularly, Bishop Thorlak (the Holy) is said to have performed countless miracles[1] which are listed in at least three different books. He heals a man with epilepsy and an eye disease, and a woman with acute blindness and other neurological symptoms, which actually might be a very early report of multiple sclerosis. Some of the better-known doctors (*læknir*) are also mentioned.

Poems

The Nordic poet, the skald, was a highly ranked man, and kings and noblemen tried to hire the most famous for their court or household. The poems were usually epics written in an extremely difficult manner, with very strict rules and rhymes. These technically difficult constructions, rhythm and rhyme, made it easy to remember the poems even if they were not written down. The oldest poems or lays were created in the 8th or 9th century, but not written down, as we know them today, until the 12th and 13th centuries.

The most famous of all Icelandic authors, Snorri Sturluson (1178–1241), wrote *Kringla Heimsins* (history of the Norwegian kings) and a textbook for poets, *Edda* (around 1220). This "how-to-make-it" book gives examples of all types of rules for the construction of a poem. Snorri quotes freely from a large collection of poems that he had at his disposal. These old poems were later "lost", but in 1643 the Icelandic bishop Brynjulfur Sveinson found a small leather book with 45 pages (8 were lost) where nearly all the poems Snorri had used as examples were found. This book was called *The Old Edda*. Brynjulfur Sveinsons' manuscript had been copied in the late 13th century, i.e. after Snorris' *Edda*. From other sources, we know that the original poems were written before 900—probably in Norway. The *Edda* poems have nearly the same position in the tradition of the Nordic people as the Vedas for India and the Homeric poems for Greece. With a few additions to the Brynjulfur Sveinsons version, *The Old Edda* contains about 30 long poems. All of them tell about gods and heroes and provide moral and practical advice.

Hávamál is a poem attributed to Odin the Highest. Of the 164 verses, verse 137 is a collection of 9 rude old medical receipts:

Rathome ther, Loddfáfnir,	Hear thou, Loddfáfnir,
enn thú ráth nemir,	and heed it well,
nióta mundo, ef thu nemr,	learn it, 'twill lend the strength
ther muno góth, ef thú getr:	follow it, 'twill further thee:
1. *Hvars thú ol dreccir,*	when ale thou drinkest,
kiós thú thér iarthar megin.	invoke earth-strength,
2. *Thviat iorth teer vith olthri,*	for earth is good against ale,
3. *enn elthr vith sóttom*	'gainst ague, fire,
4. *eic vith abbindi,*	'gainst straining acorns,
5. *ax vith fiolkyngi,*	'gainst witchery, steel,
6. *holl vith hyrogi,*	'gainst house-strife, the elder,
7. *heiptom scal mána qvethia,*	'gainst hate, the moon,
8. *beiti vith bitsóttom,*	'gainst the rabies, alum,
9. *enn vith bolvi rúnar.*	'gainst ill luck, runes.
10. *Fold scal vith flóthi taca.*	For earth absorbs the humours all.[2]

The translation of these prescriptions has always been difficult. Linguists get into trouble because they do not quite understand the medical references, and doctors cannot cope with the etymological problems.

The first point to note is that the lines were not written at the same time. The original verse (as understood by the other verses around this one) consists of the first lines and the last. The verses start with the general statement from Odin to Lodfáfnir to follow his advice. In line 1 of 137 the advice is to use earth if he has drunk too much beer, or rather, if he has drunk bad, contaminated beer—a very common occurrence in those days. The use of earth as an anti-toxic substance is well documented (*terra sigilata*, *terra sigilata cimbrica*, *terra norvegica antiscorbutica*, etc.). From another source (a medical book from 13th century Iceland) we read: "*-ok er manni gefinn olyfjansdrykkr, thá drekki han thessi jordunni*" ("If a man has got a toxic drink, he should drink this earth"). Previous to this statement the earth is described as "having a seal with the picture of a man" ("*er á innsigli er løgth ok manns likneski er á*"), which is an accurate description of *terra sigilata*. In the time of Dioscorides, the seal on this medical earth had the picture of a goat; in Galen's time the picture was one of the goddess Diana, and later Christ was used.[2]

Within this well-accepted medical advice, later copyists have put in eight new medical prescriptions. Most of these are easily understood by doctors with a basic knowledge of medieval medicine[3,4]:

Line 2. The recommendation of earth against intoxication is repeated.

Line 3. Fire and smoke against febrile diseases are well known.

Line 4. "*Eic vith abbindi*" is word for word like the line in *Regimen Sanitatis* from Salerno: "*-ventrem dant escula strictum*". This prescription underlines many points: "Health-poems" were known in both southern and northern Europe, and perhaps *Regimen Sanitatis* was known in Iceland. From the medical point of view, the linguist's translation into English is not quite correct: acorns are not used against straining but to stop diarrhoea—or, better, to treat dysentery.

Line 5. "*Ax*" here is definitely not the English "axe" or "steel". The word "*ax*" is used for "straw" or "herb". "*Fiolkyngi*" might mean witchery, but could even be used for different "internal" diseases.

Line 6. This line will be dealt with in detail below.

Line 7. The exact meaning of this line has never been established.

Line 8. The linguist has completely missed the point that earthworms (*beiti*) were a well-known remedy against wounds. Particularly, the oleic extract (*oleum lumbricale*) was used to treat infected wounds acquired from the bite of animals (*bitsóttom*).

Line 9. Magic runes were probably used against different types of misfortune and disease.

The fifth added prescription is very controversial. A commonly accepted translation is given above, but why should "house-strife" in a Viking society be treated with a tree not growing on Iceland and hardly in Norway? The word "*holl*" (the "*o*" could be pronounced in different ways like in English: "hole" or "doll" or even "*haulvi*") is usually translated with "elder" or "hall". Used in the latter way, the line runs: "House-strife should be kept in the hall (within the family)." In *Biskuppasogur (Jons Saga)* there is a passage about a man being treated for an inguinal hernia. The hernia is called "holl", probably pointing to the fact that there is a defect in the abdominal wall, a "hole". The umbilicus is in another text called "nafla-holl".[2]

The other important word in this line is "*hyrogi*". The translation is based on "*hy*", like "*hi*", i.e. the place where hibernating animals sleep during the winter. The meaning of "*rogi*" is not known, but it has been accepted that the word is similiar to "rage". The result of these rather distant associations is "house-strife". "*Hy*" has another meaning, even in some contemporary Norwegian dialects, namely "thin hairs" or "mould". The only known complete copy, from late 1300, of *The Old Edda* is full of misprints or wrongly copied words. We know this because quotations from *The Old Edda* come from different sources. Verse 137 is not known in any other version, and the word "*hyrogi*" is not found elsewhere in Nordic literature. Could it be a misspelling? The drunken (?) monks that copied the old books hardly understood what they were writing. Some linguists suggest that "*rogi*" should have been written as "*rogr*" or "*rugr*", which means rye. The large Icelandic–English dictionary from the late 19th century (Cleasby-Vigfusson) suggests "bearded rye" for "*hyrogi*". Written and understood in this way the prescription should run: moulded rye against holes/ruptures/wounds. To a medical reader that makes sense: the haemostatic effect of badly kept rye—i.e. rye infected with *secale cornuutum* = ergotamines—was known in the Nordic area! *Ignis sacer* (see Chapter 3) was well known to medieval man, but "mouldy rye" as the reason for the contracted peripheral arteries—ergotism—was not recognised before the end of the 18th century. The use of secale-infected grain is mentioned only briefly in the literature to which I have access: Dragendorf, in his *Heilpflanzen*, states without references that secale was used in ancient times as "*Webenbeförderndes Mittel*" and "*Hemostatikum*". Secale is derived from the Latin name of the "bearded rye", *secale cornutuum*, the winter form of *claviceps purpurea Tulasne*. Höfler in *Altgermanisches Heilkunde* writes that "*der Genuss verschiedener Getränke aus Planzensaften sowie das Mutterkorn*" were used as abortives.[2]

The conclusion is that the constrictor effect on blood vessels, so intensively used in our century against migraine, was known to Nordic medieval doctors. The prescription probably began in the 9th or 10th century and is the first medical use of ergot alkaloids that I have come across.[4]

The Lays of the Skalds

There are a large number of poems in the Nordic literature written by well-known authors or "skalds", some of whom were prominent and powerful political persons of their time. Their lays were made in praise of the kings, political events and the deeds of heroes. One of the most colourful skalds was Egil Skallagrimson (*c.* 910–990), who even has his own saga, *Egils Saga*. He was a tall man with a large head and was extremely ugly. He was a notorious killer (he killed his first man when he was six in a "ball game"!), pirate, ambitious politician and—in the end—a respected judge! Above all, he was a gifted poet. He was the typical representative of the resistance against the new Norwegian king and his family. He fought very effectively against the son of Harald Fairhair—Eirik Bloodaxe. Egil was born in Norway, but fled to Iceland, where he died as an old man. His life, his poems and the saga give us two interesting medical points.

After a violent life, he settles in Iceland. There one of his sons dies of a possible infectious disease, and soon afterwards the other son drowns in an accident at sea. The old killer develops a depression well described in the saga: after the funeral he goes to his bedroom, shuts the door and refuses to eat and drink for three days. They then send for his daughter, who arrives and goes into the same room as her father, stating that she, too, wants to die. But then she starts to eat and later drink, talks to her father and persuades him to do the same. With this psychiatric type of treatment he is brought back to life and writes the most impressive poem in the Nordic literature: *Sonatorrek*, an elegy in 24 verses describing the disaster of losing two sons:

For sorg eg fær'kje svevn um natti	The sorrow keeps me sleepless
Kann ikkje halda hovudet uppe	I can't keep my head erect
Eg minnet deira frå munnen ber ut	From my mouth their memories float
sveipt i skaldskaps-skrudet dyre.[6]	Wrapped in precious poetry.

The unexpected here is that in this story of blood and violence, we suddenly find the most accurate description of a reactive depression and its effective psychological treatment, both in prose and poetry.

At the very end of *Egils Saga*, the author tells us that Egil has an unsteady gait and nearly falls. The women laugh at him, and he recites:

Stiv eg går og stabbar	I stumble stiff around
skalle ottast falla.	afraid my head tilts forward.
Lite eg høyrer, og liten er	I hear little, and small is
lem som til lyst var laga.[6]	the organ that was made for lust.

The neurologist probably interprets Egil's difficulties as a polyneuropathy, with unsteady gait and impotence, he speaks of "insensible and cold feet" and is nearly blind and deaf. Then, in a postscript, the author tells a strange story about the exhumation of Egil's bones. After his conversion to Christianity a church was built on Egil's farm, and they moved his grave into the new churchyard. The story runs:

> The skull was an exceptionally large one. It was ridged all over on the outside like a scallop shell. They wanted to find out how thick it was, so Skapti (the priest) picked up a heavy axe, swung it in one hand and struck as hard as he was able with the reverse side of the axe, trying to break the skull. But the skull neither broke nor dented on impact, it simply turned white.

This recalls the clinical features of osteitis deformans, i.e. Paget's disease. The hard skull with the irregular surface, the greater-than-usual (for polyneuropathy) affection of cranial nerves (blind and deaf), the leonine appearance of Egil and a possible polyneuropathy or peripheral vascular deficiency all fit well with James Paget's (1814–1899) description of the disease that bears his name. But Queen Victoria's surgeon will have to share the honour of the first description of the disease with the author of *Egils Saga* about 700 years earlier.[7]

The Sagas

The sagas deal with dramatic events in the lives of kings and local chieftains or the fate of families or communities. Very little is mentioned of medicine except wounds and lesions received in battles or the laconic "Died in *sotteseng* (sickbed)". A few persons are labelled "*læknir*", a word that very much resembles today's Scandinavian "*læge*" (*da*), "*lege*" (*no*), "*läkare*" (*swe*), which means a medical doctor. By following various "*læknir*" in different sagas, we suddenly find a whole dynasty of doctors, one of whom even has his own saga: *Hrafns Saga Sveinbjarnarsonar*. We will follow this dynasty in more detail because it gives an idea of the training and the professional standards of the medieval Nordic doctor.

The story starts with Snorri Sturluson's *Saga of Magnus the Good* from *Kringla Heimsins*. Snorri says that king Magnus, after the big battle of Hlyrskog Heath (in Denmark) in 1043 (where the king achieved an overwhelming victory), "...ordered the wounds of his men to be bound; but there were not so many doctors in the army as were necessary, so the king himself went around, and felt the hands of those he thought best suited for the business; and when he had thus stroked their palms, he named twelve men, who, he thought, had the softest hands, and told them to bind the wounds of the people; and although none of them had ever tried it before, they all became afterwards the best of doctors." Snorri then cannot resist telling the reader that not all of these doctors were Norwegian: two were from Iceland and one was "Atle, the father of Bárd the Black from Selårdal". It is obviously important for Snorri to mention this fact. Then, when one is reading other sagas, the family of Bárd the Black is often mentioned in connection with the practice of medicine. In one part is this statement: "By God's blessings the art of medicine came into the family of Bárd the Black (*kyn Bárdar Svarta*)" (*Sturlungasaga*).

The persons whose names are in bold are all referred to as "medical doctors" or "*læknir*", but for two of them there are more detailed descriptions of their medical abilities: Hrafn Sveinbjørnarson has his own saga and Hrafn Oddson's record is told in *Biskuppasogur* (*The Saga of Bishop Árni*). It is obvious that at the time when Snorri Sturluson wrote *The History of the Norwegian Kings* (first part of the 13th century), the medical dynasty of Bárd the

KYN BÁRDAR SVARTA

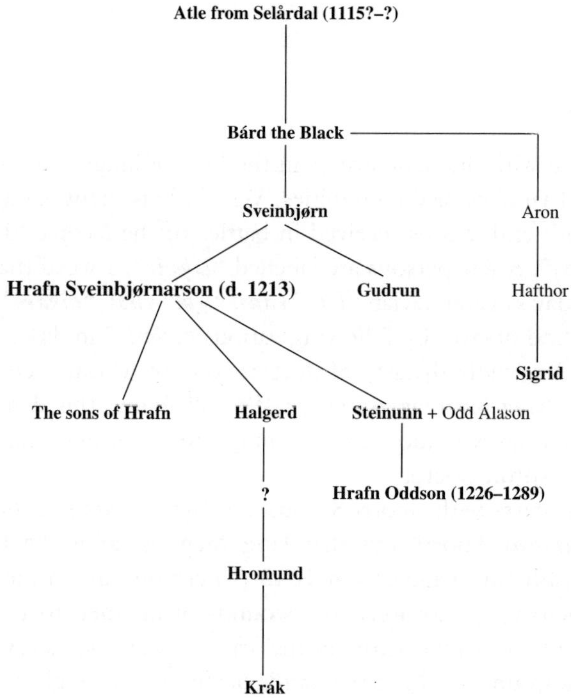

Black was well known. We then understand why Snorri found it worthwhile to mention that Atle was the father of Bárd. *Hrafns Saga* tells of his fight with Thorvald Snorrason, the son-in-law of the great historian Snorri Sturluson. The hero in the saga is Hrafn, and the villain is Thorvald. Hrafn is killed by Thorvald and his men in 1213. Only a small part of the Saga tells of Hrafn's education and medical practice. His family was influential and wealthy. Hrafn was trained in theology, law, medicine, and languages, and he probably spoke and wrote Latin. He was also a good sailor, swimmer, archer, swordsman and poet. We know that he made a long journey, probably in the 1190s: first to Norway, then to England (Canterbury, to visit the shrine of St Thomas), to "Iliansborg" (St Giles in Provence), to Santiago de Compostella in Spain and to Rome. We do not know how long he stayed in Italy, or whether he visited Salerno—at that time the best-known medical school in Europe. But as he belonged to a well-known "medical family", it would be strange if he did not visit the centre of medical wisdom of that time.

Hrafn practised medicine without taking fees. The saga presents four case histories:

One man suffered from generalised oedema and Hrafn cauterised him on the head, chest, and between the shoulders. The three other stories are remarkable in many ways:

A woman came because she probably had some kind of depression or fits. Hrafn performed venesection in her arm called "*thjotandi*" ("the humming blood vessel"). It can be inferred that some kind of auscultation was performed, since a venous hum may sometimes be heard in the elbow. The Salerno school taught that the veins in the neck and in the arm were the same and came from the head or brain. Hrafn probably opened the cephalic vein, as recommended by the Salerno school: "*Cephalicam venam incidimus propter capitis causam, et propter maniam et epilepsiam.*"

A man called Thorgils suffered some kind of fits; "several men had all they could do to hold him when the attacks came on him". Hrafn cauterised him in several places on the head, and the saga claims that the man was cured. Cauterisation was a very common type of treatment for different diseases, including epilepsy.

The fourth case reports on a man who could not pass urine because a stone had fallen into the bladder-neck and blocked the urethra. Hrafn treated him for some time in his house, without much success. He then called for the priests and the wisest men of his household. He asked them what they thought might happen to the man if he was left alone. They all said that he would surely die. Hrafn said then that he would take action on their advice. Then the text runs:

"-thá for hann hondum um hann, og kendi steinnsins i kvidinum og	"-then he passed his hands over the man, and felt the stone in his bladder
færdi framm i getnadar lim hans svo sem mátti og bat sijdann firer ofann med hárthrædi so ad eigi skylldi upp thokast. Enn odrum thrædi batt hann firer framann steininn og bad hann ad aller skylldi syngja fimm sinnum pater noster their jnni voru. Ad hann veiti giordina, sijdann skar hann á med knijfi um endilángt og tok burt ij steina. Sijdann batt hann smirsl vid sárid og græddi svo hann vard alheill.	and pushed it into the penis as far as he could and tied then above it with a thread of hair so that it should not slide back. And another thread he tied in front of the stone and asked all those present to sing five pater nosters. When they had done that, he made a lengthwise incision with a knife and removed a stone. Then he bound the wound with liniments, it healed and the man became completely well.[8]

The operation described was very risky and technically extremely advanced for the time. Even more surprising is the fact that this operation, written about in the saga by a layman, is described similarly, word for word, in one of the most popular textbooks on surgery used in the Salerno school. The book is *Liber Pantegni*, attributed to Constantinus Africanus (1045–1087), but probably translated by him from the Arabic version of the works of Paulus of Aegina (625–690). In *Liber Pantegni* the operation is described in this way:

> *At si lapidus parvus fuerit in virgam ceciderit, ligetur virga a parte inferiori, et si non posit conducendo foras extrahi, icterum a superiori parte ligabitur et in medio cum ferro incide et lapidem extrahes.*

Hrafn might have learned this operation from a book (*Liber Pantegni*?), but, remembering his long tour visiting different centres in Europe, it would have been rather strange if he had not visited a place where medicine was taught and advanced operations and treatments were performed.[3]

Conclusions

(1) The medieval Nordic doctors were well aware of the most advanced medical methods of the time. Some had probably visited the best centres of medical teaching, such as the Salerno school. Medical knowledge and medical instruments were kept within families and passed on form generation to generation.

(2) Their methods for treating epilepsy and many other conditions were not based on superstition or magic, but were "scientific" or "evidence-based", in the best meaning of these words in a medieval society.

(3) "Health-poems" were known and used to give medical advice, in accordance with the best medical knowledge in contemporary Europe.

(4) Part of their medical knowledge was unique, such as the use of the haemostatic effect of ergotamine.

(5) Some of the saga authors show an impressive ability to describe medical conditions and their treatments.

References

1. *A Book of Miracles* (Corpus Codicum Islandicorum Medii Ævi, Copenhagen, 1938).
2. P. Terry, *Poems of the Elder Edda* (University of Pennsylvania Press, Philadelphia, 1990).

3. F. Grøn, Bidrag til den norrøne lægekunsts historie, *Tidsskr Nor Lægeforen* **27**, 1–56 (1907).
4. I. Reichborn-Kjennerud, Lægerådene i den eldre Edda, *Maal og Minne* 1–57 (1923).
5. J. Grier, Ergot, *A History of Pharmacy* (The Pharmaceutical Press, London, 1937).
6. *Egils-soga*, transl. by Leiv Hegstad (Det norske samlaget, Oslo, 1927).
7. T. Hardarson and E. Snorradóttir, Egil's or Paget's disease? *Br. Med. J.* **313**, 1613–4 (1996).
8. A. Tjomsland, The saga of Hrafn Sveinbjarnarson, *Islandica*, *XXXV* (Cornell University Press, New York, 1951).

Chapter 23

The Poetry of Henry Head[1]

Christopher Gardner-Thorpe[2]

Poetry—The Best Words in the Best Order

In 1953 Randall Jarrell (1914–1965), poet, children's story writer, novelist and poetry critic, wrote "When you begin to read a poem you are entering a foreign country whose laws and language and life are a kind of translation of your own"[3] and "Today poems, good poems, are written almost exclusively by born poets."[4]

Poetry by doctors is nothing new. John Keats (1795–1821)[5] is one of the best-known doctors who wrote significant poetry, but by no means the only one. He studied medicine at Guy's Hospital in 1815 and attended the lectures of Astley Cooper (1768–1841). His notebook is at the Keats House Museum in Hampstead. He qualified as a medical practitioner in July 1816 at Apothecary's Hall at Blackfriars in London but did not proceed to surgical finals. He died less than five years later, aged 25, and was buried in Rome in February 1821. He wrote,[6] presumably of tuberculosis:

I see a lily on thy brow
With anguish moist and fever dew;
And on thy cheek a fading rose
Fast withereth too.

Neurological poems appear from time to time and some perhaps are less euphonious than Keats'. In 1927 a series, *Disrespectful Ditties*, was published by the editors of *Round the Fountain*, a journal at St Bartholomew's Hospital in London. The first verse of "Parkinson's Disease"[7] reads:

Poor Pa Parkinson very seldom smiled;
Always apathetic and never really riled,
Vacuous his features as any in Debrett's.[8]
Poor Pa Parkinson, rolling cigarettes.

"Thomsen's Disease"[9,10] reads:

One sunny afternoon in May,
After a long and tiring day,
Dr and Mrs Thomsen lay
Quiescent in the heather.
At length, addressing Mrs T.,
He said, "I think, Penelope,
The time has come for you and me
To stagger home together."
She said, "I quite agree with you;
We are much too old to bill and coo.
The air is getting chillsome too;
Get up, we mustn't linger!"
But he, before her very eyes,
Directly he essayed to rise,
Discovered much to his surprise
He couldn't stir a finger.

Although by nature rather mean,
They taxi'd home to Turnham Green
(Since luckily his wife had seen
A public telephone near).
He was so braced to find that he,
In this unknown myopathy
Had made a new discovery,
And called it "myotonia."

The next day, walking down the Strand,
He met a pal, who seized his hand
And said, "Why, this is simply grand
Let's go and have a jorum."[11]
But, though his throat was very dry,
He found however he might try
He could not free his Musculi
Flexores Digitorum.

This fell disease, so I've been told,
Appears to take a strangle-hold
When persons are exposed to cold,
Like sailors, or night-watchmen;
And, though the thing is rather rare,
That irritating symptom where
The grasp retains whatever's there
Is often seen in Scotchmen!

War poetry is especially poignant. Wilfred Owen (1893–1918), a poet from Shropshire, wrote of those wounded in the War:

Disabled[12]

He sat in a wheeled chair, waiting for dark,
And shivered in his ghastly suit of grey,
Legless, sewn short at elbow. Through the park
Voices of boys rang saddening like a hymn,

⋮

And later:

Now, he is old; his back will never brace;
He's lost his colour very far from here,
Poured it down shell-holes till the veins ran dry,
And half his lifetime lapsed in the hot race
And leap of purple spurted from his thigh.

And again:

Now, he will spend a few sick years in institutes,
And do what things the rules consider wise,
And take whatever pity they may dole.
Tonight he noticed how the women's eyes
Passed from him to the strong men that were whole.
How cold and late it is! Why don't they come
And put him into bed? Why don't they come?

Henry Head (1861–1940) and His Family[13–15]

Henry Head was born[16] on 4 August 1861 at Stoke Newington in London.[17] From an early age Head wished to study medicine and in 1890 he qualified at University College in London. He lived at 6 Clarence Terrace, London NW.[18] He was a natural teacher and became a Fellow of the Royal Society in 1899,[19] FRCP in 1900, and in 1919 he was appointed Consulting Physician to the London Hospital.

Thomas Hardy (1840–1928) may have influenced Head's poetry. In 1901 Head wrote a poem, published in *Destroyers*[20]:

Spring Death

In memory of J.W. who died on Active Service in 1901

I will beat forth my sorry to the sun,
For dumb and cold I sit at home with grief.

Eddies of spring-tide through the dark limbs run
Of this foul city, over park and square
Ripple in golden leaf.
Each solitary tree, once dank and bare,
Poised in a fluttering skirt of gauzy green,
Whirls to the rhythm of awakening earth;
Through murky lane and highway throbs a clean
Bass note of birth.

The chestnut spreads her fingers to the breeze,
Adorned with perfumed candles for the feast.
Once more the little murmurs haunt the trees,
And all that buds is cast a pall of sleep.
From grimy bonds released,
Over the churchyard paling, lilacs peep,
Each golden leaflet quick with gentle rain,
And all the world that once was tired and old,
Decked out with new desires, grows young again,
Lilac and gold.

But death has stripped me bare of all desire:
An outcast from earth's generous festival,
I go to warm me by the altar fire,
Whereat we worshipped. Happy little shrine—
Soft garlands on the wall,
The music and the laughter and the wine,
Talk, like a fountain pulsing to the blue,
To fall in rainbow droplets on the grass,
Warm human joys—they shall my heart renew,
They cannot pass.

What shadow haunts that dear familiar room
And, like a night-bird poised on silent wing,
Hovers upon the violet-scented gloom?
Our instruments of joy lie untouched there
And, scarcely whispering,
We say not what we would but all we dare,
Quelling the tumult of forbidden tears;
No more to wander with the roving throng,
Bowed by resentment for our numbered years—
Our years of song.

Together through the blue transparent nights,
Together through the hum of London streets,
Our path was like a garden gay with lights,
Tall lilies among tulips gold and red;
Where with insistent beats
Love called, and all the world a-trysting sped.
Beneath the whispering plane-trees passion burned,
Glowed like illumined green in every breast,

Then piping happy songs we homeward turned,
Turned home to rest.

Over the house-top climbs a cowslip moon,
To join the expectant company of stars,
New-risen—And I little care how soon
My feet turn homeward by familiar ways.
No fellowship unbars
That narrow dwelling, where the measured days
Pass, and leave naught to show that they are fled.
I am grown weary, and to me alone
Love pipes a foolish tune, for thou art dead,
And youth is gone.

In 1904, at the age of 42, Head married Ruth Mayhew. She wrote novels and also *A Simple Guide to Pictures by Mrs Henry Head*.[21] Ruth later wrote (in 1916) on Henry James and in 1922 she compiled an anthology of Thomas Hardy's writing[22] for which Henry wrote an introduction.[23] Mrs Kitty Ionides, a friend of the family, wrote[24]: "... where I often stayed presided over by Mrs Head, much conversation and laughter although in those days I was sometimes overawed by the highbrow, as it would now be called, of Henry's conversation with Ruth Mayhew on early French poetry. He married

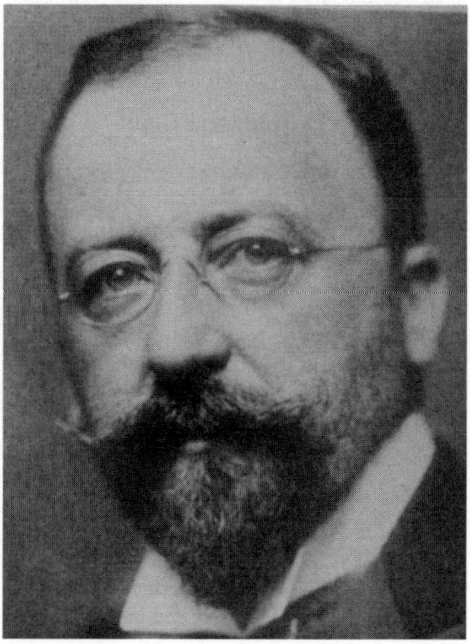

Fig. 1. Henry Head.

her later and they were extremely happy.... I always remember Mrs Head with a small lace cap and her portly body tightly encased in black satin and a cameo brooch at the throat. She was one of the most wonderful personalities I have ever known, full of insatiable love of life and human beings to whom she gave her wise and untiring help.... The beauty of the lines given in her exquisite voice was memorable.... All the fun and laughter at the dinner table was entirely devoid of malice. Indeed none could have lived in her presence. At a dinner party in my house in London Mrs Head was seated on my future husband's right hand and in a pause of the conversation I heard her turn her rather loud voice to say 'I always wear Henry's pyjamas on board ship. They are so much easier when I climb up to my bunk.' I imagine they were talking of foreign travel."

In 1910 Head lived at 4 Montagu Square in London.[25] He first became interested in aphasia in 1910 while investigating the sensory effects of cortical lesions. During the First World War (1914–1918), Head became Civilian Consultant to the Empire Hospital for Officers at Vincent Square.

Pat Barker, winner of the 1995 Booker Prize, has in *The Trilogy*[26–28] brought Head's name to the forefront again. During the First World War, Head's friends included Siegfried Louvain Sassoon (1886–1967), well-known First World War poet and writer of prose, whom Head treated as a patient. It was said that Sassoon wanted to penetrate the callous complacency of the civilian, and Sassoon's poems "Died of Wounds"[29] and "Does It Matter?"[30] refer particularly to this.

Does it Matter

Does it matter?—losing your legs?....
For people will always be kind,
And you need not show that you mind
When the others come in after hunting
To gobble their muffins and eggs.

Does it matter?—losing your sight?....
There's such splendid work for the blind
And people will always be kind,
As you sit on the terrace remembering
And turning your face to the light.

Do they matter?—those dreams from the pit?....
You can drink and forget and be glad,
And people won't say that you are mad;
For they'll know you've fought for your country
And no one will worry a bit.

Head knew other First World War poets, including Robert Graves (1895–1985), who was impressed by Head's scientific integrity, and Robert Nichols

(1893–1944), who thought Head an authority on Leonardo da Vinci (1452–1519).

In 1919 Head published *Destroyers and Other Verses*,[31,32] an 88-page octavo, of which only 500 copies were published and which included these six poems and four previously unpublished, dedicated to his wife:

To her
without whose touch the
Strings would have been
Mute.

Head acknowledged the *Yale Review* (Newhaven, Connecticut) for "I Cannot Stand and Wait", "Destroyers" and "Died of His Wounds", *The English Review* for "Homing Wings" and "The Price", and *The Dublin Review* for "To Courage, Seated". The poetry appears in four groups. First are the 1914–1918 poems, namely "I Cannot Stand and Wait", "Homing Wings", "Paris, April 1916", "The Price", "Destroyers", "Died of His Wounds", "Epiphany", "To Courage, Seated", "Elan Vital" and "Pegasus", and these are followed by *Songs of La Mouche*. Four pages of text discuss Elise K., better known as Camille Selden, who was born at Saxony in 1829 and died at Rouen in 1896. She associated with Alfred Meissner (1822–1885), the Austrian poet and playwright who wrote about those whom she had met in Paris and whose poems she translated into French. Head also discusses Heinriche Heine (1799–1856), perhaps the last of the Romantic poets. Meissner went to Paris to save Heine's works from destruction by his wife. Here Head includes poems of Meissner and Heine.

After these, there appear two further collections, *Seedtime and Harvest*[33] and *Sun and Shower*.[34] Head may have taken the title of the former from the quotation he gave from the Bible[35] and from Hardy at the end of the introduction to Ruth's anthology on Hardy: ". . . while the earth remaineth, seed-time and harvest, and cold and heat, [and] summer and winter, and day and night shall not cease" and where he concluded that "this might serve as a motto for this Anthology, and is the real philosophic thread upon which Thomas Hardy has strung his splendid achievements."[36]

Two other volumes of verses are said to have preceded this and two to have followed.[37]

Head sent his first poem to the neurosurgeon Harvey Cushing (1869–1939), who published it in the *Yale Review* in 1916[38]:

I Cannot Stand and Wait

How can I serve who am too old to fight?
I cannot stand and wait

With folded hands, and lay me down at night
In restless expectation that the day
Will bring some stroke of Fate
I cannot help to stay.
Once, like the spider in his patterned web,
Based on immutable law,
Boldly I spun the strands of arduous thought,
Now seeming naught,
Rent in the sudden hurricane of war.

Within my corner I will take my place,
And grant me grace
Some delicate thing to perfect and complete
With passionate contentment, as of old
Before my heart grew cold.
This in the Temple I will dedicate,
A widow's mite,
Among more precious gifts, obscured from sight
By the majestic panoply of state.
But when triumphal candles have burned low
And valorous trophies crumbled into dust,
Perchance my gift may glow,
Still radiating sacrificial joy
Amid the ravages of moth and dust.

There are similarities to Sonnet 16 (or 19, depending upon the publisher) of John Milton (1608–1674), on his blindness[39]:

When I consider how my light is spent,
Ere half my days, in this dark world and wide,
And that one Talent which is death to hide,
Lodg'd with me useless, though my Soul more bent
To serve therewith my Maker, and present
My true account, least he returning chide,
Doth God exact day-labour, light deny'd,
I fondly ask; But patience to prevent
That, murmur, soon replies, God doth not need
Either man's work or his own gifts, who best
Bear his milde yoak, they serve him best, his State
Is Kingly. Thousands at his bidding speed
And post o'er Land and Ocean without rest:
They also serve who only stand and waite.

Head's "Homing Wings" was published in 1916[40]:

Homing Wings

Poised like the black-winged swallow born to roam
And find a living in the ambient air,
We sacrificed our home
For unpolluted realms of natural law.
Must we despair

Because the neutral tissue of our dreams
Dissolves like ravelled mist before the heat,
And at our feet
The radiant prospect of this ancient land,
Grey hamlets, happy fields, sequestered streams,
Unconquerable stand?
E'en the world-wandering bird suspends her nest
Beneath the overhanging cottage eaves
In fecund rest;
And breezes ocean-born
In brooding oaks scarce stir the crumpled leaves,
Where poppies flame among the ripening corn.
So we return to worship homely things,
That filled our baby hands, ancestral springs
Resurgent and intense
Stirring the reverent heart
Of childhood's innocence.

And "Paris, April 1916":

Paris, April 1916

"*Ils vantaient notre esprit, jamais notre endurance.*"

How silent are the streets of this grave town;
Discordant vanity is swept away,
And mourners everywhere pass up and down,
Sombring the radiance of an April day.
Here all men wear the inward, brooding look
Of a young mother, when her time is near,
Devoid of fear.
She knows the agony of hope still-born
And, once before, her body racked and torn
Was at the last denied its victory.

How can we understand,
Whose land inviolate was clogged with dreams?
They with a single purpose are imbued,
That like a mighty river onward streams
In multitudinous channels ruthlessly,
Past tangled isles and barriers of sand,
Until its irrestible waters roll
To their triumphal goal,
With all-embracing, silent fortitude.

Next was published "The Price", in 1917[41]:

The Price

Night hovers blue above the sombre square,
The solitary amber lanterns throw

A soft penumbra on the path below,
And through the plumed pavilion of the trees
A solemn breeze
Bears faintly from the river midnight bells;
While at this peaceful hour my spirit tells
Its tale of arduous joys,
Pain conquered, Fear resolved, or Hope regained,
Swift recognition of some law divine,
Shy gratitude that could not be restrained,
All these were mine,
And so, supremely blest,
I sink to rest.

Through labyrinthine sleep I grope my way,
Feeble of purpose, sick at heart, and sure
Some unknown ill will lead my steps astray,
Till, cold and gray,
The dawn rays through my shuttered windows steal
And with closed eyes I thank my God for light,
For the fierce purpose of another day,
When work and thought forbid the heart to feel.

"Destroyers" was published in the *Yale Review* in 1917[42]:

Destroyers

On this primeval strip of western land,
With purple bays and tongues of shining sand,
Time, like an echoing tide,
Moves drowsily in idle ebb and flow;
The sunshine slumbers in the tangled grass
And homely folk with simple greeting pass,
As to their worship or their work they go.
Man, earth, and sea
Seem linked in elemental harmony,
And my insurgent sorrow finds release
In dreams of peace.

But silent, gray,
Out of the curtained haze,
Across the bay
Two fierce destroyers glide with bows a-foam
And predatory gaze,
Like cormorants that seek a submerged prey.
An angel of destruction guards the door
And keeps the peace of our ancestral home;
Freedom to dream, to work, and to adore,
These vagrant days, nights of untroubled breath,
Are bought with death.

"Died of His Wounds" apeared in the *Yale Review* in 1918[43]:

Died of His Wounds

Death set his mark and left a mangled thing,
With palsied limbs no science could restore,
To weary out the weeks or months or years,
Amidst the tumult of a mother's tears
Behind the sick-room door,
Where tender skill and subtle knowledge bring
Brief respite only from the ultimate
Decree of fate.

Then, like the flowers we planted in his room,
Bud after bud we watched his soul unfold;
Each delicate bloom
Of alabaster, violet, and gold
Struggled to light,
Drawing its vital breath
Within the pallid atmosphere of death.

That valiant spirit has not passed away,
But lives and grows
Within us, as a penetrating ray
Of sunshine on a crystal surface glows
With many-hued refraction. He has fled
Into the unknown silence of the night,
But cannot die till human hearts are dead.

And "Epiphany":

Epiphany

No starry candles lit this festal time,
And round our Twelfth Night there was none
Who did not mourn a husband, brother, son
Gone in his prime;
Not with the customary pomp of death,
With sick-bed ritual and with flickering breath,
But like the blossom of tempestuous May,
In one night swept away;
And of its radiance no memorial seen
Beyond the empty place where it had been.

So we stand sorrow-laden at the feast,
Where wisdom knelt in homage to a child,
And three world-weary pilgrims from the East
Laid at His feet
Gold, and a healing balm, and odours sweet.
We too must bring our offering, pay the price
To gain the gold of sacramental peace
Where doubts dissolve, insurgent longings cease,
And sorry is sublimed in sacrifice.

The next poem, entitled "To Courage Seated", was published in 1918[44]:

To Courage Seated

We wandered through the chill autumnal Park,
And spoke of courage and the youthful dead,
And how the boldest spirit may be cowed
By indiscriminate terror. Overhead,
The moon rode high on her predestined arc,
Steadfast through tidal waves of sombre cloud.
Like vast antennae, search-lights swept the sky,
When, suddenly, as if in swift reply,
Out of the south, with jets of luminous smoke,
And coughing clatter, hidden guns awoke.

And we fell silent at the thought of death.
We were too old to leap with panting breath
Into the turmoil of the bloody strife,
And dance upon the razor-edge of life
To fame or to oblivion. We must wait
Like senators of old, with folded hands,
In silence, seated, for the stroke of Fate.
One boon alone an ardent soul demands,
To die before its passion waxes cold,
Enthusiasm fails, or Love grows old.

And "Elan Vital":

Elan Vital

All things that live and grow are full of hope.
The slender primrose on the woodland slope,
Tangled and overgrown,
Unfolds its crumpled florets one by one
To seek the sun;
The snow-bound crocus thrusts an amber cone
Through frozen earth; even the fallen elm
Fringes with tender green its ancient bole.
But Death exacts a toll
From Beauty, Courage, innocent Desire,
And tempests overwhelm
The fruit-tree blossom, trumpled in the mire,
Sweet harbinger of unfulfilled delight.

When terror keeps the watches of the night
And childhood's faith is gone
And passion spent,
We stagger to our feet and stumble on
In pain, in sorrow and bewilderment
Impelled to hope by man's instinctive soul.

"Pegasus" was published around the same time:

Pegasus

The wind is still; from far and wide the air
Resounds with Sabbath bells, calling to prayer,
And from the vast, unfathomable blue
Hums a propeller's penetrating drone.
We stand enchanted, and our eyes pursue
An aeroplane that climbs the summer sky
To drift alone
On mountainous clouds of ever-virgin snow,
Suspended like a black-winged dragon-fly,
That turning gleams,
Dove-gray and silver in the morning beams;
Or like a dead leaf, loosened from a height,
Spins in its perilous flight.
We catch our breath like children at a show,
Of martial music and heroic deeds,
On every glittering incident intent,
Forgetting for a time terrestrial creeds
For joy that man now rides the firmament.

After the Great War

Head retired from the London Hospital in 1919 with the first symptoms of Parkinsonism, and shortly afterwards, at the suggestion of Siegfried Sassoon, went to live in Dorset as a neighbour of Thomas Hardy,[45] who wrote much of his poetry in the last few years of his life. Hardy died soon after and Annie Mitchell, a cook at Max Gate in 1913 and 1914, recalls of Hardy: "He tottered rather than walked and as he was 73 that was to be expected. He spoke very quietly. You had to listen very attentively to what he was telling you."[46] Did he have Parkinsonism too?

The Heads moved to Hartley Court near Reading. Was Henry Head related to Thomas Hardy, perhaps a distant cousin? Hardy's grandmother was named Head (see Appendix).

It was probably from Dorset that in 1926 Head published his great two-volume work *Aphasia and Kindred Disorders of Speech*.[47,48] Speech is tied up with thinking and single words are meaningless. The speechless patient not only cannot speak aloud but he cannot propositionise internally. He cannot say anything to himself and therefore has nothing to write. He concludes that there are no centres for speaking, reading, writing or other forms of behaviour comprised in the normal use of language. Two aspects of language are the formulation of thought and its skilful expression. "The superb logician may

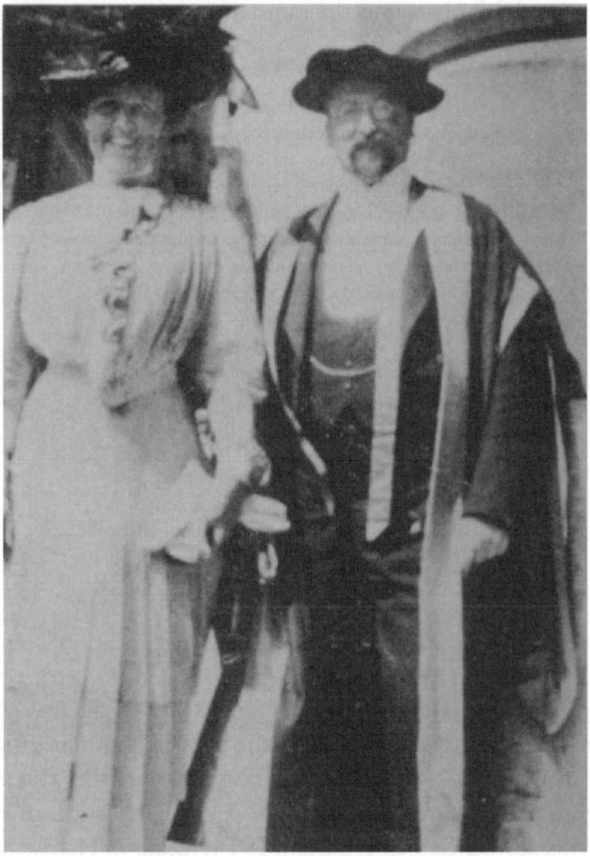

Fig. 2. Henry and Ruth Head.

have difficulty in expanding his ideas and we are familiar with the practiced speaker whose words are jejune (scanty, unsatisfying to the mind) of thought."

In 1927 Head was knighted. Ruth Head died in 1939 and not long afterwards, on 8 October 1940, Henry Head died at Hartley Court, near Reading. He was aged 78 and had been immobilized by Parkinsonism for many years, with great difficulty in speaking though his mind was still alert.[49]

Russell Brain (1895–1966), distinguished neurologist at The London Hospital and President of the Royal College of Physicians, wrote: "Had Henry Head not adopted medicine as a profession, he might have been equally distinguished as a writer." We may agree that he was such. Head's bibliography was published in Henry Head's centenary.[50] A good accolade to Head is the Henry Head Centenary Edition of the journal *Brain*.[51]

Adrian Head, cousin of Henry, paints and writes poetry, including:

Sonnet

Men in their wisdom fight for various things,
For freedom by their lights, for trade and soil
For flags of silk, for commissars and kings,
And break the thread of progress and of toil
To lay their corpses in some alien mud,
Offer youth's splendid courage as a foil
To shroud the picture of their streaming blood
That runs so gladly in defence of oil.
I'll die again if duly called upon
And sift the truth from all contending claims,
Tread with my heart where better men have gone;
But let no man, over my last remains,
Say then that once again the gods of war
Took pen and wrote "The mixture as before."

Henry's only escape from the house and wheelchair were the daily drives. Adrian had asked him whether he had any early recollections which he felt were indicative of his later development; Henry's answer was that he had been told (but did not recall) that when in the nursery he liked to be given a bowl of water and a brush and to watch the water run down the window when put on with the brush, and that he would spend ages watching this. Adrian went on to say that he did not know what it would portend apart from his acute observation—but the nanny involved must have been a most patient soul and very tolerant of mess! Adrian wrote his 16-year-old tribute:

To Cousin Henry (FRS LRCP MD)
Oct 8th 1940

Joyful must thy spirit be
From thy trammelled body free,
In the wider open space
Where such bindings have no place
In pure immortality.

There can there be no iron nor wood
To bind the limbs that never stood
Great must be thy joy indeed
To see those limbs and thine e'er freed
By the Doctor who is good.

Great was thy endless toil on earth
To mend the limbs that see rebirth
And nerves of muscle, body mind

Great is thy joy, these whole to find
For which thy toil was of such worth.

What greater toil than thine of love?
May thy spirit stay above
Those who following seek to find
What thou hadst ever in thy mind
Seeing all whole, at last, in love.

Mind and body of all e'er freed
Thy seeing this here was not decreed
But greater than thine has been no strife
And then last nourished the plant to life
That found in thy fertile brain the seed.

Conquerors must rise and fall again
But their glory lasts for a moment and then
They are gone in a dimness that lasts for ever
But thy works of good are forgotten never
For thou shalt be known as a server of men.

Randall Jarrell wrote:

> Anyone who has spent much time finding out what people do when they read a poem, what poems actually mean for them, will have discovered that a surprising part of the difficulty they have comes from their almost systematic unreceptiveness, their queer unwillingness to pay attention even to the reference of pronouns, the meaning of the punctuation, which subject goes with which verb, and so on; "After all," they seem to feel, "I'm not reading *prose.*" You need to read good poetry with an attitude that is a mixture of sharp intelligence and of willing emotional empathy at once penetrating and generous.[52]

Appendix

A family tree[53] shows that Thomas Hardy's great-grandparents were James Head and Mary Hopson. James died in May 1772 and four months later his daughter, Mary Head (1772–1857), was born. She was baptized at Fawley in Berkshire, due south of Wantage. She was orphaned on 8 May 1779, when Mary Hopson-Head was buried. Mary had a younger brother, William, baptized on 25 April 1779 without mention of a father or a second marriage, so William was probably illegitimate and he was buried on 2 May 1779, a day or two before his mother's death. Mary was the niece of a Henry Head who was churchwarden at nearby Chaddleworth. The effect of all this on Mary must have been considerable. Reference may be made to this in Hardy's *Jude the*

Obscure. Jude's first name is given as Fawley and his surname as Head. One of the alternative surnames for Jude is Hopeson. Scenes of the novel are placed in Berkshire and the name of the widow Edlin is taken from a Fawley family appearing in the registers.

Mary had an illegitimate child by John Reed and the child was baptized at St Mary's, Reading, in 1803 at the age of six or seven years, rather like Tess, and the story has other similarities since Mary was also incarcerated in the Bridewell at Reading for three months for stealing a copper kettle.

Mary made good and married Hardy's grandfather, Thomas Hardy (1778–1837). At some stage she moved to the cottage at Bockhampton. Their children were James, John and Thomas.

Thomas (1811–1892) married Jemima Hand (1830–1904) and their child was our Thomas Hardy. In 1837 she was widowed and was styled Mary Head Hardy. The name of Mary Head is preserved in *Marygreen* and *Bridehead*.

Thomas Hardy wrote before the Boer War and, in about 1887, the last verse of Tess's Lament[54] reads:

It wears me out to think of it,
To think of it;
I cannot bear my fate as writ,
I'd have my life unbe;
Would turn my memory to a blot,
Make every relic of me rot,
My doings be as they were not,
And gone all trace of me!

In 1885 Thomas Hardy first slept in the house that he built, Max Gate in Dorchester. There he had many visitors, including Robert Louis Stevenson,[55] who wrote the poem inscribed on his grave in Western Samoa:

Under the wide and starry sky
Dig the grave and let me lie:
Glad did I live and gladly die,
And I laid me down with a will.

This be the verse you grave for me:
Here he lies where he long'd to be;
Home is the sailor, home from sea,
And the hunter home from the hill.

Acknowledgements

I am indebted to many who have helped with this work; in particular, to Adrian Head for his kindness and generosity and for his permission to publish some of his thoughts and poetic works.

Notes and References

1. Based on a paper read at The Mansell Bequest Symposium on the Neurology of the Arts, held at The Medical Society of London on 30 April and 1 May 2001.
2. MD, FRCP, FACP, Consultant Neurologist; Exeter Neurosciences and The Peninsula Medical School, Royal Devon and Exeter Hospital, Barrack Road, Exeter, EX2 5DW, UK. E-mail: cgardnerthorpe@doctors.org.uk
3. Randall Jarrell, Poetry and the Age (1953). In: The Obscurity of the Poet, *Penguin Book of Twentieth-Century Essays*, selected by E.N. Hamilton (Penguin, Allen Lane, 1999), p. 269.
4. Randall Jarrell, Poetry and the Age (1953). In: The Obscurity of the Poet, *Penguin Book of Twentieth-Century Essays*, selected by E.N. Hamilton (Penguin, Allen Lane, 1999), p. 270.
5. R. Richardson, Medical museum: Keats's notebook, *Lancet*, **357**, 320 (2001).
6. J. Keats, *La Belle Dame Sans Merci* (1920). In: Other Men's Flowers, by A.P. Wavell, *The Penguin Poets* (Penguin, Middlesex 1960), pp. 138–9.
7. Gemini, *St Bartholomew's Hospital Journal*, Jun. 1922.
8. Debrett publishes several guides to the aristocracy and gentility, and the behaviour expected of and by them.
9. "Thomsen... suffered from it himself." (Taylor's *Practice of Medicine*).
10. A. Barnsley.
11. Large drinking bowl containing, especially, punch.
12. J. Silkin, ed., *The Penguin Book of First World War Poetry*, 2nd edn. (Penguin, 1996), pp. 194–5.
13. R. Brain, *Doctors Past and Present* (Pitman, London, 1964), pp. 100–8.
14. Dictionary of National Biography 1931–40, pp. 410–2.
15. G. Holmes, *Obituary Notices of Fellows of The Royal Society 1939–1941*, Vol. 3 (Morrison and Gibb, London).
16. Birth certificate No. 466 for 1861, Stoke Newington, Middlesex.
17. For a fuller account of Henry Head and his work, see: C. Gardner-Thorpe, Henry Head (1861–1940). In *Twentieth Century Neurology*, ed. Frank Clifford Rose (Imperial College Press, London, 2001), pp. 9–30.
18. Printed list of candidates of The Royal Society (1899).
19. Bulloch's Roll. Index of Fellows of The Royal Society.
20. *Destroyers and Other Verses (1919)*, pp. 85–7.
21. Published in 1914 by Chatto and Windus, London.
22. Works of Thomas Hardy, arranged by Ruth Head, with an introduction by Henry Head, MD, FRS (1922).
23. Pictures and Other Passages from Henry James, selected by Ruth Head (1916).
24. Personal communication from Adrian Head (2000).

25. Nisbet's Medical Directory (James Nisbet and Co., London, 1910), p. 282. *Head, H., 4 Montagu Square, W. (T. 2003 Pad.), L., 1890, FRCP Lond., MD Camb., FRS. Ed. Cambridge; Univ. Coll. and London Hosps. Phys. London Hosp.*
26. Pat. Barker, *Regeneration* (1991).
27. Pat. Barker, *The Eye in the Door* (1995).
28. Pat. Barker, *The Ghost Road* (1994).
29. *Poems of the Great War: 1914–1918* (Penguin, 1998), p. 6.
30. J. Silkin, ed., *The Penguin Book of First World War Poetry*, 2nd edn. (Penguin, 1996), pp. 131–2.
31. H. Head, *Destroyers and Other Verses by Henry Head MD FRS* (Humphry Milford, Oxford University, 1919).
32. S.G. Reich, History of neurology, *Archives of Neurology* **45**, 1257–60 (1988). This article contains a good photograph of Henry and Ruth in 1909.
33. See Appendix 1.
34. See Appendix 2.
35. Genesis 8: 22.
36. Henry Head, *The Works of Thomas Hardy Arranged by Ruth Head with an Introduction by Henry Head, M.D., F.R.S.*, p. viii (Chatto and Windus, London, 1922). *Seed-Time and Harvest* is also the title of Part I of the contents, which includes "Tess", "Mary South", "The Spring Months" and "A Ballad".
37. Some of these volumes have not yet been traced.
38. *Yale Review* **5**, 540 (1916).
39. Milton, "On His Blindness", *The Penguin Book of English Verse*, ed. John Hayward (Penguin, 1963), pp. 147–8.
40. *The English Review* **23**, 99 (1916).
41. *The English Review* **24**, 3 (1917).
42. *Yale Review* **6**, 473 (1917).
43. *Yale Review* **7**, 307 (1918).
44. *The Dublin Review* **162**, 129 (1918).
45. It is interesting to consider why Head moved there. Robert Gitting's biography of Hardy does not clarify this fully; the first volume, *Young Thomas Hardy*, was published in 1975, and the second, *The Older Hardy*, in 1978; Heinemann of London were the publishers and later Penguin.
46. Monograph **65**, 397.
47. Macdonald Critchley wrote on Head's contribution to aphasia in *Brain*, **84**, 551–60 (1961).
48. *Aphasia and Kindred Disorders of Speech* (Cambridge University Press, 1926).
49. Death certificate No. 380, Registration District of Wokingham in the County of Berkshire. Registered 9 October 1940.
50. Pages 39–41.
51. 1961, *84, part IV*.

52. Randall Jarrell, Poetry and the Age (1953). In: The obscurity of the poet, *Penguin Book of Twentieth-Century Essays*, selected by E.N. Hamilton (Allen Lane, Penguin, 1999), p. 270.
53. *Monograph 28*, pp. 18, 19, 33, 34.
54. D. Wright, *Thomas Hardy: Selected Poetry* (The Penguin Poetry Library, 1978), pp. 200–1.
55. J. Stevens Cox, *72 Monographs on the Life of Thomas Hardy* (The Toucan Press, Beaminster, Dorset).

Chapter 24

Silas Marner, George Eliot and Catalepsy

F. Clifford Rose

Introduction

Some years ago, a television film producer, making a film about Silas Marner, asked me to advise how the actor should portray catalepsy. I read (or it may have been re-read) *Silas Marner*, the novel written by George Eliot which was published in 1861. It was the third of her seven most famous novels (Table 1).

Silas Marner

In this novel, Eliot describes "a male, middle-aged weaver (who) suffered from attacks of catalepsy". Silas was a linen weaver who was forced to leave the village where he was born, having been accused (wrongly) of thieving. He had "protuberant eyes" due to myopia, which "really saw nothing very distinctly that was not close to them".

A detailed description of Silas Marner's attacks (Table 2) is given by a witness in the book:

Table 1. George Eliot's novels.

1859	*Adam Bede*
1860	*The Mill on the Floss*
1861	*Silas Marner*
1863	*Romola*
1868	*The Spanish Gypsy*
1871	*Middlemarch*
1876	*Daniel Deronda*

Table 2. Silas Marner's attacks.

Middle-aged male
Triggers: tension, prayer meetings
Diminished consciousness
Eyes fixed
Limbs stiff
Sudden recovery
Cold and faint afterwards
Amnesic for events

> One evening. . .he saw Silas Marner leaning against a stile with a heavy bag on his back, instead of resting the bag on the stile, as a man in his senses would have done, and that on coming up to him he saw that Marner's eyes were set like a dead man's, and he spoke to him and shook him, and his limbs were stiff, and his hands clutched the bag as if they'd been made of iron; but just as he had made up his mind that the weaver was dead, he came all right again, like, as you may say, in the twinkling of an eye, and said "Good-night" and walked off.[1]

Later Eliot writes:

> Some said Marner must have been in a "fit"—a word which seemed to explain things otherwise incredible but the argumentative Mr Macey, clerk of the parish, shook his head and asked "if anybody was ever known to go off in a fit and not fall down".[1]

The length of the attack seems to be against the diagnosis of epilepsy:

> . . .he had fallen at a prayer-meeting into a mysterious rigidity and suspension of consciousness which, lasting for an hour or more, had been mistaken for death.[1]

Its occurrence at a prayer meeting could be a point in favour of sleep epilepsy, but the length of the tonic phase is much longer than in the usual epileptic attack.

The author later indicates that depression might have been a factor in the provocation of attacks:

> He was arrested, as he had been already since his loss, by the invisible Wand of catalepsy, and stood like a graven image, with wide but sightless eyes, holding open his door, powerless to resist. . . . When Marner's sensibility returned, he continued the action which had been arrested and closed his door, unaware of any intermediate change, except that the light had grown dim and he was chilled and faint.[1]

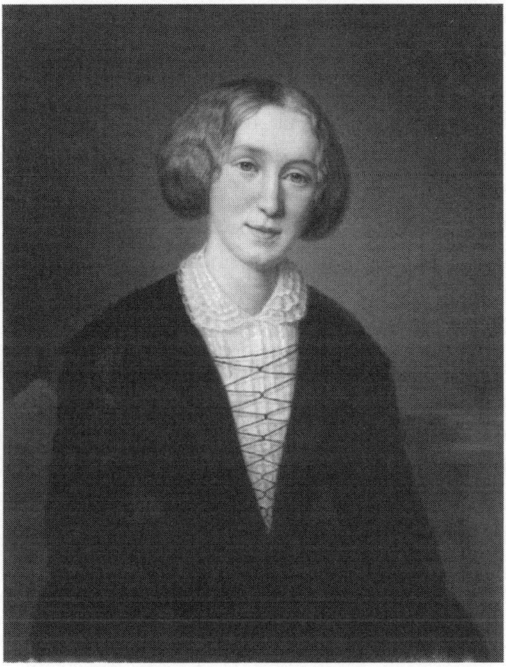

Fig. 1. George Eliot.

There is no indication of how long the lack of awareness persists but Marner clearly does not wish to discuss his illness:

> He had not mentioned to anyone his unconsciousness of the child's entrance, shrinking from questions which might lead to the fact he himself suspected—namely, that he had been in one of his trances.[1]

The treatment recommended in the novel would not be accepted today:

> Silas had taken to smoking a pipe daily during the last two years, having been strongly urged to it by the sages of Raveloe, as a practice "good for the fits", as this advice was sanctioned by Dr Kimble, on the ground that it was well to try what could do no harm—a principle which was made to answer for a great deal of work in that gentleman's medical practice.[1]

The questions that arise from George Eliot's case history of Silas Marner are: What is catalepsy? How did George Eliot know about it? Did Silas Marner have it?

Eliot was born on the 22 November 1819 at South Farm, Arbury, Warwickshire, which is south of the Midlands, just over 100 miles to the north-east of London. Her real name was Mary Anne (or Marian) Evans but she dropped the "e" from "Anne" when she signed her name in the register as a bridesmaid at her sister's wedding in 1837 (Figure 1).

To her publisher on the 24 February 1861, in a letter regarding *Silas Marner*, she wrote: "...I should not have believed that anyone would have been interested in it but myself...if Mr Lewes had not been strongly attested by it.... It came to me first of all, quite suddenly, as a sort of legendary tale, suggested by my recollection of having once, in early childhood, seen a linen weaver with a bag on his back...."[2] Her publisher (John Blackwood), in a letter to his wife, wrote: "*Silas Marner* sprang from her childish recollection of a man with a stoop and expression of face that led her to think that he was an alien from his fellows."

The question of where she learned about catalepsy might be answered by her contacts with the medical profession. The earliest was when her sister married a medical practitioner, Dr Edward Clarke, in 1837. Herbert Spencer, the famous philosopher, was knowledgeable about biology, and was a "good friend" who lived in the same house at 142 Strand, which Eliot left in October 1853.

In 1854 she met Dr John Elliotson at a party.[2] He was a well-known physician with an interest in such neurological syndromes as Parkinson's disease. She met the most famous neurologist of that period, Hughlings Jackson, socially in Cambridge, but this was after *Silas Marner* was written in 1861. It is more likely that she had learned about the condition from George Henry Lewes,[a] her partner who had been a medical student, and later wrote on physiology. Together they had met du Bois Reymond[2] in Germany, and he, as a neurologist, would have known about the condition.

Eliot had a lifelong history of chronic violent headaches with vomiting, which she associated with "hysteria": "...at a party...oppressive noise that accompanied the dancing" created in her an illness of such intensity that "I regularly disgraced myself.... The consequence was headache, and then that most wretched and unpitied of afflictions, hysteria...."[3] Karl states: "The headaches, which continued with varying degrees of severity for her entire lifetime, are some indication of a tense, nervous, or, as she says, hysteria-prone person. Yet the headaches cannot be identified merely as the result of tension or conflict...(but)...also showed some positive function, in that they gave her a reason to retreat. If the headaches were truly migraine, they were often severe

a. Lewes, born in 1817, earned his living as a writer and journalist. After his death in 1878, Eliot, who had lived with him for 25 years, endowed a research fellowship in Physiology.[4]

enough to send her into retirement for long periods of time. Suffering excruciating pain, she felt transported into another dimension, not only of pain but of experience, in which she became ultra-sensitive to sound, light, movement." "...At the end of August 1852...Violent headache and sickness reflected the depression of spirit she felt on resuming her work in the Strand...sitting in the dark room at the back of No. 142...October...she shook off her headaches, which were probably due to eyestrain and anxiety...." The associated nausea and photophobia are characteristic of migraine, although the provocative factor may well have been anxiety and depression. There seems little doubt that George Eliot suffered from migraine all her life.

Catalepsy

The classification of epilepsy (Table 3) developed by Galen (*c.* 110–200 AD) and his successors distinguished three conditions under this general term: (1) an idiopathic form, located in the head; (2) analepsy, originating in the stomach; and (3) catalepsy, which was associated with fever and mental disturbances.[5] Caelius Aurelianus (6th century AD) also stated that fever was characteristic of catalepsy and absent in epilepsy whereas frothing from the mouth and nose was present in epilepsy but not catalepsy (Table 4); this distinction was maintained until the Middle Ages but virtually disappeared with the Renaissance.[5]

To quote Temkin[5] again: "It is, of course, quite possible that in making catalepsy a form of epilepsy, one of the original meanings of the word *catalepsis* (i.e., "grip") rather than the name of a disease has been used."

Table 3. Galen's classification of epilepsy (2nd century AD).

1. *Idiopathic*:	located in the head
2. *Analepsy*:	originating in the stomach
3. *Catalepsy*:	fever and mental disorder

Table 4. Caelius Aurelianus (6th Century AD).

	Epilepsy	Catalepsy
Mouth foaming	+	–
Fever	–	+

Arnold of Villanova (*c.* 1234–1311) in *Brevarium practicae medicinae* (1482), as translated by Von Storch and Von Storch,[6] kept to Galen's classification of epilepsy and reserved the term "catalepsy" "for attacks originating in the more remote limbs, whereas the majority included in this category of attacks originating in all parts other than the stomach."[5] These attacks began in an extremity where the sufferer experienced some form of sensory alteration.[7]

This division should have been put to rest by Nicholas Culpeper's *The Compleat Practice of Physick* of 1655 (mainly a translation of Lazarus Riverius[8]). In this he writes: "There is in Galen, and almost all Authors, a threefold Epilepsy. The first is that which hurts the Brain, the second is that which hurts the brain in which the Disease is by consent from the stomach, the third is when the disease is sent from other parts of the body to the head: And these have their proper names; the first, as being chief, is called Epilepsia; the second Analepsia; the third Catalepsia: But (by Galen's leave) that division is superfluous...."[5]

The term was much used in the Middle Ages, but was dismissed in the English translation (1722) of Boerhaave's *Aphorismi*:[9] "Catoche, Cotochus, or Catelapsis, is that Disease in which the patient becomes of a sudden unmoved, void of feeling, and retains the same Posture and Action of all Parts of the Body which he was in when the Disease seized him first (Table 5). NB This doth happen so seldom that there is hardly one Physician in ten, who in fifty years Practice shall happen to see it. Galen in fifty years practice saw but one." In spite of this, the term was still used by Hughlings Jackson and lumped together with delirium and somnambulism.[10]

Neurologists of the late 19th century gave varied definitions of catalepsy. Wilks[11] included "if a limb be placed in any position there it will remain", a description more in favour of catatonia (*flexibilitas cerea*). Grainger Stewart[12] also thought that it was the same as catatonia, stating that "prolonged rigidity of muscles characterises epilepsy".

Under the rubric of "Trance and Catalepsy", Gowers[13] begins with the following statement: "A curious group of diseases have for their characteristic the occurrence of a state of sleep-like unconsciousness, which is called 'catalepsy' when it is accompanied by a peculiar plastic state of the limbs, and

Table 5. Boerhaave (1709).

Sudden loss of movement
Void of feeling
Retains posture

Table 6. Gowers (1885).

Age 6–30 years
Females more than males
Induced by hypnotism
Hysterical subject
Plastic limbs
Flexibilitas cerea

'trance' or 'lethargy' when this condition of the limbs is absent. These conditions are most common in the subjects of hysteria.... They may often be induced by the methods termed 'Mesmerism' and 'hypnotism'. Spontaneous catalepsy has been met with in both sexes and at most ages, from six to thirty, but it is most frequent in the female sex and in early adult life..." "It...has been said to occur in epilepsy, but its connection with the latter disease is very doubtful."[13] The attacks may be preceded by "headache, giddiness or hiccough...commonly with loss of consciousness.... The muscular system passes into a state of rigidity...at first considerable and movement is resisted; but after a short time the limbs can be moved, and then remain in any position in which they may be placed...as if the limbs were made of wax, and hence the condition has been termed *flexibilitas cerea*." (Table 6)

The term "cerebellar catalepsy" was used by Babinski: "The patient is made to lie on his back, his thighs flexed, on his abdomen, and the legs lightly flexed on the thighs, the feet facing out slightly away from each other." The term used by Babinksi has long been forgotten and is no longer considered to be a feature of cerebellar disease. Another report, in 1918, showed a state of inability to move which persisted for ten minutes. Neither Oppenheim nor Dejerine believed in it, while Bing also confused it with catatonia.

In the last century Kinnier Wilson[14] considered that catalepsy was a state of sustained motionlessness with or without clouding of the sensorium and concluded that it was usually hysterical. Lennox,[15] in his two-volume treatise, gives two entries for catalepsy in the index. On page 296 we read under the heading of "Arrest of Motion—and of Mentation": "Some cases are what the ancients termed catalepsy." The literal meaning of this is "to be seized under (or below)". Under the rubric of "Trance—catalepsy"[15] he points out that these terms indicate an immobility longer than that associated with cataplexy or sleep paralysis, and it is "not so quickly reversible and attended perhaps by some clouding of sensorium. Catalepsy implies some muscular fixation, even a *flexibilitas cerea*. The seizures of Silas Marner were of this nature."

Table 7. Lennox (1960).

Longer immobility
Sensorial clouding
Flexibilitas cerea
"There seems no use for 'catalepsy', a term which implies a condition other than epilepsy"

Lennox goes on to state that "clearly, Boerhaave's definition, if the immobility is transient, would apply to the motionless seizures of psychomotor epilepsy". An illustrative case history is George Eliot's Silas Marner, whose hoard of gold vanished during one of his trance-like "cataleptic seizures." Lennox concludes that "there seems no use for 'catalepsy', a term which implies a condition other than epilepsy." (Table 7)

Yawger[16] reports a 27-year-old male who had drop epilepsy since the age of 6 years. He "suddenly developed a cataleptic attack which lasted eight days"; it "began with mutism and then passed rapidly into stupor with loss of bowel and bladder control. At the beginning of stupor there was generalised rigidity and this was so marked that it was only with difficulty that the extremities could be bent. Two days later the rigidity yielded to catatonia so that the extremities remained in any position placed until they fell from exhaustion and gravity." This might well have been a case of hystero-epilepsy, one of the commonest causes of admission to a neurological hospital in that period.

There is often confusion between catalepsy, narcolepsy and cataplexy; the last term was introduced by Adie. Kinnier Wilson[14] states "that both narcoleptic and cataplectic attacks may comprise a component which corresponds to the usual conception of catalepsy or trance".

Temkin[5] concludes: "The inclusion of catalepsy among the types of epilepsy is one instance of nosological confusion." If it ever existed, catalepsy as described was very rare and has now vanished from the neurological scene.

Other Victorian Writers

During the mid-19th century, there were several references in novels relating to epilepsy and catalepsy, although the two were often confused (Table 8).

George Eliot was not alone among Victorian novelists in writing on catalepsy.[17] Catalepsy is mentioned in the novel *Berenice*, by Edgar Allan Poe

Table 8. Victorian novelists.

1839	Poe	*The Fall of the House of Usher*	"lingering smile"
1844	Poe	*The Premature Burial*	stimulates death
1857	Flaubert	*Madame Bovary*	magnetism restores life
1859	Dickens	*A Tale of Two Cities*	"convulsionists"
1861	Eliot	*Silas Marner*	stiff limbs
1883	Collins	*Heart and Science*	"partial catalepsy"
1918	Bennett	*The Pretty Lady*	"luxurious catalepsy"

(1809–1849), written in 1835. Poe describes a progressive physical and mental disorder which "makes it plausible for her to appear dead".[18] Her cousin describes it as "a species of epilepsy not infrequently terminating in *trance* itself". The cousins become engaged and, as her illness worsens, Berenice loses her beauty. One morning she has seizures and in the evening she appears dead and is buried. In *The Fall of the House of Usher*, Poe describes the condition of Madeline of Usher:

> The disease which had thus entombed this lady in the maturity of youth had left as usual in all maladies of a strictly cataleptical character. The mockery of a faint blush upon the bosom and the face, and that suspiciously lingering smile upon the lip which is so terrible in death.[19]

What Poe meant by "strictly cataleptical" may never be known but the flushing of chest and face is not typical of epilepsy, nor is the *risus sardonicus*, which is more indicative of *rigor mortis*. She makes her way out of the coffin and meets her brother, who probably knew she had not really been dead. Poe was obviously fascinated by the possibilities of being buried alive as it featured in another of his stories, "The Premature Burial". In this he writes of prolonged cataleptic seizures which might be the consequence of being buried alive rather than its cause. When the fear goes, the catalepsy is cured. In this story, he writes in the first person: "For several years I have been subject to attacks of the Singular disorder which physicians have agreed to term catalepsy in default of a more definitive title." This description is not epilepsy, and how the patient survives before the days of intensive care, a trance that lasts for weeks or even months, is difficult to understand. Even more puzzling is that "the closest scrutiny, and the most rigorous medical tests" fail to establish any distinction between this state and "absolute death". The failure of this distinction cannot but be attributed to the novelist's imagination.

Catalepsy, trance and lethargy, lasting for days or weeks, are really examples of spontaneously developed mesmeric sleep in hysteric patients or subjects of incipient insanity. . . . "It is in this condition that the lay journals find agreement for their stories of premature burial."[20]

In *Madame Bovary*, Gustave Flaubert (1857) writes "about catalepsy, and the wonders of magnetism" and "bringing her back to life". This is indeed confusion produced by ignorance.

In *A Tale of Two Cities*, Charles Dickens (1859) writes of "members of a fantastic sect of consvulsionists, and were even then considering within themselves whether they showed foaming rage. . . and turn cataleptic on the spot. . . ." Although we are in the dark as to what he meant by "cataleptic", the rest would fit in with hystero-epilepsy.

In *Heart and Science* (1883), Wilkie Collins (1824–1889) talks of "partial catalepsy", but other than writing "there is no saying when the change may come" there is little to show his exact meaning. Catalepsy is also mentioned in Wilkic Collins' *Poor Miss Elemia* (1872).

Even early in the 20th century, Arnold Bennett still used the term. In *The Pretty Lady* (1918), he writes: "Leaving a small ring of gas alight in the gas stove, she sat down all dirty on a hard chair in front of it and fell into a luxurious catalepsy." The inference is that little more was meant by the use of the term than simply a deep sleep.

Tennyson

Alfred Tennyson (1808–1892), whose father, brother and cousin had epilepsy, talked about catalepsy as "weird seizures" in his long narrative poem "The Princess", in 1847. It was "an amorous polemic on the rights of women".[22] The author refers to catalepsy but it is not until the fourth edition, several years later, that reference is made to "weird seizures", which were manifested as "derealisation experiences".[18,23] When the Prince meets the Princess, she has two seizures where she "appears to him as a shadow". He next goes into battle "in a dreamy state". Wounded, he "experiences his recuperation period as a continuation of the seizure". The seizures ceased when the two came together. The court physician diagnosed the attacks as catalepsy. Tennyson possessed a copy of Quincy's medical dictionary (1804), which defined catalepsy as "a sudden suppression of movement and perception where the body is immobilised ('freezes') in its present position". Those seizures can last from a few minutes to a few hours, after which the sufferer is amnesic for the event as if they awoke from sleep.[18] These episodes described by Quincy are more like catatonia and differ completely from the Prince's attacks, where his change in perception is short-lasting and he feels like a shadow in a dream surrounded by ghosts; he is unable to distinguish reality from illusion. It is likely that Tennyson's description is more like epilepsy, possibly with a temporal lobe origin. Tennyson's father's epilepsy was probably of the temporal lobe type even though his doctors diagnosed catalepsy. This may have been the source of Tennyson's knowledge of the term "catalepsy".

It seems likely that catalepsy was in common parlance in the 19th and early 20th centuries. As in the common saying nowadays of "I nearly had a fit", it does not indicate a specific neurological entity. Certainly Silas Marner's attacks cannot be recognised as a specific disorder. It could encompass a variety of different symptoms from several disorders.

The Beginnings, the End and a New Beginning

There has been much confusion regarding the term "catalepsy", not only its meaning but also in relation to other similar-sounding syndromes such as catatonia; this is a psychiatric syndrome that can include mutism, stupor, negativism, mannerisms, echolalia, echopraxia and excitement (furore).

The term "catalepsy" appears to have arisen phoenix-like in recent years. In a literature search of the past ten years, the number of references with "catalepsy", surprisingly, was well into three figures. The reason for this is that biological psychiatrists have used the term in their experimental animal studies for a specific righting test: "The typical catalepsy test consists of placing an animal into an unusual posture and recording the time taken to correct this posture. This time is regarded as an index of the intensity of the catalepsy."[24] Some have defined catalepsy in laboratory animals as "a failure to correct an externally imposed posture",[25] which fits in with the traditional *flexibilitas cerea* or waxy flexibility of catatonia.

In view of this confusion, the term "catalepsy" should be defined on each occasion of its usage. The advice I gave to the film producer mentioned in the opening sentence of this chapter was "follow George Eliot's description", which advice Ben Kingsley, who acted the part of Silas Marner, took.

References

1. G. Eliot, *Silas Marner* (Thomas Nilson, London, 1861), pp. 8, 9, 11, 191, 222.
2. G. Haight, *George Eliot: A Biography* (Penguin, London, 1992), pp. 136, 341.
3. F. Karl, *George Eliot: A Biography* (Flamingo (Harper Collins), London, 1996), p. 40.

4. E.M. Tansey, George Eliot's gift to medicine, *Trans. Med. Soc. London*, 15–24 (1988).
5. O. Temkin, *The Falling Sickness*, 2nd edn. (Johns Hopkins Press, Baltimore University, 1971), pp. 120, 133, 202.
6. E.P. Von Storch and T.J.C. Von Storch, Arnold of Villanova on epilepsy, *Ann. Med. Hist.* **10**, 251–60 (1938).
7. M.J. Eadie and P.F. Bladen, *A Disease Once Sacred* (John Libbey, Eastleigh, England, 2001).
8. Lazarus Riverius, *The Compleat Practice of Physick*, Nicholas Culpeper (and others). Being Chiefly a Translation of the works of L. R. London, 1653.
9. H. Boerhaave, *Aphorismi* (Leyden, 1709).
10. J. Taylor, G. Hemes and F.M.R. Walshe, *John Hughlings Jackson's Selected Writings* (Arts & Boeve, Nijmegen, 1931).
11. S. Wilks, *Lectures on Diseases of the Nervous System* (J. and A. Churchill, London, 1878).
12. T. Grainger Stewart, *An introduction to the Study of the Diseases of the Nervous System* (Ball and Bradfute, Edinburgh, 1884).
13. W.R. Gowers, *A Manual of Diseases of the Nervous System* (J. and A. Churchill, London, 1885), pp. 946, 948.
14. S.A.K. Wilson, In: Ninian Bruce A. (ed.), *Neurology* (Edward Arnold, London, 1940).
15. W.G. Lennox, *Epilepsy and Relaxed Disorders* (Churchill, London, 1960), p. 476.
16. N.S. Yawger, An epileptic with cataleptic attacks, *J. Neuro. Mental Dis.* **492** (1915).
17. G.D. Perkin, Catalepsy, *J. Neurol. Neurosurg. Psychiatry* **59**, 86 (1995).
18. P. Wolf, Epilepsy and catalepsy in Anglo-American literature between romanticism and realism: Tennyson, Poe, Eliot and Collins, *J. Hist. Neurosci.* **9**, 286–93 (2000).
19. E.A. Poe, *Complete Stories and Poems* (Doubleday and Co, New York, 1906).
20. G.H. Gould and W.L. Pyle, *Anomalies and Curiosities of Medicine* (1896), Philadelphia reprint (Sydenham, New York, 1937).
21. B.H. Wright, Tennyson, the Weird Seizures, in *The Princess*, and *Epilepsy Literature and Medicine* **6**, 61–76 (Johns Hopkins University Press, Baltimore, 1987).
22. I. Ousby, *The Cambridge Guide to Literature in English* (Cambridge University Press, Cambridge, 1993).
23. P. Wolf, *Epilepsie und Katalepsie in der angelsachsischen Literatur Romantik und Realismus: Tennyson, Poe, Eliot and Collins*, Epilepsie-Blatter, 7, Suppl. 2, 11–14 (1994).
24. P.R. Sanberg, M.D. Bunsey, M. Giordano and A.B. Norman, The catalepsy test: its ups and downs, *Behav. Neurosci.* **102**(5), 748–59 (1988).
25. J.L. Saver, P. Greenstein, M. Rontal and M.M. Mesulam, Asymmetric catalepsy after right hemisphere stroke, *Movement Disorders* **8**(1), 69–73 (1993).

Index